The Praise Keeps Coming . . .

"We know we eat too much. We want to stop, but we can't—it's simply too hard to resist all the high-calorie food out there. That is the problem. With *The 'I' Diet,* we have a way to actually regain control of our appetites."

—David A. Kessler, M.D., former FDA Commissioner and author of *The End of Overeating*

"Perhaps the most comprehensive approach to eating for effective weight control . . . explains how natural hardwired instincts to eat in response to hunger, availability, caloric density, familiarity and variety, which served us well in Paleolithic times (and until the mid-20th century), have been compromised by changes in the kinds, amounts and constancy of foods in the modern world. . . . The book guides readers to alternative approaches to fulfilling the demands of these instincts in ways that can help them lose weight and, at the same time, adopt a more wholesome, nutritious and healthful eating style."

—Jane E. Brody, *The New York Times*

"Humans evolved with powerful survival instincts that regulate our food intake. Dr. Roberts combines her extensive experience with sound science to help readers work with these instincts rather than fight them. Everyone will gain practical insights from these pages."

—Walter Willett, M.D., Chair, Department of Nutrition, Harvard School of Public Health, and author of *Eat, Drink, and Be Healthy*

"What I have learned from Dr. Roberts' magical diet is that I can eat until I am full as long as I am eating the right foods, in the proper amounts. I had absolutely no clue before going on the 'I' Diet which foods were good for my weight and which were not. But now I do, and my waistline—and my heart—will be forever grateful. I recommend *The 'I' Diet* to anyone who has struggled with weight gain or obesity and has given up hope. This diet will change their life."

—Henry Louis Gates Jr., The Alphonse Fletcher University Professor, Harvard University

and coming . . .

"Call it the high-brow diet. The creation of Susan Roberts, a professor of both nutrition and psychiatry at Tufts University . . . it combines both areas of Roberts' expertise in an attempt to retrain dieters' brains. . . . Roberts' philosophy of eating tackles the two main reasons why dieters fail—hunger and deprivation. . . . [Her] dieting program is focused on reprogramming hunger away from the needs of our early ancestors (who ate whatever they could get, whenever they could get it) and toward the reality of modern life (the constant availability of tasty, fatty foods). In this way, the diet addresses the fact that feeling satiated is a complex brain function, and that food instincts are really just an outdated survival mechanism that makes us fat. This is *The 'I' Diet*'s Darwinian element—helping us evolve to meet the reality of supermarket aisles packed with 36 varieties of cookies."

—Hannah Seligson, *The Daily Beast*

....

"A breakthrough approach helps take hunger and cravings out of the weight-loss equation—so slimming down feels absolutely effortless!"

—*Woman's World*

....

"A scientifically sound diet plan that could help you lose weight without feeling deprived. If weight loss has been a struggle for you because you rely on willpower, learning about your eating instincts may be the secret you have been waiting for."

—Kathleen M. Zelman, *WebMD*

....

"[T]ranslates years of research and laboratory work with overweight volunteers at Tufts into an eight-week program designed to help readers reteach their bodies how to control hunger without feeling deprived."

—M.E. Malone, *The Boston Globe*

....

"An honest, straightforward and helpful guide for people who wish to lose weight sensibly and safely and then keep it off. The "I" Diet is scientifically sound and easy to implement. I highly recommend it."

—F. Xavier Pi-Sunyer, M.D., Professor of Medicine, Columbia University, and Director, New York Obesity Research Center, St. Luke's–Roosevelt Hospital

and coming . . .

"Finally, an easy-to-follow plan for healthy and permanent weight loss based on science! If you don't lose weight after reading Dr. Roberts' book, I suggest you read it again."

—William J. Evans, Ph.D., the Jane and Ed Warmack Chair in Nutritional Longevity, University of Arkansas for Medical Sciences

"In *The 'I' Diet,* Susan Roberts translates over 20 years' experience conducting nutrition studies into a practical prescription for weight loss. Whereas many diet book authors focus simplistically on just one factor, she shows us how many aspects of the modern food environment gang up against our biology—and most importantly, what we can do about it. Her eight-week program, based on the latest scientific insights into nutrition and psychology, provides wise guidance along the road to long-term weight management. I recommend *The 'I' Diet* with enthusiasm."

—David S. Ludwig, M.D., Ph.D., Director, Optimal Weight for Life (OWL) Program, Children's Hospital, Boston, and author of *Ending the Food Fight: Guide Your Child to a Healthy Weight in a Fast Food/Fake Food World*

"A must-read book for anyone interested in losing weight and/or keeping it off. Based on the latest cutting-edge research and presented in a clear, concise way . . . *The 'I' Diet* artfully blends sound science with a practical road map for weight loss."

—Eileen Kennedy, D.Sc., Dean, Friedman School of Nutrition Science and Policy, Tufts University

"This clearly written book doesn't promise magic. It does something better: It arms you with the tools to create a diet that you can enjoy and stick with for life. And Dr. Roberts' recipes are terrific."

—Susan K. Fried, Ph.D., Professor, University of Maryland School of Medicine

"A real paradigm shift. . . . This truth-telling book, written by an international authority on human nutrition, offers a fresh approach to an old problem. Full of innovative strategies, *The 'I' Diet* shifts the emphasis from the failed diet wars to eating behavior."

—Michael Goran, Ph.D., Keck School of Medicine, University of Southern California

and coming.

"Susan Roberts, a top-rate expert, has crafted her studies into an innovative program that offers new ideas and a plan designed around both health and weight loss as goals."
—Kelly D. Brownell, Ph.D., Professor of Psychology, Epidemiology and Public Health Director, Rudd Center for Food Policy and Obesity, Yale University, and author of *Food Fight*

....

"Sue Roberts is dead-on with the five food instincts she describes. Drawing on solid research evidence and filled with specific and creative 'how to's' for managing these instincts, *The 'I' Diet* is an eating plan I will recommend to others . . . and use myself!"
—Megan A. McCrory, Ph.D., Purdue University

....

"Drawing upon her extensive experience in obesity research, Roberts, with coauthor Sargent, has written a highly readable and eminently practical guide to losing weight and then maintaining the loss. This is a great example of how science should inform public policy, as well as individual behavior."
—Robert Russell, M.D., Editor, *Nutrition Reviews*

....

"With approaches tested at the highest critical level, this book should set a new standard in educating readers on the science and practice of weight management and control."
—Irwin Rosenberg, M.D., Chair, Food and Nutrition Board of the National Academies of Science

....

"This book expertly organizes and interprets scientific studies, turning them into small, understandable pieces of information that can be readily applied to even the busiest life. The abundance of practical tips and delightfully fresh recipes make reading this book a must for any person desiring to lose weight and keep it off."
—Mel Heyman, M.D., M.P.H., Children's Medical Center, University of California, San Francisco

the "i" diet

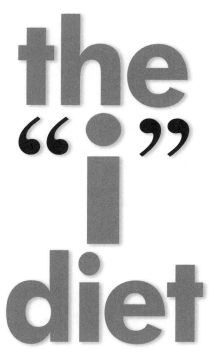

the "i" diet

Use Your **Instincts** to Lose Weight— and Keep It Off—Without Feeling Hungry

Susan B. Roberts, Ph.D.
Winner of the American Society for Nutrition's E.V. McCollum Award

and Betty Kelly Sargent

WORKMAN PUBLISHING • NEW YORK

The "I" Diet is a safe, scientifically structured weight-loss program. Nevertheless, we recommend showing this plan to your doctor for confirmation that you are healthy enough to start this diet. We also recommend that you have your doctor monitor your progress and health during weight loss.

The voices and stories of volunteers in our research studies are heard throughout this book. Except in the Preface, names and details have been changed to protect privacy.

We are grateful for the permission to include the following recipes: Lentil Vegetable Soup (page 149) from *Cooking Jewish* by Judy Bart Kancigor; Crisp Fennel Salad (page 176) from *Celebrate!* by Sheila Lukins; Haddock with Tomato-Cumin Sauce (page 201), adapted from Diane Forley's recipe in *The Anatomy of a Dish;* and Seafood Stew in Tamarind Broth (page 204) from *BowlFood Cookbook* by Lynne Aronson and Elizabeth Simon.

Library of Congress Cataloging-in-Publication Data is available.

ISBN 978-0-7611-5874-5

Originally published in 2008 as *The Instinct Diet,* now with new material.

Workman books are available at special discounts when purchased in bulk for premiums and sales promotions as well as for fund-raising or educational use. Special editions or book excerpts also can be created to specification. For details, contact the Special Sales Director at the address below, or send an email to specialmarkets@workman.com.

Design by Janet Vicario with Yin Ling Wong and Jen Browning
Cover photography and "after" photos in the Preface by Tracy Powell
Wardrobe styling by Ellen Silverstein
Photo on page xx courtesy of Professor Gates

Workman Publishing Company, Inc.
225 Varick Street
New York, NY 10014-4381
workman.com

WORKMAN is a registered trademark of Workman Publishing Co., Inc.

Printed in the United States of America
First printing December 2009

10 9 8 7 6 5 4 3

For

John and Diana,
and all the research volunteers I've had the privilege of
working with over the years at Tufts and M.I.T.,
and research volunteers everywhere who selflessly
give of themselves so that nutrition science can advance
S.B.R.

For
Elizabeth,
James, Izabela and Xavy
B.K.S.

Contents

Success!

A Preface to the New Edition

The publication of the original *Instinct Diet* was a watershed moment for me. After 17 years of exacting, often challenging (and sometimes tedious) weight-loss research in my lab at Tufts University, I was convinced that I could give people a better way to lose weight—and really, truly keep it off—than they could find in other diets. And by helping others with a problem I had struggled with myself, I was also hoping to heal the wounds of my own painful history.

Here's the backstory: I grew up in England in a family that loved food. My parents were overweight,

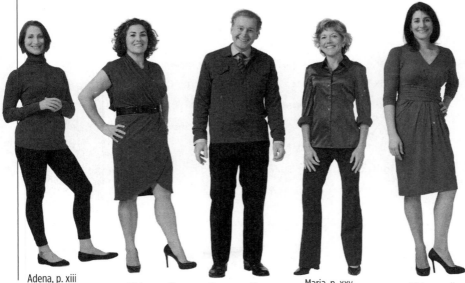

Adena, p. xiii

Alicia, p. xviii

Dave, p. xxii

Maria, p. xxv

Niki, p. xxvii

so were most of my siblings and so was I. To make matters worse, I was also the kid who came in last at every track meet, the adolescent with the tummy, the girl who always looked just a little bit different. Then, in my teens, I got sick with mononucleosis. Illness is not a weight-loss method I'd ever recommend, but I would be lying if I didn't admit I was thrilled that my recovery was accompanied by the loss of all those extra pounds. No surprise, keeping the weight off after I got my health back was a real challenge, especially since I was working part-time as a chef.

When it was time for college, I decided to major in nutrition, and it was always the obesity lectures that interested me most.

After graduation, I did research in Africa and then returned to the University of Cambridge to earn my Ph.D. in nutrition. It was there that I met my wonderful husband, John. When he was offered a position at Harvard Medical School (where he's now a professor of cell biology) and I was invited to M.I.T., we moved to Boston. What a great decision that turned out to be! I had landed in the center of nutrition research in the United States. And the Tufts Human

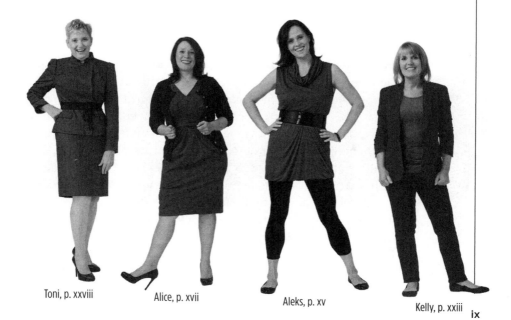

Toni, p. xxviii   Alice, p. xvii   Aleks, p. xv   Kelly, p. xxiii

Nutrition Research Center, which I moved to soon afterwards, is the epicenter of it all.

It was at Tufts that I started my weight-control research program on obesity, as well as on protein, carbohydrates, fat, the Glycemic Index, fiber and everything else I could think of. After publishing nearly 200 scientific papers and reading several thousand research papers by other scientists, I realized something essential. All the studies agreed that five things affect our eating behavior: *hunger,* the *availability* of food, the *variety* of food, the *familiarity* of food and how rich or *calorie-dense* the food is. The consistency of the findings was startling, since most topics in nutrition have as many opinions written about them as there are scientists writing them. Not here. There was striking agreement that these five variables have predictable effects on what and how much we eat and what we enjoy. And then I had my own eureka moment—these are our *basic food instincts.* I knew I was onto something and went about proving I was right by focusing my research on the five instincts—why we have them, how they work, how we can *use* them to control our weight. And so the Instinct Diet began to take shape.

My Big Dream

Over the years, I saw volunteers in my lab achieve amazing results. They lost up to 50 pounds, without any additional exercise or drugs. They experienced minimal weight regain after a year. They saw great health improvements, most notably substantial decreases in cholesterol levels and blood pressure. But the most important outcome was that they felt *great.* They would chatter on about how happy they were, wondering aloud what the "magic" of the diet was. I knew the only magic was our own biology and realized that it was now time to write a book. I wanted people everywhere to learn what I had learned, to benefit from what I had seen in my lab and to experience that sense of magic firsthand.

That was my dream: pretty big stuff, I thought. But the reality of publishing the book was much more exciting.

Dr. Roberts

I had decided not to limit its scope to my lab research, but to take the best from my program and merge it with the very best stuff from other research worldwide. And I discovered that the "I" Diet (that's what everyone calls it) works even better than I had predicted; indeed, people who followed the program were getting results more remarkable than those I had observed in my lab. Instead of losing 4 pounds in two weeks, dieters were losing an average of 7 pounds and in some cases as many as 10. And rather than shedding 10 to 15 pounds in eight weeks, the "I" dieters were losing 16 pounds on average and sometimes 20 pounds or more.

As the success stories poured in, I came to realize the import of what was happening. I had known that my diet would work—it's based on the very best science and it delivers real results—but it does it *so much faster* and *with much less hunger and better craving control* than I had ever imagined. Meaning? The "I" Diet is actually a *healthy* crash diet; if you follow it, you will lose weight and fat as fast as is humanly possible without in any way compromising your health. And if you make this way of eating part of your life, you will keep that weight and fat off forever. Of course, you don't have to lose weight as fast as possible. The great thing about a diet that actually works and produces rapid weight loss if you follow it to the letter is that you can, if you prefer, follow it at a leisurely pace for reliable slow weight loss.

What Really Happens

All this makes the paperback *"I" Diet* an even more exciting venture than the original hardcover. (We decided to change the name of the book not only because, as I said, everyone on the plan calls it the "I" Diet, but also to emphasize the fact that this is a diet that speaks to the "I" in each of us—one food instinct may trigger me to overeat, while you may respond to another.) Now I get a chance to share some of the successes that people have achieved on *this* diet—not the diet I had so carefully tested in my lab, but the one that now exists in the real world. And here's where I get to brag. Most diets (particularly those featured on TV) simply lie to imply success or boast about their best weight losses and warn in small type that results may not be typical. But with the "I" Diet, even average success is fantastic.

Follow the "I" Diet and you can honestly expect:

✽ To lose, on average, 7 pounds in the first two weeks. If you follow the program to the letter, you may lose up to 10 pounds.

✽ To lose, on average, 16 pounds in eight weeks. If you're diligent, you can lose up to 21 pounds. Worst-case scenario, *even if you have failed to lose weight on other diets:* at least one pound a week. "I" dieters typically achieve their dream weight (for the people featured in this chapter, this meant losing an average of 30 pounds).

✽ To drop two clothing sizes in eight weeks.

✽ To lose plenty of belly fat and reduce your waist size. (Other diets promise this but usually don't deliver.)

✽ To avoid the dieting plateaus that have made you give up in the past.

Beyond all that, you'll end up with what many people feel is even more important than their first-ever weight-loss success: a new and healthier relationship with food. "I" dieters feel in control, often for the first time in their lives, and actually lose the cravings that once made weight loss impossible. Because they're truly satisfied, they're not tempted to eat empty calories. Stop for a moment and think—really *think*—about what this means. Feeling satisfied is much more than not feeling hungry; it means you actually don't feel tempted to eat any more than you've eaten. That is *huge*.

Now, I am a scientist, so I have to tell you that the weight you'll lose on the "I" Diet is not all fat; that would be impossible. The human body is capable of losing about 3.5 pounds of fat per week, and that's if you eat nothing at all (an unsustainable and very dangerous idea). Most dieters have to get rid of excess body water at the beginning of weight loss, and seeing it come off makes for an exciting start. The really important key to success, however, is keeping it up, not "getting stuck" after a week or two; that's when most dieters quit, and why most diets fail. In every report that I've received from "I" dieters, not a single person has hit a plateau before reaching his or her goal weight. And often they achieve their first goal sooner than they hoped and then go on to set another goal and achieve their dream weight! Everyone just keeps losing more until the weight is right.

And then there's the food. Missing favorite foods and good meals is one of the reasons many people give up on dieting. Not having time to make healthful meals is yet another stumbling block. Those realities motivated me to develop the "I" Diet recipes. As a former chef and working mother who still loves food and cooks every single day even though time is short, I designed almost all the recipes in the book, and seeing people's passion for "I" Diet foods has been wonderful. It means that we finally have a diet that's sustainable for life.

Even with all this good news, I have still had to confront a healthy dose of skepticism fed by the crazy media drumbeat that portion control and calorie counting are the main things that matter. When you've tried several diets and found them all hard, it takes a leap of faith to believe that this new diet is different, transformational and simply better. But I hope you *will* believe me. Give it a try. Put yourself on my menus without making substitutions or changes for just a week and experience the difference first-hand. But first, listen to the stories of some people who did just that.

"I" Diet Success Stories

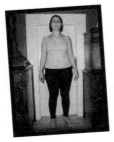

Adena

Age: 39

Height: 5′2″

Marital status: married

Profession: psychologist

Weight loss: 18 pounds in nine weeks; current total loss of 25 pounds

Clothing size: down from 10/12 to 4/6

Adena describes herself as a lifetime yo-yo dieter. She lost her first 30 pounds when she was only 13 and then bounced up and down without ever reaching the weight she wanted. Her goal, when she began the "I" Diet, was to finally get to the weight she wanted and stay there. And that's what she's done.

"This is by far the best and easiest diet I've ever been on," Adena says. "It started working for me right from day one, and I never did plateau—something that had always held me back in the past. Part of what makes Instinct so special is that it's based on science; as a scientist myself, I know how important that is. In just nine weeks, I went from 138 pounds to 120. In the next few weeks, I reached my lifetime goal and have kept to it almost effortlessly.

"The most exciting thing for me about the 'I' Diet is that I don't have to feel hungry; in fact, when I get hungry, I know it means I'm supposed to have something good to eat. This is such a change from other diets I've tried, when I found myself thinking about food all the time. I've never before seen a diet plan that genuinely keeps you satisfied. This is the reason I know that the weight I've lost will not come back.

"The biggest surprise is that my cravings have changed radically. I crave the foods I'm now eating instead of the fatty, sugar-filled foods I used to eat. When I wake up, I'm excited about eating my 'I' Diet Soda Bread and peanut butter for breakfast. I think I might be a little addicted (if there's such a thing as being a *little* addicted) to that bread as well as to the Masala Tea. I have them both every day, and I'm feeling happier and more energetic than ever before.

> ❝ Now I crave what I'm *supposed* to eat. How amazing is that! I'm a lifelong member of Weight Watchers, but I'll never go back—for the simple reason that this diet works better and is much easier. ❞

"The real payoff came when I tried on my old size 10 and 12 pants and realized that none of them even remotely fit. I hightailed it down to the Gap and tried on some nice-looking 8s and 10s (just in case). They didn't fit either. So I rushed back to the racks, picked out several size 6s, slipped on a pair and—*voilà!* There I was. Just like back in high school. I was so excited, I was almost speechless—and that's pretty unusual for me.

"I've been on the 'I' Diet maintenance plan for several months and feel like I now have a life plan for staying healthy and thin. It was scary at first, because I've been a dieter for almost 30 years and that was part of who I was. But the 'I' Diet plan is so healthy and flexible that it fits right in with my lifestyle even though I don't really cook much and love to feel full. By the way, I've now stocked up on size 4/6 jeans and skirts and dresses because I'm finally confident that my dieting days are over."

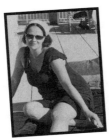

Aleks

Age: 34

Height: 5'11"

Marital status: newlywed

Profession: events organizer

Weight loss: 21.5 pounds in eight weeks; current total loss of 35 pounds

Clothing size: down from 14 to 12 and then 8

Aleks has always suffered from emotional eating. When she was stressed, she would eat. When she was sad, she would eat. Sometimes when she was just a little tired or bored, she would also eat. All that has changed. She has finally squashed the triggers that caused her to crave unhealthy, fatty foods . . . and she looks better and feels happier than she ever has in her life.

"It seems like I've been overweight all my life," Aleks says. "I have so many memories of growing up in Poland and eating lots of thickly buttered bread and fatty meats with heavy sauces. Most of the kids my age were normal-size, but I was always the tallest and always on the heavy side. Then when we came to the States, I was trying to escape the pain of my father's death and the loss of the country that was so dear to me. That's when my emotional eating really started. And that's when I fell in love with fast food. Eventually, I just accepted the fact that I was heavy— a big-boned girl, as some of my friends put it.

"I have always tried to control my weight in the privacy of my own home, but the 'I' Diet is the first diet I felt comfortable going on. It's so healthy and science-based, and I'm just amazed by the results. I found it refreshing to learn about cravings, about what makes us feel full and why, and especially the fact that we can rewire our brains in order to control our cravings and actually feel attracted to healthy, slimming foods.

"It took a little getting used to at first. There were nights when those old cravings would crop up, but after only two weeks the combination of feeling full and satisfied and being able to eat the great desserts made them completely disappear in about two weeks. It's clear to me now that I spent years overeating just to feel satisfied, stuffing myself with large portions of unhealthy foods, nibbling on appetizers, eating when I felt down . . . and I did all that while blaming myself for being weak.

"I weigh myself every day, and it's such an incentive to see the scale moving down almost every time I get on it. Sometimes I backslide a little, but I always forgive myself and go right back to the Stage I menus for a day or two so that nothing is lost—except a little more weight, of course.

> **❝What a sense of freedom to know that my emotions don't have to go hand in hand with my weight. ❞**

"The best thing about all this is that now I realize that losing weight is not the unattainable goal I always feared it was. I can eat mindfully, and I have control over what I eat—even over what I crave. My adorable, skinny husband is happy with the diet, too. He loves the recipes. Once in a while I'll make a little extra pasta for him to eat while I have a salad, but most of the time we enjoy the same foods and he keeps telling me what a great cook I am.

"What a relief it is to know that I'm capable of being comfortable in my own skin. I'm wearing clothes that I never thought I could fit into, and I'm so happy about the way I look.

"The 'I' Diet has helped me change my life."

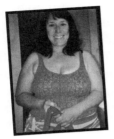

Alice

Age: 50

Height: 5′4″

Marital status: married with three school-age children

Profession: career consultant

Weight loss: 29 pounds in seven months—and still coming off!

Clothing size: down from a tight 16 to 10/12

A lice is a woman to whom success has always come naturally—in just about every area of her life. Weight control was one goal that seemed to stay beyond her reach. Now that sense of failure about her weight is behind her.

"I'm not sure why," Alice says, "but no matter what diet I tried, nothing seemed to work over the long term. Then I tried the 'I' Diet, and it was like a miracle. Part of it is because this diet makes sense intellectually. It's not just some fad. It's based on real science, and that really appeals to me. The whole concept makes complete sense.

> 66 Because I feel so satisfied and no foods are banned, there is no desire to cheat. Now that I understand the role my instincts were playing in what I ate, I don't feel guilty anymore. The 'I' Diet has let me off the hook. 99

"Now I have a whole new way of thinking about food. It's not about willpower. It's about my instincts and and using them to help me lose weight instead of letting them undermine all my best efforts. My kids love this food as well. They understand why fiber is so important. They don't skip meals, and they no longer eat junk food because they're 'starving.'

"This diet has been transformational for me. I know that sounds a little 'out there,' but I honestly feel more hopeful about life. I feel healthier. I feel more in control of what I eat. And my goals are finally being realized because I've been freed from the frustration of ineffective dieting. This is the very first time in my life that I don't feel guilty about my weight. I realize that I wasn't being weak, I was just giving in to some very powerful instincts that I had no idea even existed. What a joy to finally get this and to be able to do something about it.

"It's also interesting that I'm happy to talk to other people about this diet, not embarrassed to admit that I'm on a diet, as I was in the past. With other diets, I would mistake emotional eating for real biological hunger. I'd crave chocolate ice cream after dinner and dream about baked potatoes stuffed with cheese and butter. Now I don't do that because no foods are banned on the 'I' Diet. As long as I don't go overboard, I can satisfy my new, *healthier* cravings anytime I want to.

"With other diets, I would gain back all the weight I'd lost plus some extra pounds almost the minute I stopped. Not so now. I've been losing weight slowly and steadily, and I have absolutely changed the way I feel about food and the way I relate to it. It's even possible to go off the 'I' Diet for a few days if you're on vacation and get *right back on* and still continue to lose weight. It is completely realistic and in tune with the real-life issues that confront busy working mothers. I still love eating and eating well—and that's just what I'm doing on this diet. The difference is that now I'm in charge of what I eat, not the other way around. I'm just sorry this amazing diet wasn't available years ago."

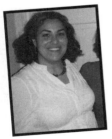

Alicia

Age: 35
Height: 5'2"
Marital status: married; mother of toddler
Profession: law firm investigator
Weight loss: 19 pounds in seven weeks; 30 pounds in five months
Clothing size: down from 16 to 10

Alicia lives such a busy life—a demanding career, a happy married life and a two-year-old daughter—that it's hardly surprising that watching what she eats is a challenge. But even before life got hectic, Alicia was gaining weight every year. Her eating was out of control. With the 'I' Diet, she finally has a handle on her eating habits. She's lost more weight than ever before, and she knows that the weight she lost this time will stay lost forever.

"The 'I' Diet is unlike any diet I've ever tried," Alicia says. "And I've tried them all: South Beach, Weight Watchers (several times), Jenny Craig, Atkins and dozens of diets of my own design. Nothing worked. I was *always* unsatisfied, and I found it hard to believe that this didn't happen with the 'I' Diet. Well, the first two days were a little tough to get through hunger-wise, but since then I have not felt hungry as long as I stick to my menus.

"In the past I always blamed myself for having uncontrollable food cravings. I was a pizza fanatic, and potato chips and chocolate-chip cookies had a hold on me like there was no tomorrow. Now I know it wasn't willpower that was lacking; it was just that I didn't understand my instincts. Now I get it, and I can walk right by the high-calorie foods that derailed me on other diets.

"It only took a few days of following the start-off menus for those longings to go away. Now I rarely think about those snacks and sweets, and when I do, I feel kind of repulsed by them.

> **"** My cravings used to be out of control. I'd stuff myself with pizza and chips and cookies and crackers. Now that's all gone. **"**

All that fat and sugar and salt! Yuck! Occasionally I lapse and have another binge if I'm traveling and get hungry, but afterwards I feel physically terrible, and it's easy to get right back to instinctive eating. That's unlike any diet I was ever on before, when getting back on the wagon seemed like torture.

"The other thing I like so much about this diet is that the recipes are delicious. My husband agrees on that one. Our personal favorites are the 'I' Diet Soda Bread, Instant Hot Cereals, Thai Chicken Salad, Tanzanian Chicken Kebabs, Mexican Lettuce Wraps and the Chicken Parm. I've never seen a diet with recipes that even come close to these.

"The 'I' Diet does take a little planning, but it's not difficult and the payoff is huge. In just eight weeks I went from 184 pounds to 165, and I recently just reached my dream weight of 154. I'm excited about a new future in which I can control—and enjoy—what I eat.

Henry Louis Gates Jr.

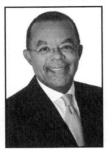

I was introduced to Henry Louis Gates Jr., The Alphonse Fletcher University Professor at Harvard, by Angela De Leon, a Ph.D. student in Nutritional Biology at the University of California at Davis, who is also Professor Gates' fiancée. He wanted to lose just 10 pounds, but he faced particular challenges: a strong hunger instinct, a great love of good food, and a never-ending stream of fancy dinners and parties to attend.

Since he lives down the street from my lab at Tufts, our first meeting took place at his house. I was struck both by his genuine motivation to lose weight and by his failure to make it work after he turned 50. He complained that his pants had grown too tight, and he found even a slightly bulging tummy embarrassing. His kitchen was stuffed with evidence of his failed attempts—many kinds of commercial frozen dinners, an array of "healthy" soups and oatmeals. But the fact was, he couldn't manage to lose weight despite these attempts.

I started by asking him what and where he likes to eat, because I know that diets only work if people enjoy the food. First problem: This is a man who typically eats out five nights a week at the best restaurants in town. And when he isn't in town, he's doing the same thing someplace else! I also learned that he's a real foodie. Giving up great dinners, juicy hamburgers for lunch (with potato chips!), Indian food and several glasses of wine nightly just wasn't in the cards.

So we got started. I threw out the frozen dinners, soups and oatmeals, and got him eating "I" Diet food. (Because his fiancée lives on the west coast and because he is so very busy, he took the extraordinary measure of hiring someone to make up my good and easy recipes for him.) I also designed a hamburger especially for him (check out the results on pages 264–65) so he didn't miss something he loved. And it worked. It worked so well that he got rid of the 10 pounds sooner and more easily than he dared hope, then realized he actually wanted to lose another 5 and went on to do that as well. Between late February and July 1, even with all his traveling, he lost 15 pounds, without giving up wine, potato chips or bread (well, he only eats my bread, which he calls "Sue Bread"). Today, he's bought a whole new wardrobe to accommodate his new waistline (three inches smaller and no longer counting) and is maintaining his weight without effort.

"At first, I was skeptical that dieting required anything more complicated than portion control," Professor Gates says today. "I never really eat that much, but I was eating the wrong things—like lots of pieces of whole-wheat bread slathered with butter to go with my coffee while I wrote at home in the mornings. I would try to nibble my way through the morning until I got really hungry. Then I would eat a turkey sandwich from the deli, or a burger with fries or chips. And then, in the evenings, a dinner out with friends or colleagues, prefaced by a Cosmopolitan, and the meal accompanied by three or four glasses of a fine red wine. Sigh. I thought all calories were the same, so I attributed those ever-tightening trousers to dieting being something difficult. What Sue made me realize was that I didn't understand how food is processed; nor did I understand what to eat, how to eat and when to eat. I had no idea that eating so much "healthy" bakery-baked whole-wheat bread and butter was killing me, even before I made my way into Harvard Square to down my favorite deli sandwich and chips. Sue is quite a tough taskmaster, though, and convinced me to try it her way. I was so amazed that I felt full and lost weight the first day that I e-mailed her with my weight loss. And I e-mailed her every day with my results until I hit 15 pounds.

"I think the most important reason the 'I' Diet works for me is that it makes me totally full and satisfied. I eat huge amounts of food, several times a day. I stay satisfied for hours, and then eat again—without guilt!—when I get hungry. And you know what? I never, now, worry that what I'm eating is going to make me gain weight. I cannot tell you what a psychological relief that is. Eating guilt-free is where it's at; no-stress eating, I call it. This diet is based on science, the science of my very own digestive system.

"The food is delicious and spicy, and that's important to me. I have enjoyed 'I' recipes for hamburgers, Indian food, North African food, Italian food, chili, black bean soup, oatmeal, breakfast rolls, and there's even room for chips and wine and English cheddar cheese on homemade crackers with chutney! When I was losing weight, I actually used to take 'I' Diet dinners in little Tupperware containers with me to my friends' homes and also to my favorite restaurants. It may sound hard to believe, but I would ask them to heat up the dishes for me. And each restaurant did! They would put them on plates, add a garnish and serve each course with whatever my friends had ordered. (I wouldn't recommend this technique if you're going to a restaurant where they don't know you.) And I drank two glasses of wine each night; sometimes, well, maybe three, including that Cosmopolitan, after my weight loss had securely begun. One extra benefit was that this also saved me a lot of money! Anyway, the main value of this was that I could lose weight while still keeping my friends company. The bread, too, is fantastic. I love real bread, not the air-filled supermarket stuff, and Sue's is incredibly satisfying. In fact, I keep encouraging her to market it nationwide and think it's so important for keeping my weight on track that I take some with me on business trips so I can have an 'I' breakfast and lunch in whatever city or country I happen to be.

"Another thing that made this diet work for me is that it was so effective that I didn't have to stay on it all the time. I ate 'I' Diet meals when I could, but when I wanted to ignore the menu I did, and then got back on the diet the next day. It still works for me. Today I'm weight-stable and feel better than I have in years. And I think I look fantastic, but you could check with Angela about that!"

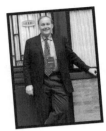

Dave

Age: 52
Height: 5'11"
Marital status: married with two young children
Profession: professor and businessman
Weight loss: 50 pounds in six and a half months
Clothing size: dropped five pants sizes

Dave is one of those rare academics who is so smart and in so much demand that he has appointments in two institutes, not just one. He has also seen much success as a businessman, and he has a wonderful family that adores him. The one area where success eluded him was weight control. With a strong history of weight problems, Dave tried and tried to keep off the pounds, primarily with an exercise program that would impress any fitness instructor. But he could never manage to avoid weight gain, let alone sustain weight loss. Now all that is behind him, and he says the "I" Diet allowed him to become the size he wanted to be when he was 19!

> ❝ The 'I' Diet has enabled me to become the person I've wanted to be for a very long time. My doctor says it has added 10 years to my life. ❞

"I just can't believe it," Dave told me. "I have struggled with weight my whole adult life. Every year I would work hard to take off a few pounds, only to end up putting on a few—and sometimes more than just a few.

"Starting on the 'I' Diet, and indeed staying on it, has been a pleasure for me. This diet is easy to follow, satisfying and, just as so many 'I' dieters say, I never feel hungry. Walking around feeling satisfied has changed my whole outlook on life. That's pretty incredible, considering that I've had food issues since I was a teenager.

"I'm also very attracted to the science that this diet is built on. It's much easier to avoid the environmental temptations that so often stand in the way of effective weight loss when we know how to control the food triggers our instincts respond to.

"I have not felt this healthy for years. I'm now cycling to work and going farther and faster than ever. Old friends whom I haven't seen for a while are amazed and want to know what has finally worked for me. The 'I' Diet has changed my life, and I have no doubt that I'll be able to stay on the maintenance plan forever.

"Everything in the book is self-explanatory; it makes weight loss seem almost effortless. There is no more struggle, and the menus in the book couldn't be easier to follow. My doctor is thrilled and says I've added at least 10 years to my life. My family is pretty happy to hear that, too. And you can guess how I feel about it."

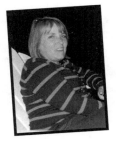

Kelly
Age: 45
Height: 5'2"
Marital status: married with three children
Profession: teacher
Weight loss: 19 pounds in eight weeks; current total loss of 25 pounds
Clothing size: down from 10/12 to 4/6

Kelly is a super-busy teacher with a husband and three young children to care for when she gets home from school. She had lots of doubts about the "I" Diet in the beginning, not the least of which was whether it really was new and better. As a health-conscious fitness enthusiast and soccer coach for a local team, she thought she knew every last thing about healthy eating and doubted that this diet could tell her anything she hadn't heard before. Two days into the program, she became a convert. And now she loves the compliments she keeps hearing from her husband and friends.

"I really didn't think this was going to work," she says, but she lost seven pounds the first week on the diet and after that there was no stopping her.

"What appealed to me most was that the menus are all clearly outlined in the book, so I didn't need to think about meal planning. Also, I could easily adapt them to appeal to my husband and the kids, so we had no problems there. My kids actually love the recipes, which means I can diet and they become more adventurous eaters.

"I started out at 150 pounds, a lot for my five feet two inches, and I was bursting out of my size 10 dresses, soon to become a size 12. Then I lost 10 pounds in the first two weeks on the 'I' Diet, and even though much of this was probably water loss, I was so encouraged that I never looked back.

"This is not just another fad diet. This is a diet that works. Even though I was eating delicious foods like No-Fuss Pizza (yes, I can even eat pizza with my family and not feel deprived), John's Pasta Supper, Chicken with Warm Peanut Sauce and German Rolls, the weight kept sliding off. And like so many of my friends who have used the diet, I was never hungry and felt genuinely satisfied, even at the start. Also, my cravings for snacks and less healthy foods have completely disappeared. And even though I worried about plateauing, it never happened until I was the weight I wanted to be.

> **"** I like to think of the 'I' Diet as a lifestyle change, not a diet. Good-bye, cravings. Hello, healthy choices. My mood has improved 100%. I wake up every morning with a smile and look forward to plunging into my day. **"**

"Now I'm on the weight maintenance program and make healthy choices, and I even prefer these nutritious foods to the chemical-filled stuff I used to crave. Some meals we eat 'I' Diet food just because it's great food and easy to prepare, and other times I eat other stuff, and that combination keeps my weight down. I'm much more aware of what I eat now, and this has not only made a big difference for me, it's also good for my husband and children. We are all feeling better and more energetic, and now when I go into school with my new size 4/6 body, I just love the way people look at me and smile, wondering what I've been doing to look so terrific."

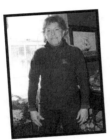

Maria

Age: 51
Height: 5'1"
Marital status: married with three children
Profession: investment banker
Weight loss: 19 pounds in eight weeks; current total loss of 29 pounds
Clothing size: down from 8/10 to 2

Maria grew up in a big Italian-Lithuanian family; eating massive six-hour-long meals at holiday time was not unusual for them. Still, she managed to keep her weight in line with a lot of exercise and a good helping of willpower. Then she had to give up running because of a hip injury and her weight spiraled out of control.

"My mother believed that food is love," Maria remembers. "Part of that philosophy is wonderful, but the extra inches around the tummy part is anything but. I really started packing on the pounds about three years ago when I couldn't run anymore. I went from running about 25 miles a week to *nada,* and since my husband and I both work, we began to rely on packaged meals and lots of processed foods. Big mistake. I went from a size 4 to an 8/10 in what seemed like a matter of weeks. And then there was my dear mother, who used to bring wonderful baked goods to our house every weekend. We always devoured her cakes because they had been prepared with so much love and we certainly did not want to hurt her feelings. But then she passed away. It was a sad time for all of us.

"About a year after my mother's death, I decided things had to change. My cholesterol had shot up, as had my husband's, so we decided to try the 'I' Diet. Within days, the way I looked at food did a 180-degree turn. I went to a theater group dinner that first week, and suddenly the Caesar salad looked as if it had been dressed in motor oil. Even the pasta looked unappetizing. I couldn't believe that my tastes had changed so quickly. Great recipes like Arista Chicken and Baked Salmon with Lemon-Dill Sauce actually tasted better to me!

"I also noticed my energy and stamina increasing and my mood improving. I started sleeping better and was able to run a little. Even the tension in my neck and shoulders started to go away. After eight weeks, I was down 16 pounds and back into my size 4s. But I was on a roll at that point. I kept going and eventually lost every ounce I wanted to—29 pounds in all. Actually, I've recovered an entire closetful of formerly nonwearable clothes—you know, those you hold on to, just in case. My physical transformation was so quick that I didn't feel exactly like 'me' until suddenly it felt normal to be thin and younger again. And I relish the hugs my husband and I give each other now that we can squeeze closer together than we have since our wedding day.

> ❝ After my first two days on the 'I' Diet, my body adjusted to the new foods and I was never hungry again. The way I looked at food did a 180-degree turn. Now I love how I feel. I have the tools to manage my weight for the rest of my life. ❞

"And then there's this: I had three orthopedic surgeons tell me my running days were over and that I needed a hip replacement. After losing all that weight, I'm running 25 miles a week and feeling great . . . without surgery.

"Thanks to the 'I' Diet, I now have the tools to manage my weight for the rest of my life. It's such a good feeling to know that I can stay thin and healthy and fit while enjoying good food and good wine. I love the way I feel now, the way I look now, the way I eat now. This would make my mother very happy."

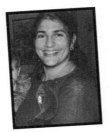

Niki

Age: 37

Height: 5'9"

Marital status: married with two children

Weight loss: 22 pounds in eight weeks; current total loss of 40 pounds

Clothing size: down from 14 to 8

Niki had the problem so many women have. She gained a lot of weight when she was pregnant with her first child, then gained more with her second and has had a difficult time getting back to her healthy weight. She was getting discouraged when she discovered the "I" Diet.

"This diet resonated with me," she says. "Being able to understand my food instincts helped me figure out how to work with them so I could change the unhealthy way I had been eating.

"I gained 60 pounds when I was pregnant with my first child, and I was a complete flop at losing the extra weight. After my second child was born, the weight just seemed a part of me. My energy was low, my clothes didn't fit and I was not happy with the way I looked.

"On the 'I' Diet, I went from 198 to 176 pounds in just eight weeks. I never felt better or had more energy, so I kept going and lost every pound I had gained with the children. This is so different from the diets I tried before. I would always plateau before I got anywhere and then gain the weight right back as soon as I stopped. Not this time. The way I think about food has completely changed. My brain has changed, I guess, and it has made such an immense difference in my life.

"One of the things I really like is how good it has been for our kids. I was worried that having a dieting mom would create problems, but the opposite has been true. Our children

> **"** My husband loves this diet as much as I do. Who knew you could lose so much weight so fast? Now I can keep up with the kids all day long. I don't know who's more surprised, them or me. **"**

are very young, just two and four, and they're starting to enjoy vegetables for the first time as a result of my diet. We have them every day now, instead of just a couple of times a week, and I think they would be upset if they didn't see a little broccoli or some carrots or tomato slices on their plate.

"The 'I' Diet has not only taught us to eat healthy foods; it has also helped us to understand why the foods we used to eat had such a hold on us and to get a grip on appropriate portion sizes. It has also helped me kick what I never recognized as a sugar habit. I used to start the day with two teaspoons of sugar in my coffee. Then all day I'd drink 'fruit water,' which is loaded with sugar, and sweets were a staple in my diet. Now I've stopped most of that, although I do allow myself an occasional dark chocolate snack. This lack of excess sugar makes me feel great, super-energized, happier, more even-tempered.

"This diet has changed my life. Because we love the food and it's so easy to prepare, weight control has become something that happens automatically in my family without an uphill struggle."

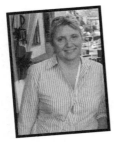

Toni

Age: 57

Height: 5'9"

Marital status: married with two children

Profession: executive director of a human services agency

Special health consideration: cancer survivor

Weight loss: 14 pounds in eight weeks; current total loss of 31 pounds

Clothing size: down from 14 to 10

Toni, who had battled cancer, has a busy life filled with work, teenagers and a husband with his own medical problems. But she was also an unconscious eater; she would eat whenever food was available or she was under stress or a party beckoned. All previous diets had failed because she never thought about food except when she was eating it.

"I used to eat because food was in front of me," Toni recalls. "It was that simple. In the past, when I went on a diet, I would always be hungry, so of course the diet never lasted very long. I would plateau and then put the weight right back on again. The amazing thing about the 'I' Diet is that you never feel hungry when you're on it. I ate all the time and felt positively full, which was fantastic. I just didn't think that was possible. But it is, and the 'I' Diet proves it.

"Dr. Roberts has taught me to value myself and my body by taking the time to plan for three daily meals and two snacks that make me feel full and satisfied so that weight loss is possible. And I had no idea how important fiber is. What a revelation it was the day I arrived at a breakfast meeting already full from a fiber-rich breakfast at home; I could sit and sip my coffee while others were tearing into the pastries and cakes and doughnuts. (I must admit I felt a little superior.) Over and over again during the past eight weeks, I've been able to walk away from temptations. And I'm proud to say I've gone from 185 to 154 pounds and have lost several dress sizes, too.

"The food is very good, but what I value most is finally being in control. At nine o'clock every evening, I have a cup of tea and that's my shutoff valve. As long as I can work in a little something sweet every day, I'm just fine. Then I conclude the day with my tea ceremony and let the stress drift out of my life. So much has changed for me: I used to be an emotional eater, but after losing 31 pounds I'm proud to say that's behind me.

> **❝**I never realized that hunger was my problem—because I always ate when I was hungry! Now I know how to stay more satisfied, and weight loss has become, if not easy, then actually possible. As long as I can have a little something sweet at the end of the day, I'm a happy camper.**❞**

"When I discovered the 'I' Diet, I felt that the angels had been listening. My relationship with food is now completely transformed. Thank you, angels. Thank you."

Do you believe in magic?

Now it's your turn. As I said before, the "I" Diet may not be magic, but it's the next best thing when it comes to weight loss . . . if you'll give it a shot.

So, how to begin? What I have learned in the lab, and from the wonderful "I" dieters who have been willing to tell their stories, is that most people do far better on my ready-made menu plan. It's simply the best way to learn the more structured eating habits and food choices that are necessary for weight loss. Still, some people don't want to follow menus that aren't their own but are ready to take our good science and adopt it to control their weight in their own way. That's why *The "I" Diet* offers menus and recipes to get you started but also explains everything you need to know to design your own individualized approach to hunger-free weight control. (Be ready to give my menus a second chance if you find you want to lose more weight than your own plan will allow.) By the way, I've added a few new recipes for this edition, starting on page 261. I simply couldn't stop myself from doing more kitchen experimentation!

I would love to know what you think. You can give me your feedback at www.instinctdiet.com. I look forward to hearing from you.

With thanks and best wishes,

Susan Roberts
Autumn 2009

PART I

THE BIG PICTURE

in•stinct (in'stingkt) *n* **1a.** the innate aspect of behavior that is unlearned, complex, and normally adaptive **b.** a powerful motivation or impulse
I (ī) *pron* **1a.** used to refer to oneself as speaker or writer **b.** the self, the ego
—The American Heritage Dictionary
of the English Language

CHAPTER 1

Our Five Basic Food Instincts

The Key to Permanent Weight Control

P icking up this book means you want to lose weight. It also means you have in your hands everything you need to actually do just that, even if weight control has eluded you in the past despite your best efforts. Why? Because the "I" Diet works. Just give it a try. You will lose weight healthily . . . and you will lose it forever.

If you're like most dieters, this may sound impossible. You have undoubtedly tried lots of diets: high-protein, low-carbohydrate, low-fat, liquid, grapefruit, cleansing. You've counted points, bought your food pre-packaged, gorged on steaks, slurped cabbage soup till you were green. And then you've blamed yourself for not being able to lose much weight or for gaining it right back. Speaking as a weight-loss researcher who has published nearly 200 research studies on weight control, I am here to tell you that the problem was not with you, but with the ineffective ways you were cutting calories. The "I" Diet will put you back in control.

Let's start with some things you *won't* experience on the "I" Diet. You won't get stuck on weight-loss plateaus, the reason many if not most dieters give up. (No more feeling like a failure when your scale doesn't move or actually inches up.) You won't have to exercise as part of the diet (though you should for your health). And best of all, you won't feel hungry; rather, you will feel full and *satisfied* all day long.

fiction: Lack of exercise keeps us from losing weight.
fact: Wrong.

Exercise is great for our physical health and state of mind, and for preventing weight gain in the first place, but it has a disappointingly small effect on weight loss. When it comes to shedding pounds, it's what and how much we eat that counts most. Normally sedentary people who add 60 minutes of exercise to their daily schedule might be able to lose about six pounds of body fat in about six months. But how many of us can put aside an hour every single day for exercise? Even if you could cram 30 minutes of vigorous daily exercise into your busy schedule, you'd probably lose only three pounds over a six-month period. So don't allow yourself to believe that exercise is a panacea for weight problems. This kind of thinking may keep you from focusing on what you put in your mouth.

Now for what you *will* experience. Sustainable, sometimes rapid weight loss: an average of 7 pounds (and up to 10 pounds) in the first two weeks. If you keep at it, you will lose up to 20 pounds in eight weeks. And then, if you want, you can go on to lose much more. Let me repeat, *this is all weight that you can keep off.* Many diet programs boast inflated claims, but among honest programs the "I" Diet is uniquely successful because its new approach to hunger reduction allows you to lose body fat as fast as the human body safely can. And it does this by combining the very best weight-loss science from around the world with genuinely delicious, easily prepared food. Most diets just address calorie reduction, even if they pretend otherwise, which means their food plans prove ineffective. Just cutting calories is a recipe for hunger—and eventual diet failure.

The "I" Diet eliminates your triggers and cravings. And, most importantly, it takes away hunger, allowing you to keep your calories down day after day.

How It Works

Five basic food instincts are responsible for our continuing survival against all odds. We know this from studying human history and from all the consistent findings of modern research into our eating patterns. These instincts can be our downfall unless we understand them and start to work *with* them. Our instinctive eating behavior falls into these categories:

✳ **Hunger** We need to *satisfy* our hunger. We like feeling full. We see this instinct in newborn infants, and we know this is not something they have learned; it is an innate need that will help to ensure their survival.

✳ **Availability** We eat just because the food is there. And— here's the thing to watch out for—we want to eat more when more food is there for the taking.

✳ **Calorie density** We love to eat and we love food, especially when it's loaded with calories. This is true in every culture.

✳ **Familiarity** We enjoy eating foods that are familiar to us. We associate these foods with feeling safe and comforted, and we have triggers that can drive us to eat them again . . . and again.

✳ **Variety** We are instinctively attracted to a variety of foods, and we eat considerably more when we're presented with more choices.

These food instincts are basic to who we are. We cannot change the fact that we have them, but we can learn to manage them. Just follow the "I" Diet carefully for a few weeks while your brain begins its job of reprogramming itself. When it comes to successful, permanent weight loss, almost nothing is more helpful than working with the innate biology that controls what we eat. Spiders spin webs because they are spiders, and we humans eat the way we do because we're human. It's time to embrace the true nature of human eating behavior to make weight control easier. That's what the "I" Diet is all about.

> **Our biological instincts play a key role in *what* we eat, *how* we eat, *when* we eat and *how much* we eat.**

Which Instincts Challenge You the Most?

Certain food instincts can be more difficult to manage than others. For example, have you found that hunger keeps you from trying to lose weight? Or that you can't pass by a bowl of potato chips without stopping to gobble up a handful or two? Your answers to the questions below will help you spot those instincts that are apt to give you the most trouble and therefore need extra consideration.

INSTINCT	HALLMARK
Hunger	Do you get hungry when you try to lose weight?
Availability	Do you eat more when portions are large or food is free?
Calorie density	Do you love high-calorie foods like chocolate, salty snacks, French fries or mac and cheese?
Familiarity	Do you still crave the foods your mother used to cook, or lose control and overeat when you're happy, upset or stressed?
Variety	Do you buy different kinds of chocolate, chips, cookies or ice cream (rather than just one kind of each)?

Dieting by Instinct

Once you become an expert on your own instinctive eating behavior, you'll find it easier to lose weight and keep it off. The next five chapters describe each food instinct in detail and explain exactly how your instincts affect your eating habits. The rest of the book is devoted to showing you lots of ways to put what you've learned into practice. If you want to get rid of some excess pounds as soon as reasonably possible, I strongly urge you to follow our eight-week menu plan in Stages I and II, rather than going it on your own. If, however, you want to learn how to prevent weight gain, lose a few pounds gradually or simply have more control over food and eating, reading up about your food instincts will help you achieve your goal as you discover new ways to make small but effective changes in your daily life. Stage III of the program will also show you how to avoid weight gain.

Since *The "I" Diet* is much more than a "what to eat" diet book, you'll find valuable "how to eat" instructions in each chapter. For example, you'll be introduced to the four proven ways to cut hunger and learn how useful they can be in different situations. You'll also start retraining your taste preferences so that, before you know it, you'll be loving the foods that make it easier to control your weight. You'll find out how to cope with temptation by taking charge of your food environment and by eating in structured ways that actually reduce your cravings. And here's the big payoff: You'll learn how to make simple changes in your daily routine that will help you feel more satisfied and reduce cravings by literally changing the neurological activity going on inside your head.

Stage I

This stage of the "I" Diet lasts just two weeks. It works because the composition of each nutritious meal suppresses hunger and the variety of foods you eat is deliberately restricted to help you get a good start on managing your instincts. Each daily menu lets you choose between Simply Good meals, made from foods you can pick up at your local supermarket or deli, and a complete line of Home Cooking recipes for preparing wonderful dishes from scratch. Both options include regular and vegetarian meals. Within each day, you can mix-and-match no-cooking with home cooking suggestions and meat with vegetarian choices.

You'll get to enjoy lots of tasty lean protein sources like skinless chicken breast and good (monounsaturated and polyunsaturated) fats like olive oil as well as appetite-satisfying carbohydrates like high-fiber cereals and apples in carefully balanced amounts, but all within three different daily menus repeated throughout the two weeks. You will also be encouraged to eat different vegetables and fruits and even some nuts, cheese and a very special type of dessert that will keep late-night munchies in check. What you won't get to eat, only for these first two weeks, is refined (white) carbohydrates. No alcohol, either, because it not only adds calories but also encourages cheating. But don't worry, you'll be adding these back into your diet in Stages II and III, once you're better able to cope with them.

fiction: With the right diet, you can lose 15 pounds in two weeks . . . and keep them off.
fact: No, you can't.

Let's say you normally consume an average of 2,500 calories a day. Even if you decided to stop eating altogether, you could lose only about three pounds of fat a week, and it goes without saying that this would be an unhealthy and even dangerous thing to do.

So how do some diets *appear* to deliver much faster weight loss? The reason is very simple. When you lose weight, you lose body fat *plus* water and a bit of muscle, so that just a pound of fat loss can show up on your scale as two or three pounds of weight loss. And if the diet is much lower in sodium or carbohydrates than your regular diet, you'll lose even more water, so your weight loss could actually appear to be as high as 15 pounds in two weeks. The trouble is, it's impossible to go on eating like that for very long, and the water weight will come right back with your first non-diet meal.

As long as you follow the "I" Diet plan, and that plan is supplying fewer calories than your body needs, you'll be losing fat every day with minimal water loss—as fast as sustainably possible. By the end of the eight-week program, you will have genuinely lost up to 20 pounds and should be able to keep those pounds off permanently.

Stage II

During this six-week stage of the menu plan, you'll get to eat a greater variety of foods and include more of the familiar tastes that you enjoy. The seven days of menus, which repeat each week, will help you develop good food habits and good meal routines. In fact, it's usually at about this time that my volunteers at Tufts talk about the magic of their diet. They don't understand how they can be eating so much, feeling so satisfied, really enjoying what they eat and still losing weight.

I don't want you to eliminate any food groups in Stage II, because your instincts can be satisfied only if you eat a wide variety of foods. Just as in Stage I, however, the foods you eat and the balance of those foods are carefully organized to keep hunger down and satisfaction up. By the end of Stage II, the *typical* "I" dieter has lost 16 pounds and is looking great and feeling better.

Stage III

This stage is the rest of your life. You'll learn the skills that you need to keep your weight down permanently. This is an important formal step in the "I" Diet program, not just an afterthought. *A different set of skills is needed to prevent weight regain.* These skills range from planning your own weight maintenance menus to keeping track of calories or making some general changes to what you eat so that you don't have to count anything but can still keep calories down and weight off. You can pick the approach that works for who you are and the life you lead.

Instincts at Work

Success for a Dress

When Anne came into our lab, she had a specific goal in mind— she wanted to celebrate her 20th wedding anniversary by renewing her vows with her husband at a family party the following year. Problem was, she had her heart set on wearing the dress she wore at her wedding but she'd put on 40 pounds since that happy day. "Food was Mom's way of saying she loved us," Anne said. "I was surrounded by barbecue, buttery mashed potatoes and home-baked apple pie from the time I was a little girl. And I've been eating the same things ever since." Clearly, familiarity was one of Anne's biggest challenges. With this in mind, we got started. One year later, Anne had lost 46 pounds and looked gorgeous at her ceremony, wearing the same satin gown she'd worn so many years before.

Losing Weight, Gaining Life

The "I" Diet is a life-changing program that is also a plan for rapid weight loss if you want it to be. Although some of the early drop in weight may be due to water loss, you can lose up to 20 pounds of mostly fat-weight by the end of eight weeks and the *typical* weight loss is 16 pounds. This will make a huge difference in inches and in your clothing size. Furthermore, the "I" Diet menu plan is so nutritious that you can always go back to Stage I and start all over again. Of course, you should never begin a diet without an okay from your doctor, but once you have the go-ahead, you can repeat the "I" Diet for greater weight loss. And since most of the weight you'll lose will be fat (not water or muscle, as in so many fad diets), it won't come right back on with your first non-diet meal. You'll find that our weight maintenance program will be a big help in keeping those pounds off permanently. I know, everyone says this is impossible, but it's not. I'll show you why it's not and how to do it.

Along the way, you'll also discover that you don't have to grit your teeth and suffer to lose weight. You can actually *enjoy* the process, rather than just wait for the end result. I'm glad to report that many "I" dieters have lost substantial amounts of weight and have been happy and healthy while doing so. Because of the scientific underpinning of the "I" Diet program, there is every reason in the world to believe that it will work the same way for you.

CHAPTER 2

Hunger
The Need to Feel Full

H unger is the one food instinct everyone is aware of—even people who have never dieted and don't realize how overpowering it can be. And most people who have dieted a time or two *know* they need a lot of help with this basic instinct. In fact, hunger is one of the two major reasons people give for abandoning a diet (the other is that they miss their favorite foods). If you're hungry, you can't keep calories down enough to sustain weight loss.

What foods should your diet contain to make hunger easier to avoid while you try to lose weight? Some diet gurus plug a low-carbohydrate, high-protein regimen as the one solution. Others say a high-carbohydrate and low-fat combination works best. Still others insist none of this matters and it's only calories that count. Now it's time for this confusion to stop! The truth is, there's no such thing as a holy grail when it comes to dietary composition and weight loss—but what you eat does make a huge difference.

Learning to control the signals that control your food instincts is one of the most valuable things you can do to make dieting easier. For example, if you eat at regular times, your body learns not to expect food at other times. I always recommend three meals and two snacks every day during weight loss (although if you're a person who really doesn't snack much, you might find that one snack is enough to keep you hunger-free). You don't have to be slavish about these regular meals. It's important that they fit your lifestyle and make eating more enjoyable, not less. If you like to sleep late on the weekends, it's fine to skip breakfast. Just make sure this becomes a regular weekend ritual so that it fits into a pattern that your body will learn to anticipate and enjoy.

In fact, your body uses several different signals to tell your brain that you need food, and this means there's more than one way to eat in order to control those signals. Once you understand this central fact, dieting can actually become much easier and much more enjoyable. In this chapter, you'll learn different ways to make hunger control easier (by eating the right food, spread out evenly over three meals and two snacks daily, always accompanied by a low-cal drink), but first we'll explore the way our brain "sees" food and what it has to do with our eating habits.

Why We Feel Hungry

There are three different but connected areas of the brain that compose what I like to call the food brain. The *hunger/satiety* center, located in the hypothalamus, receives signals from various parts of the body and responds by giving us our sensations of hunger or fullness. In communication with the hypothalamus, the *pleasure* center in the cerebral cortex recognizes different tastes of food, and the *reward* center in the midbrain secretes dopamine and other chemicals that make us feel good. Blood levels of glucose and fatty acids, as well as hormones such as ghrelin from the stomach and leptin from fat cells, are just some of the signals originating in the body that our brain is constantly monitoring. There are also nerve signals originating in the stomach and intestine that activate our food brain, along with numerous "gut hormones" that reach the brain through both blood and nerve signaling.

Every component of the food brain is also linked to the senses, so that the sight or smell of appetizing food initiates a series of responses called the cephalic phase of digestion. The autonomic nervous system springs into action, and here's what happens:

✸ Saliva production doubles.

✸ Gastric secretions increase to prepare for digestion (causing a gurgling stomach).

✸ Stomach muscles relax, creating a bigger stomach volume that will need more food to fill it before it registers as full.

✸ The pancreas secretes the hormone insulin even before there is food in the stomach. The insulin surge causes blood glucose to drop, which in turn causes hunger to increase.

✸ Gastric motility increases to push incoming food along quickly so it's digested sooner.

These physiological responses promote a negative cycle of overeating, and then overeating again, by speeding up the digestive process so that we end up being hungrier again, sooner. Controlling the signals transmitted to our food brain from our body and to sensory centers is the key to getting *all* our food instincts, including hunger, working for us.

The Illusion of Willpower

Do you ever find yourself in front of the fridge without realizing you were headed that way? Welcome to your subconscious, the principal controller of your need to eat. In fact, as discussed by Harvard psychologist Steven Pinker, using the subconscious brain is essential for survival skills because the conscious brain can't be entrusted with them. This is why weight control simply can't be left up to willpower, or the exercise of conscious control over conscious mental processes. Willpower has its place in decisions about food choices and the like, but if we try to use it to control hunger and desire after our instincts have been revved up, *forget it!*

Hunger-Fighting Meals

Hunger is, by and large, a meal-by-meal sensation. In other words, you need to consider each meal and snack as an individual event, rather than thinking about what you eat over the course of a whole day. You don't have to add it all up to see if you ate, say, enough fiber for that day—just think about whether each meal and each snack gives you what you need to satisfy your hunger. Because there are several ways to feel satisfied and delay the return of a growling stomach, you can choose a particular hunger-suppressing food combination at one meal and a different one at the next.

Obviously, you can't eat everything you want and still lose weight, but you do have several good options to make satisfying meals every day. Our own studies and those of other scientists around the world show that there are *four* effective ways to accomplish this. The diets that focus on just one of these ways soon lead to temptation and cheating; in other words, they fail to provide the variety of nutrients and flavors that you need to keep your food instincts satisfied as you restrict calories to lose weight. Using all four ways, outlined below, makes good practical sense since each one is particularly helpful in specific situations. For example, fiber is a great addition to home meals, allowing you to eat some normal foods and still lose weight, while the high-protein, low-carbohydrate combination is a great option for maintaining your diet when you're eating out or far from home.

Fiber, Fiber Everywhere

Fiber is extremely helpful both for losing weight and for keeping it off. Our research at Tufts has shown that people who eat 35 to 55 grams of fiber per day feel more satisfied during weight loss and lose more weight than those who eat less than that. As shown in the chart on the facing page, the typical American diet includes only about 15 grams of fiber a day, not even close to the recommended level for weight maintenance, which is 25 grams per day for women and 35 grams per day for men.

There are several different types of fiber, and all seem to help weight control. *Insoluble dietary fiber* forms a sludge that provides bulk from

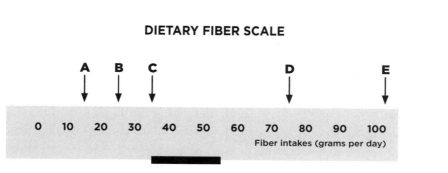

DIETARY FIBER SCALE

The optimal range for weight loss

A = Typical North American fiber intake.

B, C = Recommended intakes for women and men who don't need to lose weight.

D = Typical intakes of members of the Caloric Restriction Society, a group dedicated to achieving longer life through staying thin.

E = Estimated intake of our Paleolithic ancestors.

the top of your GI tract to the bottom. Examples include cellulose and the fibers in wheat bran, corn bran and rice bran. *Soluble dietary fiber* dissolves in water to form a thick gel, giving you a lot of bulk quickly (think of oatmeal and how full you feel for 30 minutes after eating it). This kind of fiber is found in foods like beans, fruit, vegetables and cereals containing oats and barley. The "I" Diet includes a variety of foods containing both insoluble and soluble fibers for their metabolic benefits. *Purified* and *synthetic fibers* such as inulin and guar gum are something else again. Food manufacturers often use them, but they're not classified as "dietary" fibers because they're not part of intact foods. These fibers probably have some benefits for weight control and are sometimes used in the "I" Diet menus in amounts that compensate for their possible lower effectiveness.

A particular advantage of high-fiber foods is that they can be added to a meal containing regular foods so you can eat things that would otherwise work against weight loss. For example, the "I" Diet cereal desserts

Great Sources of Dietary Fiber

¼ cup General Mills Fiber One cereal

¼ cup Kellogg's All-Bran Extra Fiber cereal

⅓ cup cooked pinto or other beans

10 Spicy Sesame Cracker Chips (page 182)

1 cup cooked green veggies, such as steamed broccoli

⅔ cup raspberries or blackberries

6 dried black mission figs

1 large apple

Each serving contains 5 to 6 grams of fiber. A single serving per meal added to your usual diet will help give you a total of 8 to 10 grams per meal.

(page 236) are high in fiber, making it possible to have foods like pizza and even ice cream on the menu. All the menus in Stages I and II have plenty of fiber with each meal, totaling about 35 to 45 grams per day. For people who get especially hungry, high-fiber cereal is a "free" food on the "I" Diet and gives extra fiber for extra fullness. In fact, fiber is such a great diet aid that even if you're not ready for a formal diet plan, it can still help you lose weight. See the list on this page for foods you can add to your regular diet. Since this will help you cut portions of other foods, it's likely you will lose some weight without trying too hard.

I want to emphasize that it's important to have fiber with most meals, rather than trying to pack a huge amount of fiber into one meal a day. So, by all means, have a bowl of high-fiber cereal (rich in insoluble fiber) mixed with a few raisins, nuts and seeds (containing soluble fiber) for breakfast, but try to keep up the good work with a large bean salad or a side of fiber-enriched bread for lunch and then complete your day with one of our high-fiber cereal desserts.

Do be sure to drink six to eight glasses of water daily when you eat more fiber to get the full benefits of the fiber and to prevent constipation. (Fiber needs water to work correctly in the intestines; indeed, its water-holding property is part of why it makes you feel more satisfied.) The relatively high intakes of fiber in the "I" Diet menus are perfectly safe. As shown in the scale on the previous page, our Paleolithic ancestors ate about 100 grams a day, so an intake of 40 grams or so is nothing that the human body isn't prepared to receive. Just don't increase your intake too rapidly. (In Chapter 8, you'll learn how to gauge your present fiber intake and how to get it up to satisfying levels safely.)

The High-Protein, Low-Carbohydrate Combo

Proteins have been shown to be very satisfying and to slow the return of hunger. Unlike refined carbohydrates, they don't induce big fluctuations in blood glucose, one of our hunger signals. Also, proteins are digested slowly, sending nutrients into the bloodstream over a period of hours (not minutes, like many carbohydrate sources) and may also have beneficial effects on hunger-making hormones like ghrelin.

That's why a piece of grilled fresh fish (research studies show that fish is especially satisfying, even by the standards of high-protein foods) or half a chicken breast with a side of green vegetables or a salad are good examples of high-protein meals that keep hunger at bay for several hours. High-protein, low-carb meals are also extremely practical when you're eating out. You can go to a restaurant and have half a lean entrée with a side salad and a glass of mineral water and keep to your diet without making a public fuss about it.

Proteins without carbohydrates get dull. Carbs on their own can be fattening. Mix them up—and eat them anywhere, with pleasure.

The trouble with high-protein diets is that they can get really boring. If you try to stay on a high-protein diet meal after meal, week in and week out, the temptation to cheat may get stronger and stronger because your variety instinct is clamoring for attention. This is why high-protein meals are included in the "I" Diet as one of several options rather than the only way to eat.

"Good" *and* "Bad" Carbohydrates

The Glycemic Index (GI), originally used in research on treating diabetes, measures how much a particular food increases blood glucose in the two-hour period after eating. Foods with a high GI value cause a big rise in blood glucose; low-GI foods, only a small rise. The significance here is that low-GI foods have been shown to suppress hunger extremely well because the more stable blood glucose produced by these foods tells our food brain

Typical Glycemic Index Values

Glucose (standard value)	100
Carrots	16–92
Chex cereal	86
Rice Krispies, Corn Flakes	82
Baked potato	80
Watermelon	80
White rice	40–75
Oatmeal	42–75
Honey	72
White bread	70
100% whole-wheat bread	70
Sucrose (table sugar)	60
Baked beans	56
Oat bran bread	56
Coarse wheat bread	53
Cheese pizza	50
Banana, ripe	50
Cherries, fresh	46
Pumpernickel	46
Apple, raw	40
Garbanzo beans, cooked	40
Orange, fresh	40
Coarse barley bread	37
Grapefruit, fresh	25

that all is well and we don't need to eat again yet.

Many things affect GI values. The more a food is cooked, the higher its GI. The riper a plant or the more finely ground a grain, the higher its GI. On the other hand, the presence of fat or acid lowers the GI. But don't worry about any of that. Just remember that refined and finely ground cereals and starches, which are digested relatively quickly, usually have a substantially higher GI value than coarsely milled and whole cereal grains, nuts, fruits, legumes and non-starchy vegetables. Here's another way you might think about it: Unrefined, whole, chunky, lightly cooked and sour foods almost always have low GIs.

It's really worthwhile to include some low-GI foods among the options in your menu plan, not only for their benefit in reducing hunger but also because they provide the carbohydrates your body needs. We do seem to instinctively crave carbohydrates, and any plan that doesn't have a way to give you some carbs in a healthy form will be fundamentally unsatisfying after a while. This is why low-GI foods like legumes (chickpeas and kidney beans, for example) and low-carb bread (not really that low in carbs, but low GI) are important members of the "I" Diet food group. In addition, we recently discovered that the quality of weight loss is better on low-GI diets because even if you don't lose more weight, *there's more body fat in the weight you do lose.* And as shown in our studies at Tufts with Taso Pittas and also in similar studies by David Ludwig at Harvard, people who start out with high insulin secretion do better on low-GI diets, losing more weight more easily.

Even though low GI is generally good, it's possible to go *too* low. And if you do, you may find that carbohydrates with very low GI values are less appetizing and tempt you to cheat. Just picture yourself eating plain boiled wheat kernels, instead of wheat kernels ground up into coarse flour and made into a decent loaf of bread, and you'll get the idea.

> ### Can Low-GI Foods Taste Good?
>
> Low-GI foods, when eaten alone, may not taste as good as foods with higher GI values. They're digested more slowly, so our brain learns to like them but not love them, probably because they don't release as many of the feel-good taste and reward chemicals. In our recipes, low-GI foods like beans, wheat berries, barley and green vegetables are always mixed with some fat or high-GI foods in the same meal to make them yummy.

The solution? Mix things up! As you flip through the menus in Part II of this book, you'll see that many of our suggested meals combine low-GI carbohydrates with some higher-GI foods for taste.

High Volume

My friend Barbara Rolls, a pioneer in research on meal volume and feeling satisfied, has shown that volunteers presented with meals whose calorie content has been secretly lowered (say, by making a milk shake with low-fat milk instead of regular milk) will eat just as much food but take in fewer calories. From my own lab, Edward Saltzman showed that volume is far more important than whether calories come from carbohydrates or fat. The mechanism that causes this isn't known for sure but is probably related to the activation of stretch receptors in the stomach or simply our perception of the "right" amount of food. When food is bulky, you feel more satisfied and your diet gets a boost.

Taken together, these results mean that a high-volume food can be either a high-carb food such as hot oat bran cereal or a high-fat food that also has a lot of water, such as stir-fried Chinese vegetables. High volume by itself isn't a magic bullet for weight loss, but when combined with

Hot Stuff

More than 20 years ago, I was introduced to the satisfying effects of hot peppers when I worked in West Africa. Most of the food there was pretty hot, but the people of one tribe in my area were renowned for making their food extra spicy and other tribes joked that they were economizing by making it so peppery that no one would need too much of it. Research has shown that this actually works. The chemical capsaicin, the hot ingredient in hot peppers (as well as in cayenne and to a lesser extent in ginger and pepper), reduces calorie intake (especially of low-fat meals) by as much as 8%.

generous amounts of fiber, it's a worthy member of the "I" Diet menu plan because it makes it easier to stop eating sooner.

A high-fiber cereal with nonfat or 1% milk makes an ideal meal for breakfast. The milk contributes to the perfection because it contains vitamin D, and new research has demonstrated that a deficiency of this vitamin can cause insulin resistance (which works against weight control and may also increase the risk of clinical depression). Another high-volume star is soup, which has been proven to be very effective in making you feel satisfied if it contains dense particles such as barley grains that slow down digestion. Still another great high-volume meal is a full dinner salad with enough low-calorie dressing for taste—tons of volume in a green or mixed vegetable salad. And when you add nice crunchy and high-substance bits on top, such as grilled chicken breast, sunflower seeds, a few nuts and carrot slices, you get plenty of chewing, which apparently also aids in feeling satisfied and full.

Mixing It Up

Each meal in the "I" Diet menu plan has at least one of the hunger-suppressing compositions described in this chapter. Some meals emphasize high protein; others, high volume and fiber; still others, low GI. Usually, several of these good compositions are added together for super-satisfying weight-loss meals.

Fine, you say, but this sounds really complicated. Will I ever learn how to get all my meals into the perfect hunger-suppressing balance? I promise

Best Foods for Keeping Hunger Down and Satisfaction Up

High-fiber cereals, e.g., Fiber One, All-Bran Extra Fiber	Mixed in "I" Diet recipes with chocolate, yogurt, milk, sugar-free ice cream, even salads.
Green and raw vegetable salads with vinaigrette or light dressing	Very high volume; lots of natural variety.
Cooked non-starchy vegetables such as broccoli, mushrooms, zucchini	High volume; high fiber.
White fish such as cod and haddock; also salmon	Low in calories, high in protein; highest satiety of any protein food.
Apples	Portable sweet-tasting snack; low in calories, high in fiber; hard to eat too quickly; wide variety.
Berries, e.g., raspberries, strawberries, blackberries	Low in calories, high in fiber and easy enjoyment. Frozen berries are a great standby.
Legumes in entrées, soups and salads	Very high in fiber and volume; wide variety; good taste (when not overcooked).
Low-carb, coarse, high-fiber, high-protein and barley breads	More filling than regular breads; high protein and higher fiber.
Nonfat and 1% milk; nonfat and 2% plain Greek yogurt; nonfat yogurt sweetened with sugar substitute	A great way to add protein to high-fiber cereal and "I" Diet Hot or Cold Chocolate (page 253). Greek yogurt is especially high in protein and delicious with fruit for breakfast.
Spicy Sesame Cracker Chips (page 182)	Good for providing that salty snack fix; high in fiber.

A Typical "I" Diet Day

Here's one of our menus, with every kind of hunger-suppressing meal and snack.

Breakfast: High-fiber cereal with granola and milk; strawberries; water, coffee/tea (high fiber, mixed GI, high volume).

Mid-morning snack: Apple and peanuts (high volume).

Lunch: Lentil soup; ham-and-cheese sandwich; frozen grapes; water, coffee/tea (high fiber, mixed GI, high volume).

Afternoon snack: "I" Diet Hot or Cold Chocolate (high volume).

Dinner: Steak, broccoli and a side salad; Ginger-Pecan Crunch or pear with caramel sauce; water, coffee/tea (protein, high fiber, mixed GI, high volume).

you, by the time you finish this book, you will know how to do it. For now, don't worry. Just follow the structured menus for both Stage I (the first two weeks) and Stage II (the next six weeks) as closely as you can to learn by good example. But before you do that, it's a good idea to learn about the other instincts that are controlling the way you think about food.

CHAPTER 3

Availability
Just Because It's There

W hen you open a bag of potato chips, do you have to keep eating down to the last chip? Or if you stick your hand in the cookie jar, do you find you can't stop yourself until you've eaten everything that was in there? If so, it's because your availability instinct has taken charge and you just can't help yourself. It's a little recognized fact that having food readily available can trigger hormonal and nervous system activity that makes us hungry—even if we've just finished a fancy five-course dinner.

Still more surprising is the recent finding that the available food doesn't even have to taste good. We'll wolf it down as if we haven't eaten for days. It turns out that we'll even overeat stale peanuts if there's a big enough bowlful within easy reach!

Food, Food Everywhere

Our instinct to eat just because it's there developed thousands of years ago. As members of the species now called *Homo sapiens sapiens*, we had to cope with the changing circumstances in the world around us. This was essential for survival, and the most successful survivors were those who ate whenever food was available. The problem for us today is the *abundance* of available food, especially if it's food that we know and like. Too often, the cephalic phase of digestion comes into play, and our metabolism is off and running before we know it. Saliva production increases, gastric acids flow, a surge of insulin creates a drop in blood glucose and we feel that we need more food in our stomach even if it's already full.

Bigger portions are a further problem because even more food is in front of you when you sit down to eat, so your availability instinct keeps you from putting your fork down when you should feel full. After summarizing all the research studies on portion size and food consumption, my lab calculated that for every 1,000 calories added to your plate on top of what you need, you'll most likely end up eating about 190 of them. That doesn't sound like a lot, but doing this just once a day for a year can cause a weight gain of many pounds. It's easy to blame our mothers for telling us to clean our plates, but in fact most of us do this pretty instinctively with no encouragement at all.

You're not just being weak when you can't help eating something because it's sitting in front of you. Your availability instinct is telling you to go right ahead!

On top of our biology, there's a purely practical reason for being drawn to large portions. Our notion of what's normal in terms of serving size has been skewed by the obscenely large portions served in restaurants. And when portion sizes are routinely several times what we actually need, the internal signals that we rely on to tell us when to stop eating become confused. In a study conducted by Brian Wansink at Cornell, soup bowls were refilled surreptitiously so that none of the participants knew how much they were consuming (because the levels in the bowls never went down). The surprising result was that, on average, the participants ate 76% more soup but estimated that they had eaten only 5% more!

Good Bad Popcorn

n a study at Cornell University, 158 moviegoers were offered free popcorn in return for answering some questions about the theater after the movie. Half got fresh popcorn in 120-gram (4-ounce) or 240-gram (8-ounce) buckets. The other half got stale popcorn in the same-size buckets. After the movie, the containers were weighed to see how much everybody ate.

Average amount eaten (in grams)

Fresh popcorn, small size	59	Stale popcorn, small size	38
Fresh popcorn, large size	86	Stale popcorn, large size	51

The moviegoers who were given a large bucket of stale popcorn ate almost as much as those who were given a smaller bucket of fresh popcorn. This doesn't mean they liked it. They just ate it because it was there.

Gulp, Gulp, Gulp

Large portions also encourage what I call the Gulping Syndrome. Faced with a large plate of a favorite food, we tend to take bigger bites than we normally would and swallow them quickly without realizing what we're doing. Often we prepare the next mouthful on our fork while we're still swallowing the previous one. Studies show that even preschoolers will take larger bites if they're presented with large portions of food; instinctively adapting to their environment, they open their mouths wider and swallow faster.

Here's why the Gulping Syndrome is such a problem. When we take big bites of food, we don't give ourselves time to realize that we're getting full and we don't savor the taste enough. This means we end up eating more food simply because it takes longer for us to feel satisfied.

No Time for Taste

What we think of as taste is really 90% smell. In the mad rush of gulping down large portions, fewer of the volatile smell chemicals in food get to activate the 10 million olfactory receptors located in our nose. This loss of intense taste when large portions are eaten in big bites is probably why small portions have been found to be just as satisfying as large ones. Studies show that people given small bowls for ice cream eat about a third less than if they're given large bowls but feel equally satisfied.

Be the Boss

Who's in charge of your food environment? *You* are. So it's up to you to avoid temptation by getting rid of what tempts you. This might sound like a small thing, but I promise you it can make a big difference. According to our research, being susceptible to foods lying around at home can cause a massive 40 pounds of weight gain between the ages of 20 and 55. Below are some suggestions for removing temptations from your home.

✳ **Make your available food *good* food.** Consult the Starter Shopping List on page 70 and then use the Savvy Shopper Supermarket Directory (Appendix E), which will make it easy to find all the foods that can actively help you lose weight. Put these foods where you can see them and get to them easily. Arrange fruit in a bowl, and pile up Snack Attack Packs (page 248) on the kitchen counter. Keep a bowl of cut-up celery, red peppers and other vegetables in the fridge, ready to go.

Have you created an environment of super-available foods on purpose because you love to eat and this makes it easier? Enjoying more satisfying foods *with every meal* works against temptation triggered by hunger.

✳ **Learn that less is more.** Whenever possible, buy smaller portions—even of healthy foods. No need to buy a seven-pound chicken when a four-pounder will do. Bring home only as much fruit as you plan to eat. Apply this principle to all your food purchases and you'll be pleasantly surprised by the reduced size of your grocery bill as well as your waistline.

✳ **Get rid of unhealthy foods.** I know this isn't easy, but just do it. Clean out your kitchen cupboards and check under the bed and any other place where you might have hidden stuff that tempts you. Toss out all those half-full bags of chips and crackers and the leftover cake from last night's party. If you can't bear to throw food away, or if others in your family might threaten your life if you get rid of their triple crème Saga cheese, put all the rich stuff in one cupboard or on the bottom shelf in the back of the fridge and pretend (to yourself) that you don't know it's there.

* **Write down everything you eat.** Keeping an honest record of exactly what goes into your mouth is an invaluable tool when it comes to weight loss. It's surprising how many people fall into the trap of *eating outside awareness*. Food is everywhere, tempting us all the time, and we

---

Instincts at Work

A Man and His Car

For many years, Michael had made Saturday morning trips to Boston's Italian North End to collect the warm, fragrant loaves of bread that his family loved. When he needed to lose weight, he was willing to exclude white bread from his menu plan but didn't want to give up his weekly trips. The trouble was, that bread was just too tempting as it sat in the passenger seat on the drive home, and he would start down the slippery slope of temptation by pulling off a small piece and gobbling it down quickly until a whole loaf was gone before he pulled into his driveway. Weight loss was not happening! Then Michael got an idea. The next Saturday, he put the bread in the trunk of his car, and his wife was able to stash it away when he got home. Oh yes, he began to lose weight.

---

can easily think we're eating a lot less than we really are. It's even possible to overeat when we eat nothing unhealthy. I suggest keeping a careful record of what you eat for several days before you start the "I" Diet. You may discover that casual eating is your diet destroyer. At Tufts, we find that many volunteers cut down on portion size and casual eating soon after they start recording everything they eat. In fact, writing down what they eat improves their food awareness to such an extent that quite a few of them begin to lose weight even before their diet starts.

* **Make high-calorie foods less user-friendly.** The less often you see large amounts of foods like nuts, cheese and chocolate, and the harder they are to get at, the less tempted you'll be to overeat them. You might buy nuts in the shell, for example, or limit yourself to grated Parmesan cheese (not the delectable soft blocks that you can cut nice slices from). In the chocolate

In Praise of Small Spoons

Spoon size has a surprising effect on your ability to enjoy a small portion. Dig into a quarter-cup of ice cream with a big modern dessert spoon and you'll be finished in a couple of bites. Using an old-fashioned teaspoon, however, you take about 20 bites and your dessert seems more substantial. Yard sales and antique stores are awash in tiny spoons that have only a quarter of the capacity of the modern teaspoon, so for a few pennies you can get a great diet aid.

department, try buying a chunk of Belgian chocolate and storing it in the refrigerator so that cutting off a piece to eat is a job in itself (and requires care!). Incidentally, most people are less likely to overeat dark chocolate than milk chocolate, so stick with the dark if that helps. And when it comes to alcohol (after Stage I of the "I" Diet), try refilling your glass with mineral water after the first drink so there's no place to put a refill. This works for wine, beer and mixed drinks, too. It may take a little getting used to, but it's calorie wise.

At mealtimes, don't put anything on the table that you shouldn't eat in unlimited quantities. Leave entrée dishes on a side table or countertop nearby. Put less food on your plate, and cut it up before you start eating. And speaking of plates, smaller ones make portions look bigger and seem more satisfying.

✳ **Outsmart the Holiday Binge Syndrome.** The same tricks that work during the rest of the year are especially important at holiday time. Buy less food—an 8-pound Thanksgiving turkey instead of a 14-pound one, for example. If you bake, make half as many cookies as you usually do and give away as many as you can. Include lots of fresh vegetables and fruits in your meals, and throw away or "re-gift" most of the holiday candy, cakes and other delights your friends love to shower on you. Better yet, ask for non-food gifts next time!

Out and About

The more small changes you can make to control the food environment around you when you're not eating at home, the easier it will be to avoid backsliding in the calorie department.

✳ **Limit restaurant meals.** Eat at home as often as possible, especially during Stage I. Restaurant meals contain more calories and less fiber than home-cooked meals, and the more often people eat out, the heavier they tend to be. In a study we did of 73 men and women from age 19 to 80, those who ate in restaurants only three

In one study, restaurant chefs reported that the portions they considered "normal" were two to three times the size recommended by the U.S. government!

times a month on average had fully a quarter less body fat than those who ate out once a day. It didn't matter where they ate; it was the *frequency* of restaurant meals that mattered. Partly this is because of the huge portions that restaurants serve. But a study in my lab also found that some restaurants serve even larger portions than they admit to, which is bad news indeed for those of us who want to control our weight. Some dishes had literally twice as many calories as the website menus indicated, and that didn't include the sides! Weight control is challenging enough when you know what the choices contain; it's next to impossible if you're getting hundreds of calories more than you think.

If you don't have time for home cooking, use our Simply Good menus, created mostly from prepared supermarket foods. It's very important to start reprogramming your instincts early on, and this is the best way I know to do that. When you must eat in a restaurant, never start out hungry. Remember how *Gone with the Wind*'s Scarlett O'Hara ate before she went to the big party where she first met Rhett Butler? Take a tip from a Southern belle, but keep your pre-meal "meal" light—maybe a bowl of high-fiber cereal with low-fat milk, or a small salad.

Try to gather as much nutrition information as you can about the restaurant ahead of time; check the Internet or the listing in Appendix H. Planning simple choices such as grilled chicken and a fresh green salad before you get to the restaurant makes it easier to keep calories down and say "No, thanks" to other stuff. And don't be embarrassed about being really, really picky when you order. Asking for dressing on the side is just the start here. No extra carbs, no butter on broiled fish (or a butter-laden something underneath) and an additional helping of steamed veggies are all yours for the asking.

Trick Your Brain

Available food becomes less of a problem if you pay less attention to it. You can get hungry just because of sensory information fed to your brain from your eyes, nose and mouth. When you stop the information flow, you short-circuit the hunger. What if driving past the doughnut shop every morning fills you with temptation? If driving down a different street doesn't make sense, then look straight ahead and breathe through your mouth as you pass by. Temptation banished!

✳ **Keep tempting food out of reach.** When you do eat out, take charge. Tell the waiter to skip the bread, and if your dinner companions are sharing French fries or fried calamari, ask them to keep the dishes on the other side of the table. Wine by the glass is easier to control than wine by the bottle. Also, it's a good idea to take a pass on appetizers. And if you can't resist dessert, ask for a half-portion or divide it yourself and either give the other half to someone at the table or just leave it behind.

✳ **Beware of buffets.** When a buffet is your only option, try to put together meals that are as close to those on the "I" Diet menus as possible. Scrambled eggs and fruit are good for breakfast; so is high-fiber cereal. For lunch and dinner, stick with salads and steamed vegetables plus a quarter-cup of lean meat or fish. A couple of bites of dessert are okay as long as you don't get carried away.

✳ **Skip the calories at parties.** Have some high-fiber cereal beforehand and you probably won't find it hard to bypass the greasy, low-quality foods that swamp most party menus. Keep your glass topped with mineral water.

✳ **Imagine that a tempting food is really inedible.** When you catch yourself eyeing a food full of calories, promptly imagine that there's something drastically wrong with it. For example, if you're tempted by a calorie-laden breakfast sandwich when you're buying your morning coffee, imagine that someone's hand slipped and poured a cup of salt over the eggs. Or, when you see some divine-looking macaroni and cheese in the cafeteria, imagine that the brown stuff on top is sand. This technique of mine can save you hundreds of calories every day.

CHAPTER 4

Calorie Density

Too Good to Resist

A lmost everybody loves high-calorie foods, but does this mean we're *instinctively* attracted to foods that are jam-packed with calories? You bet it does. Calories are king all over the world, in every culture. In the west, we love brownies, doughnuts, chips, cheese and hot fudge sundaes. In China, the most popular foods are braised pork bellies, meat-filled dumplings, fried dough and fried scallion pancakes—the highest-calorie foods available. Even in Africa, where calorie-rich foods are generally hard to find, people seek out the most calorie-laden things they can get their hands on, such as white bread made from imported flour, and add oil to any recipe when it can be afforded.

An affinity for foods loaded with calories was an asset during early human development, when the next meal was an unpredictable event. It made sense back then to eat calorie-rich foods because they provided

What Does "High-Calorie" Mean?

I n my lab at Tufts, we define high-calorie foods as those containing more than 40 calories per ounce. For example, fresh fruits and green vegetables typically contain 8 to 16 calories per ounce and are found at the top of the recommended food list, whereas most chips and nuts fall well below the line at 155 and 165 calories, respectively. For a list of typical calorie contents, see Appendix C.

the most energy. Today, however, our instinctive attraction to those foods stands directly in the way of controlling our weight.

The other thing to realize is that we've been blindsided. People have always loved calories, but opportunities to enjoy them have increased dramatically. Forty years ago, few people ate outside of mealtimes and regular snack times. And with the exception of an occasional ice-cream cone, almost no one ate while walking down the street. Nowadays, it's hard to make a quick trip to the mall without encountering the enticing odor of a Cinnabon (730 calories per roll). We can't undo the world we live in, but we can learn to use the best strategies that science now offers to help us avoid giving in to our perfectly natural love of calories.

That Food-Is-Bliss Feeling

C ontrary to what you might think, there is no magic in the actual taste of the high-calorie foods we love. As shown by Adam Drewnowski of the University of Washington, the story is simple. The more calories per ounce a food has, the more we prefer it. And the more we prefer it, the more tempting it looks on our plate.

We love high-calorie foods because when we eat them the reward center in our food brain releases feel-good chemicals like dopamine. Our brain is remarkably good at learning to anticipate what tastes come with what calories. We quickly learn that, say, brownies release pleasing chemicals in our brain, so we learn to like the way they taste and when we see that food again we want to gobble it up.

When people say they love food too much to diet, what they're usually talking about is food loaded with calories.

Narrowing the Gap

As far as we can tell, the human brain acts like a scale when it comes to evaluating foods and deciding which ones will be the most desirable. For example, it figures out that a cupcake with frosting (150 calories) is richer than a slice of plain bread (75 calories), so it lets us know that the cupcake will taste better than the bread. It doesn't measure absolute calories, but it assesses the relative calorie density of foods by monitoring things like changes in blood levels of nutrients and hormones. This means that whatever foods are at the top end of your personal calorie scale will taste good, even if the top end isn't very high, and that narrowing the range of calorie density can make *everything* taste good!

The "I" Diet menu plan is designed to distribute calories more evenly so that you enjoy everything you eat even with a lower calorie intake. This is achieved by 1) eliminating calorie-dense treats the first two weeks as your cravings start to recalibrate, 2) introducing low-calorie, high-fiber entrées that taste similar to those containing more calories, 3) offering treats with fewer calories and more fiber to prolong digestion and ward off hunger, and 4) adding a little fat or cheese to vegetables to increase calories and their yummy factor.

Balancing the Scales

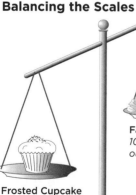

Fat-Free Salad
10 calories per ounce

Frosted Cupcake
150 calories per ounce

"I" Diet Lasagna
50 calories per ounce

Salad with Oil and Vinegar
20 calories per ounce

Before Weight Loss A cupcake will taste better than salad with fat-free dressing *because it has many more calories and less fiber.*

During Weight Loss You will enjoy both "I" Diet Lasagna and a salad with olive oil and balsamic vinegar *because there's less difference in their calorie density and fiber.*

Interestingly, it doesn't seem to matter whether our calories come from fat, carbohydrates or protein. In fact, the most popular foods are actually a mixture of all three of these. Most of us are not simply "carboholics" but "calorieholics," and our strongest preferences are for foods containing some of those rapidly digested white carbs, with a little fat and protein thrown in for good measure.

The Power of Leptin

Here's something you may be confused about now. If we instinctively love calories, how can we ever truly hope to enjoy food that helps weight loss? Won't a brownie *always* taste better?

The answer to this riddle is emerging from new research studies, and leptin is a key player. Leptin is a hormone secreted from fat cells to help control various processes, like whether you feel hungry or full. When you're overweight and overeating, leptin is secreted in excessive amounts. The more you eat, the more leptin in your bloodstream, and one of the things it does is suppress neuronal firing in both the cortex and midbrain areas where your taste and reward sensations occur. This means that when you've gained weight, you can't enjoy food as much because leptin is damping down your pleasure centers and pretty soon only really indulgent foods taste good. But as you lose weight, your leptin levels drop, your neurons are released from their leptin prison and healthy food starts to taste good. This explains something we've noticed at Tufts, which is that during and after weight loss our volunteers become more sensitive to food pleasure and lower-calorie foods taste better and better. Sure, calorie-rich foods will always taste good if you keep eating them, but when lower-calorie foods start tasting as good as those high-calorie goodies once did—why bother?

Tips for Treat Control

Learning how to enjoy high-calorie treats without overeating them is essential if you want to lose weight and keep it off. If treats have been a big part of your diet up to now, it will be important to eat them less frequently and in smaller portions.

✳ **Never eat your treat alone.** This doesn't mean you should never eat that cheese you love when you're by yourself. Just don't eat *it* by *itself*— when it's not accompanied by other lower-calorie food. When you eat your treat along with a reasonable portion of something lower in calories and higher in fiber, you'll get the delicious taste but also a feeling of fullness. If, for example, chips are your treat and you enjoy them with

> ### Sleep and Calories
>
> People who sleep 5 hours or less per night are typically 10 pounds heavier than those who sleep 7 hours or more. Sleep deprivation releases hormones that make you more tempted to eat high-calorie foods like chips, ice cream, cheese and brownies. If you're not getting enough sleep right now, see if you can reach a better balance *before* you start the "I" Diet.

a low-fat yogurt dip and some red pepper slices and celery for additional dipping, you'll end up having eaten fewer chips and fewer calories while still feeling satisfied. The same goes for appetizers of cheese and crackers and creamy dips (and even things like hamburgers, which can be quite low in calories if you enjoy a reasonably sized patty made filling with the addition of lettuce, tomatoes and pickles). You're probably used to eating these foods by themselves or with other high-calorie extras when you're hungry and end up eating far too much—sometimes a whole meal's worth of calories. If so, it's time to change, and I'm sure you can since all it takes is a little practice.

Making the most of low-calorie add-ons is also great for losing weight in a household that includes other family members. The rest of the family can still have the higher-calorie things they love, and with almost no effort you can add lower-calorie, more satisfying extras that will help you maintain control of your weight.

✳ **Apply the "sandwich" technique.** This is my variation of the don't-eat-your-treat-by-itself strategy. Using this technique, you sandwich your high-calorie mealtime and snack foods between two lower-calorie foods. For the top of the "sandwich," when you're most hungry, have something bulky and filling like a green salad with legumes, seafood and dressing or a hearty vegetable soup. For the middle of the sandwich, have your entrée and a small rich dessert like a sliver of blueberry pie. The bottom of the sandwich should always be low in calories and should signal the end of the meal—perhaps a cup of coffee or herbal tea, or a bowl of high-fiber cereal with fresh strawberries. This way, it will be easier to feel ready to stop eating before you've overeaten.

✳ **Follow the "once-a-day" plan.** With a little practice, this can work very well. The "I" Diet menu plan allows for a 100-calorie treat of your choice every day once you get into Stage II, and you can enjoy these treats to the max because you know this is your time to indulge. It's perfectly fine to skip a treat one day and double up the next so that on the second day you can indulge in twice as much of your treat (200 calories worth) or two wisely chosen 100-calorie treats.

> **Start eating high-calorie treats in moderate portions along with satisfying, lower-calorie foods and you may find yourself losing weight even before you start dieting.**

✳ **Make indulgences less indulgent.** The more you can get the tastes you love in lower-calorie, higher-fiber foods, the more you can enjoy everything you eat. Our easy, flavorful recipes are designed with this important principle in mind.

✳ **A time for everything.** Establishing regular times to eat is one of the best ways to turn your instincts into friends. I just can't stress this enough. When you get this system up and running, your brain will know that you'll be having a special chocolate dessert every Saturday evening and it will stop pestering you about dessert on Monday, Tuesday and Wednesday . . . Make a commitment to this change, and you'll see how well it works.

Don't expect too much immediately when it comes to getting the high-calorie foods you crave under better control; however, most "I" dieters experience substantial changes in temptation within two weeks of following our menus really carefully. By eating healthier food when you're hungry and sandwiching high-calorie foods into more sustaining meals, you can make real changes in how you feel about these foods. Just be patient. You'll get there. Over time, small steps will add up to great strides.

CHAPTER 5

Familiarity
Cravings and Triggers

W e love what we know, and sometimes we love it too much. It's just that simple. People enjoy eating food that's familiar to them, whether it's crayfish in New Orleans, herring in Oslo or ants in Africa. True, we start life with some basic preferences for sweet tastes over salty ones, but these "starter tastes" seem to be quickly overruled by what we eat every day. The reason we want steak for dinner instead of ants is that supermarkets all over the place have steak on sale while you'd be hard-put to find a special on toasted ants.

Instinctively, we're drawn to what we know, but what we know and therefore like is subject to change. When a new food comes on the market, we usually try it out, get used to it and end up embracing it like an old friend. Take hot dogs, for example. We had never heard of them until they were introduced in America at the Chicago exposition in 1893, and now it's hard to imagine a baseball game without them. Then there's yogurt. Fermented foods have been eaten for thousands of years, but they were not common in North America until yogurt was introduced in the late 1960s.

Playing It Safe

The foods that we already know and like are the ones that activate our familiarity instinct. Historically, this instinct kept us safe. For our Paleolithic ancestors, being cautious about trying new foods was all that stood between a good dinner and death by poison. Those who survived were the ones who instinctively ate small bites of a new berry or leaf before eating a generous amount of it. That caution kept them alive as trial-and-error taught them the difference between what was good and safe and what was dangerous. It's the same for us. As Leanne Birch of Penn State has demonstrated, even young children have to taste a new food 10 to 15 times before they begin to enjoy it.

Besides tasting little bits of new foods, we learn what's safe to eat from the people around us. As Matt Ridley has discussed in his book *The Origin of Virtue,* humans are unique within the animal kingdom in that we learn from and cooperate widely with people outside our immediate genetic family. Other species like wolves and bees also cooperate, but only within their extended family group. The efficiency of learning and specialization fostered by our widespread interactions is a major reason for our success as a species. Survival necessities like growing food take less time because they're more efficient, freeing up others of us to do things like learn to build bridges, do nutrition research, play the violin and shop!

The more you look at TV and magazine ads for food, the cozier you get with things you shouldn't eat.

The downside of learning what to eat from the people around us is that watching a next-door neighbor dig into a double cheeseburger can make us want to do the same. Even if you don't usually eat cheeseburgers, just seeing your neighbor chow down on one makes it more familiar and therefore more desirable. Advertisers take advantage of this I-know-it, therefore-I-want-it familiarity instinct. How often have you seen a TV commercial for a mouthwatering four-cheese pizza and found yourself wanting pizza for dinner that night? Too often, I'll bet. A solution to this problem: *Avoid watching TV ads for food.* Either mute the sound, change the channel or leave the room to do some dishes or feed the cat. The same holds true for magazine food ads.

Just turn the page when you see something you know would interfere with achieving your weight goal.

But let's go back to watching your neighbor eat his cheeseburger. Although it's true that this might light up your food brain, it doesn't have to work that way. Making simple changes in how you eat can get your familiarity instinct working in an all-systems-go effort geared to changing your preferences and even your cravings so that you actually want the healthy foods that help weight loss, not those loaded with fats and refined carbohydrates that just lead to overeating.

It's Not Your Fault

Remember record albums? The first couple of times you listened to them, the order of the songs might not have meant anything to you. But after a while, as each song finished, the beginning of the next one would pop up in your head. When it comes to familiarity, your food brain works the same way. Let's say you ate a luscious ripe peach when you were a child. The front part of your brain sent out signals to other parts of your brain, telling them to shoot out chemicals like dopamine that gave you a powerful sensation of pleasure. Naturally, you liked that. You ate another peach, and this time links started to form between the neurons that recognize a peach and those that reward you for eating it. From then on, every time you ate a peach, you reinforced those connections. And the more peaches you ate, the stronger the connections got, so that now you can't resist a peach when you see one.

But your crafty brain doesn't stop there. It's also busy weaving webs between the circumstances in which you ate a peach and the reward you got from eating it. In other words, it creates links between food, emotions and situations. I have a friend whose dad used to own a candy store, and every evening as a little boy he was given a treat of candy after dinner. Now my friend is a grown man with kids of his own, but he still yearns for something sweet every evening as dinner ends. Our brain also connects food with time. If you get used to eating lunch at noon, for example, you'll feel as if you need something to eat when noon comes around even if you had a large snack an hour earlier and don't really need anything else.

Stress can be a trigger, too, and make you want to eat a brownie the way you did the last time you were under pressure. Happiness can do the same thing. Or maybe you and a close friend are used to celebrating your birthdays with a dessert of chocolate cake. The next time you have a birthday with your friend, you'll feel that something is missing if the cake is overlooked.

Here's what our familiarity instinct does:

✳ It thrives on routine and teaches us to like the tastes of the things we eat on a regular basis.

✳ It teaches us to want food at the times we usually eat.

✳ It makes us want similar foods in familiar emotional situations—those times when we were especially happy or stressed or sad.

✳ It fights to keep us eating the way we always have. Like all our other instincts, *it hates change.*

And how does it do all this? By responding to our food triggers.

Don't Pull That Trigger

Food triggers can be good or bad. They're simply our brain's way of keeping all its parts talking to each other, finding associations among the different things we do so that life stays predictable and we safely repeat things we've done before.

We all have loads of food triggers, however, and often these triggers are not our friends. They create thoughts in your head, and at the same time they physically rev up your body's need to eat by stimulating the cephalic phase of digestion. Your stomach muscles relax, making your stomach larger and "noisy" as it sends out signals that it wants food. Your blood glucose drops and you feel hungry. Ivan Pavlov was awarded a Nobel Prize in 1904 for his discovery that, soon after a regimen of being fed in conjunction with the ringing of a bell, the dogs in his study learned to salivate at the sound of the bell whether there was food or not. At heart, we are all Pavlov's dogs. Even if we've just polished off a big lunch, the activation of a food trigger can make us *feel* as if we haven't eaten for hours.

The trick is to learn to break those bad habits and replace them with good ones. Each time you eat a good meal, one you *planned* to eat at a certain time, you set up a positive eating cycle. This is because your brain expects to have again what it had before. This requires some practice, since you're rewriting an established story line in your head, but repetition is all it takes. The more often you practice your new habits, the more they start to feel like comfortable *old* habits. And the more these good habits start to feel comfortable, the more weight you'll lose and the happier you will be.

Learn to Love What's Good for You

Recommend high-fiber cereals and fresh green vegetables to people who want to lose weight and there will always be some who say, *Forget it!* My job, when this happens, is to show how to introduce these healthy foods into their diet by teaching their familiarity instinct to help them begin to appreciate different tastes.

Love the Wrong Food—Get Hungry Again Sooner

Giving in to triggers doesn't just mean eating something you shouldn't eat—it may also make you hungry again sooner! Two separate studies have shown a "second-meal effect," which occurs after eating something good. One of the first studies I did at M.I.T. before moving to Tufts investigated this phenomenon. We studied a group of 19 men, both young and old. On one visit, we gave them a breakfast of French toast, syrup, ham, fruit salad and juice; on the other visit, we blended these same foods together and freeze-dried them into cookies. Their blood glucose rose almost twice as much after eating the good-tasting breakfast as it did after eating the unpalatable one. It also crashed dramatically as it came back to baseline, indicating that the good breakfast was digested more rapidly and greater hunger would be a factor at the next meal.

The "second-meal effect" is probably the reason negative eating cycles perpetuate themselves with remarkable ease. The good news is that this doesn't mean we should only eat things we *don't* like. It just means we should pay attention to other ways to control hunger, such as eating plenty of fiber.

✱ **Practice, practice, practice.** Repetition is the name of the game here, since several tries might be needed before new tastes become truly familiar and therefore enjoyed. You can't expect to like a new food the first time you try it, so have it once a week in the beginning. You don't have to eat a lot of it at first, either. Try a few bites one week, then a few more the next week, and even more the week after that. Go slow with spicy and strong-tasting foods; eating these foods too often when you're first including them in your diet might make it difficult to continue liking them. Make sure your new foods have some calories (add oil and vinegar or low-fat dressing to your salads, for example) so your food brain will adjust to them more easily.

Same but Different

A great way to retrain your familiarity instinct is to substitute a healthy familiar taste for an unhealthy one.
If you like to cook:
- Instead of mashed potatoes, try Potato Skins (page 226)
- Instead of chocolate-chip cookies, try Vanilla Spice Cookies (page 246)
- Instead of regular Alfredo sauce, try mixing low-fat Alfredo sauce with nonfat sour cream and a little 1% milk.

✱ **Build bridges.** Instead of suddenly substituting a new, healthy food you don't particularly like for an old, unhealthy but favorite standby, make a gradual transition from one to the other. For example, if your brain is hooked on high-calorie juice and you want to replace it with water, use my step-down method. Mix 90% juice with 10% water or seltzer at first. Then switch to an 80/20 mixture and move on to 70/30. Keep this up until you've reached your goal and water or seltzer or even just 10% juice is now your drink of choice. (I used to put oodles of half-and-half in my coffee, but this step-down method helped me move over to healthier non-fat milk, and now the creamy brew I used to love tastes so rich that I don't even want to drink it.)

✱ **Use your hunger wisely.** Our liking for certain foods is strengthened when we eat them to satisfy our hunger. Understanding this really matters! What it means is that we can teach ourselves to appreciate foods that are best for weight control by eating those foods when we're hungry. Conversely, by avoiding high-calorie treats when we're "starving," we gradually weaken our urge to eat them. Let your brain get a shot at increasing your pleasure circuits for good weight-loss foods. You'll need some discipline to make this work at first, but it's really worth the effort. Instead of reaching for that brownie or those cheese crackers, try substituting an apple and a tablespoon of nuts. After a while, you'll start to look forward to munching on diet-friendly foods. They'll literally make you feel satisfied and happy, which is the first important step toward taking permanent control of your weight.

Be the Boss, Part 2

Just as you learned that you can be in charge of your availability instinct, you can take ownership of your familiarity instinct. Below are some additional strategies that can work really well as long as you believe in yourself and give them time to become effective.

✻ **Create healthy rituals.** We all love having turkey at Thanksgiving or going to a barbecue on the Fourth of July. We've created food rituals around these holidays, and thinking of the foods associated with them makes us feel warm and happy. There's no reason we can't also create little everyday and weekly rituals around nutritious, satisfying foods. Make a point of serving raw veggies with a low-fat yogurt dressing as a weekday snack before dinner, or switch from pie to berries with a touch of lemon and sugar for a weekday dessert. Serve these substitutions as often as you can when you eat with family and friends, and pretty soon you'll begin to make the connection between these healthy foods and the comfort of a life in balance.

✻ **Learn when enough is enough.** Try creating your very own meal termination signal. Introduce a low-calorie food and/or a specific behavior at the end of dinner that your familiarity instinct interprets as "Eating is finished for the day." It might be a cup of herbal tea, or maybe a piece of sugarless gum or a calcium chew. For me, it's a cup of decaf tea with milk (my British background) that I enjoy in silence while I sit and relax for a few minutes; my family knows not to interrupt me unless the cat is lost or there's a fire in the kitchen. By being careful to eat nothing after your meal termination signal, you should discover that it becomes easier to ignore those late-night temptations—and eventually you probably won't even notice them!

✳ **Understand that less can be more.** Unfortunately, serving delicious food—and lots of it—is sometimes the way a mother tries to make her family feel safe and loved. But the tangled web of love and control can be a pretty unhealthy legacy for people who want to keep the cook happy and still lose weight (or even maintain their weight) at the same time. No one should ever feel that more is better, or feel pressured to eat more, or push food on others. This is the opposite of loving care.

✳ **Plan your menu and stick with it.** When you eat only planned meals and snacks at planned times, your familiarity instinct stops prodding you with those nasty old triggers that try to get you to eat at other times. And when you develop this structured food life so that you don't ever eat between well-planned meals and snacks, your cephalic phase calms right down and you experience less hunger. Your familiarity instinct wants structure. And when this instinct gets what it wants, it's less inclined to encourage you to break the rules and more inclined to help you reclaim the slim, fit body you deserve. The Stage I and Stage II menus are ready-planned for your use, or you can read Chapter 11 to find out ways to design your own menu plan.

Confront Cravings Vigorously!

Last but not least, let's talk about how to deal with cravings that can occur when your familiarity instinct is in overdrive. Cravings are the best-known problem associated with triggers and can seem like the hardest to deal with. But we've found that by following the "I" Diet menus exactly and eating only at meal and snack times, *most cravings are cured within two weeks.* People who thought they were emotional eaters realize they were simply unsatisfied and at the mercy of a few hunger-related triggers.

If your triggers are a little more stubborn, use my time-tested strategies. They can help you stop cravings once and for all. Practice them regularly for a few months, and the cravings should gradually die down and even disappear over time.

1. Tap your forehead rather than give in. One scientifically proven way to stop cravings is the "forehead tapping" technique. Since our working memory is small, we can displace craving thoughts with other mental activities, in this case a simple exercise that can be done anywhere. Just place the five fingers of one hand on your forehead, spaced apart. Tap each finger in turn at intervals of one second while

Remember, cravings only exist in your mind if you let them!

watching each one carefully as it taps. Keep repeating the exercise until your thoughts go elsewhere and the craving sensation disappears!

Alternatively, tell yourself "Not today" or "Hold on" and wait 15 to 20 minutes while you distract yourself by calling a supportive friend, drinking a full glass of water, chewing a piece of sugar-free gum, brushing your teeth, going for a walk or meditating. Keep a record of whatever thoughts and feelings you have leading up to cravings so you can recognize (and avoid) particular behavior chains that are a problem for you.

2. Be vigilant about controlling hunger. Cravings are enormously hard to control when you're hungry (because hunger is itself a powerful trigger and seems to amplify other triggers). If you're trying to lose weight, I encourage you to use our Stage I and Stage II menus rather than trying to go it alone. Remember that hunger control is important 24/7 and isn't just about eating the right foods—eating regular meals and snacks with nothing in between and pacing calories across the day are equally important.

3. Keep your eyes and nose under control. Avoid looking at and smelling tempting foods, not only to stop cravings once they've started but also to avoid triggering them in the first place. Deliberately look away when you come across foods that are out of bounds. And if you start to smell them, breathe through your mouth!

4. Eat craved foods wisely or not at all. If a craving for a particular food is very hard to control, give up that food for now before trying it again. Some people find it helpful to simply think of a troublesome food—say, white bread—as being "not food" or "garbage" or "not a food that I would ever eat." If you decide to bring back a craved food, eat only reasonable, calorie-controlled portions as part of satisfying meals when you have a supportive family member or friend present. If you find that you're able to give in only a quarter or less often as before, this is a great way to go forward.

5. Change your recipes. This is really helpful. If a taste you crave now comes with fewer calories, more fiber and more bulk, you can still enjoy it, but after a while your brain can "dissociate" this food trigger from the feeling of need and make it a less urgent sensation. The recipes in this book are designed to reduce cravings and are a great place to start!

Above all, stay positive. Believe in your ability to make weight control work. It takes a little time, and it requires repetition because you're restructuring the neurons firing around in your brain. There are days when you will backslide. Everybody does. Just accept that, forgive yourself and get on with it. You may reinforce a bad habit every now and then, but be assured that the healthy new habits you're creating will conquer those bad ones if you keep at it. And once they do, your body will start to change in ways that will astound you.

CHAPTER 6

Variety
Too Many Choices

Human evolution has been going on for about six million years. It took our prehistoric ancestors almost three million years to figure out how to use tools and another two and a half million years to discover fire. They hunted meat when it was available and otherwise gathered berries, nuts and tender shoots. Because no single food has all the nutrients that humans need, it was essential for them to eat a wide variety of foods in order to get the healthy nutrition that would keep them alive. Variety *instinctively* felt right, so they took advantage of it whenever they could.

Unfortunately, this strong survival instinct doesn't work so well for most of us in the modern food environment. Inundated with easily obtained variety of the wrong kind, we have become passive overeaters, unaware of how much we eat. Even fish and other wild creatures eat more food when they're presented with more variety, demonstrating that this instinct to fill up on variety is basic to survival. Variety is also thought to influence neurological sensations of reward, prompting us to eat more just to feel the same sense of fullness and satisfaction.

Many nutritionists say things like "Eat a variety of foods" and "There are no bad foods," but I believe that oversimplified messages like these do us a real disservice. The epidemic of obesity occurring worldwide is due partly to the simple fact that *too much* variety is available everywhere. America and Canada, in particular, are virtual experiments in how much damage toxic levels of variety can cause. The good news is that by understanding exactly how your variety instinct works, you can get it to work for you when it comes to achieving and maintaining a healthy weight. In fact, it can become one of your most valuable helpers in making weight loss easier and avoiding weight regain.

The Science Behind Variety

In study after study, variety has been shown to have a huge effect on the amount of food we eat. Because this is such an instinctive need, it increases consumption of every type of food tested, including dairy foods, sweets, fruits, vegetables, meats and nuts. If you eat a wide variety of sweets, for example, your total intake of sweets is larger than if you eat only one kind. The same goes for fruit—if you eat a wide variety, you end up eating more fruit overall. Believe it or not, this principle even applies to things like condiments, which we don't normally think of as food; the greater the variety, the more we eat. Indeed, we are so sensitive to variety that in one research study where subjects were offered three different shapes of pasta (all with the same ingredients and same taste), pasta consumption increased by 14% compared with just one shape!

Variety comes in many different guises, and all of them influence how much we eat. It can be a plate of several types of cookies rather than just one. A party platter or a dessert cart. The 150 kinds of bread in your local supermarket (I counted that many in mine!). Most of the time, this variety isn't that enjoyable, but we fall for it because we're not really conscious of what's happening to us.

Now comes the good part. While increased variety causes us to eat more, it doesn't automatically translate into more calories. This is good to know! Depending on where it comes from, variety can either increase calorie intake and cause weight gain *or* decrease calorie intake and cause weight loss. Working with my friend Megan McCrory, our lab at Tufts was the first to show this. We discovered that eating a wide variety of calorie-rich foods like entrées, sweets, fats, condiments and desserts leads to weight gain (because it means eating more calories overall). Conversely, eating a greater variety of vegetables can double or triple total vegetable consumption, which in turn reduces overall calorie intake. Greater variety in this important low-calorie food group encourages you to eat more of it, so you feel fuller sooner and can eat smaller amounts of other foods with more calories. We also showed that combining a wide variety of vegetables with a narrow variety of high-calorie food is one of the keys to permanent weight control. This is not to say that the composition of food is unimportant, but rather that variety is another way to control your weight.

Instincts at Work

Sophie's Success

Sophie came to us wanting to lose weight for her own health and to help her son, who had an emerging weight problem. At first, she resisted changing the types of foods she was eating. She didn't want to give up the variety of high-calorie meats such as sausages and salami that she was used to, nor did she want to add in too many new foods.

What got Sophie on the track to success was her discovery that variety could help! By adding a variety of satisfying foods like vegetables, legumes and high-fiber cereals, she learned to like them and her weight started coming off because she could now reduce portions of other foods to reasonable amounts. At this writing, she's lost 20 pounds and loves the way her improved eating habits are filtering down to her son.

It is *variety within the familiar* that affects how much we eat. Simply put, we have to know a food (or it has to be basically similar to something we already know) for the variety to affect us. For example, if I offered you a variety of cooked caterpillars, you wouldn't overeat them since they're unfamiliar to you even though they're a special treat in New Guinea. But if I offered you three kinds of ice cream and four different pizzas, you would eat more than if I offered you one kind of each. These are familiar foods, so more variety encourages you to eat more.

Variety recognition starts in the part of our food brain where taste recognition occurs. Here, some neurons will light up for bananas, some for chicken, some for cheese, some for broccoli, and so on. Think of this part of your brain as a nest of baby birds, each with a specific food preference. As long as the birds are asleep, everything is fine. But once you wake up one of them—say, the one that loves the taste of chocolate—that little bird will keep on squawking

Strong-tasting foods satisfy sooner. Most chocoholics can eat tons of milk chocolate but only a few squares of dark!

"Feed me, feed me" until it feels completely satisfied. If you then start eating something salty, another little bird—the salty snack lover—will wake up and squawk and squawk until it's had its fill. Nutrition scientists call this *sensory-specific satiety,* the feeling that you can stop eating because you've had enough of a particular taste. Foods that have a strong taste are thought to activate sensory-specific satiety sooner, so eating more strong flavors is probably an additional influence on how many calories you consume. In other words, if a food is really strong-flavored, you probably won't eat as much of it as you would if it had a milder taste.

Today, we can use everything that science has taught us about variety to make weight loss easier:

✳ By limiting the variety of high-calorie foods, especially at the beginning of a diet, we can feel more satisfied with fewer calories.

✳ By increasing the variety of satisfying lower-calorie foods, especially vegetables and high-fiber cereals, and eating them often and regularly so they become tastier through greater familiarity, our variety instinct stops clamoring for unhealthy foods just because they add variety. Increasing healthy variety also curtails hunger because we eat larger portions of more satisfying foods.

✳ By replacing mild-tasting foods like milk chocolate and mozzarella cheese with strong-flavored foods like dark chocolate and Parmesan cheese, we can indulge in familiar tastes but eat less while we're enjoying them.

✳ By making permanent changes in the *balance* of variety between unsatisfying high-calorie foods and satisfying low-calorie foods, we can enjoy healthy eating while more easily preventing weight regain.

Will these changes be hard? In our studies at Tufts, quite a number of volunteers worry beforehand about cutting out muffins and chips and the three kinds of chocolate candy they love, but they're quickly surprised at how good it feels to have less hunger and more control over what they eat. For them, the positive effects of balancing variety outweigh the negatives. It's also important to remember that favorite foods are not really being cut out here. By eliminating the bad, useless variety you don't really care about, you can keep the foods you actually like. In fact, you'll appreciate them all the more because they won't be competing for your attention with a sea of other unhealthy stuff.

Cutting Back

For a long time, nobody knew why liquid diets and other restrictive programs like ketogenic diets worked so well. The fact is, they cut way back on variety, which in turn cuts hunger, which in turn makes it easier to stick with a low-calorie regimen—at least for a while. Fortunately, you can achieve the same benefit with a low variety of regular foods. Stage I of the "I" Diet deliberately reduces variety to cut hunger as you start

Learn to look for healthy variety in foods and you'll be way ahead of the game when it comes to permanent weight control.

to lose weight, offering choices within each day but repeating those choices every three days. This way, you eat foods that you enjoy but in relatively limited variety. Stage I doesn't last long, so you'll be okay without a lot of variety and you can get the benefits of reduced hunger and increased satisfaction.

Continuing to keep variety in its place is one of the most important elements of Stage II even though there's quite a bit more leeway. The repeated three days of menus in Stage I just aren't interesting enough to keep you

---

Instincts at Work

Muffin, Yes. Fast Food, No.

Dana had the typical unbalanced variety of an unhealthy diet. Lunch was usually takeout from the fast-food place across the street from her office, even though she wasn't crazy about the items she brought back to her desk. What she really *did* like was a muffin with her morning coffee, so when it came time to start her diet program, she allowed herself this one indulgence.

"I learned that successful dieting comes down to figuring out what you can get away with," Dana says, "and in my case it turned out that I could keep the muffin if I gave up the stuff I didn't particularly enjoy." Dana changed her food preferences, too. "When I ordered a fast-food hamburger after not having had one for months, I could only eat half of it. It tasted awful!"

---

going forever, and the restricted variety of those two weeks will make you super-sensitive to the pleasures of *healthy* variety. Instead of jumping back to unregulated variety, Stage II increases the variety of satisfying foods that are lower in calories and higher in fiber, protein and good carbohydrates while limiting your variety of high-calorie foods. This gives you practice in eating the right balance to help rewire your food brain so that over time it becomes second nature.

By also cutting back on the high-calorie variety that just encourages overeating, you can focus on enjoying the smaller number of higher-calorie foods you love without being so tempted to overeat them. When you get to Stage II, you'll be able to use your 100-calorie-a-day free-choice allowance for anything you want, but here's a word of advice: Stick with one or two choices you really enjoy and your control over those foods will be that much easier.

A Balancing Act

Some people manage to keep their weight under control after weight loss almost exclusively by rebalancing variety. Having a smaller number of favorite breakfast foods, lunch items, dinner entrées and desserts fairly often, rather than an endless variety of less enjoyable things, probably works because you get your cephalic phase secretions under better control, reducing hunger and making it easier to eat without overeating. Remember, cutting variety is aimed not at reducing enjoyment but rather at preserving the enjoyment of things you really like and jettisoning the junk that adds calories but no genuine pleasure.

Virtuous Vegetables

Let's hear it for vegetables! Our research shows that some foods make weight loss easier, and non-starchy vegetables are at the top of the list. Not fruit. Not lean meat or dairy. The reason vegetables are so helpful is that they're high in fiber and low in calories; in other words, their composition is perfect for reducing hunger and increasing satisfaction. And because variety increases the amount you eat within any food group, there is the proven benefit of having a *variety* of vegetables.

Pick up different kinds of salad greens every time you shop—iceberg lettuce, romaine, field greens, red lettuce, Boston lettuce, arugula, baby spinach— and you'll add variety to everyday salads with no extra work.

Most people eat very few vegetables. In fact, Americans typically get more than 50% of their vegetables from iceberg lettuce, canned tomatoes, onions and potatoes (and I don't even count potatoes as a vegetable, nutritionally speaking). Anyone who sticks to this sorry list is not going to find vegetables very inviting, so getting excited about diversifying veggies is a great way to help weight control.

Don't be afraid to dress up your vegetables. Add interesting toppings, a little lemon juice or a half-teaspoon of olive oil and some salt and pepper. Because our neurons respond to calories as well as variety, just half a teaspoon of margarine, a teaspoon of grated Parmesan cheese or a handful of fresh herbs and a dash of olive oil add to the taste of vegetables and make them more appealing. And salads, of course, need to have a *variety* of delicious low-calorie dressings.

There are lots of green recipes in this book, and I encourage you to try as many as you can. We include both salads and cooked vegetables in

"I" Diet meals to add variety, thereby increasing the amount of those foods you enjoy eating. Since cooked foods are digested differently from raw foods (the cells of cooked foods tend to fall apart individually, whereas raw foods first shear into clumps of cells that have to be broken down again), combining cooked and raw foods probably also aids hunger control by spreading out the digestive process over a longer time.

Fabulous Fiber

High-fiber cereals, intact grains (whole unprocessed kernels) and legumes can make all the difference in your diet. True, these foods don't usually come to mind when you want a good meal, but often this is simply because they're eaten in such low variety that they're unappealing. Many nutritionists push beans and whole-grain breads without realizing that variety is the key to liking them more, along with eating them regularly so their familiarity makes them more enjoyable. I encourage you to *experiment* with high-fiber foods until you find some you like. High-fiber cereals are also important for weight loss, and keeping them in the cupboard helps to increase consumption. Experiment with legumes, too. If you don't like beans, you probably haven't tried a variety of *good* beans. Canned cooked beans are found in almost all supermarkets and can be made into a wide variety of delicious meals. Pinto and black beans, cannellini and chickpeas (garbanzo beans) are excellent choices. We include all these varieties and others in our recipes.

> ### Cook Up a Batch of Fiber
>
> I f you like to cook, try one of our many high-fiber recipes, including:
> - "I" Diet Soda Bread (page 160)
> - West African Bean Cakes with Spicy Dip and Green Salad (page 224)
> - Mexican Lettuce Wraps (page 194)
> - Three-Bean Salad with Fresh Herbs (page 183)
> - Chocolate-Raspberry Parfait (page 237)
> - Orange Flan (page 241)
> - Chocolate Bread Pudding (page 240)

The 50% Variety Rule

Let's look at a "normal" dinner at home: a few crackers and cheese while you're getting dinner organized, a beef casserole, mashed potatoes and green beans as a main course and ice cream with wafer cookies for dessert, followed up by a few pieces of candy afterwards. And maybe a glass of wine with your meal. That adds up to eight high-calorie items and one low-calorie item, which means that almost no one with a normal metabolism could avoid overeating.

Now let's rework that menu to make it suitable for weight maintenance with what I call the 50% Variety Rule. After weight loss, keep the beef casserole (try my new recipe, page 266), and green beans as well as the potatoes *or* the ice cream (the amount of either can be about a third of a cup). With the wine, you have three high-calorie foods—a good number. Then substitute a salad for cheese and crackers, and some fruit for cookies. Now 50% of your items are high in fiber and high in satiety, giving you a much more favorable balance. A maximum of two or three high-calorie foods like entrées, carbohydrates and desserts in any given meal and the same number of fruit and vegetable choices will give you a perfect dinner.

For a Rainy Day

Although more variety in fruits and vegetables is generally helpful for weight control, there's one important qualification here. Don't increase vegetable and fruit variety too much *within meals*. Save some variety for another meal and another day!

One or two veggies and a fruit with a regular dinner is fine. But if you have a plate of cut-up tomatoes, cauliflower, cucumber and carrots as an appetizer and then move on to broccoli with dinner and blackberries, strawberries and mango for dessert, you've used too many choices. You'll probably end up having the same things tomorrow, and pretty soon they'll start to bore you. A better strategy for increasing variety is to use the same vegetables one after the other to make an interesting week's worth of food. For example, have lots of cut-up cauliflower today, moving on to tomatoes tomorrow (good local ones with a little salt are simply delicious in summer), cucumbers the day after, and so on. For fruit, have

Tomorrow's Variety

Today's handful of leftover peas makes tomorrow's salad or soup more interesting, and half a portion of an entrée will make a great wrap if you keep low-carb tortillas on hand. For future meals, freeze individual portions of cooked fruits, vegetables and legumes to add variety—and save work!

mango today, blackberries tomorrow, strawberries the day after that. This kind of variety is a great way to keep interest high *and reduce work at the same time.*

Cutting Out Snacks and Liquid Calories

Another way to eliminate excess variety is to stay away from commercial snacks and liquids such as juice, with-sugar sodas, full-fat lattes and frozen drinks. For the most part, these are loaded with calories and deficient in fiber, and we overeat them even when variety is low—more so when there are several different kinds to choose from every time we buy. Liquid calories are sheer poison because they don't make us feel as satisfied as solid calories do and we end up having our drink on top of other things, not instead of them. If you substitute fruit and a few nuts at snack time, or my new Strawberry-Blueberry Smoothie (page 270), it's easier to stay hunger-free between meals on fewer calories.

Healthy variety is great for weight control, but save something for an occasional treat. This way, you can indulge without resorting to higher-calorie choices.

Try to reduce variety in the high-calorie foods you want to keep eating. Chips are a good example here. On our menu plan, you can eat them as part of a meal in Stage II, using your 100-calorie free-choice allowance, and we have one recipe using chips (page 265). Even so, it's best to limit yourself to one variety of the kind you like best. Whenever you shop, buy that type. Believe me—you'll eat less. This also applies to healthy but high-calorie foods like nuts. Just decide on one variety to keep at home and see how easy it becomes to restrict yourself to reasonable portions.

Spicing It Up

Intense flavors wake you right up and make you feel satisfied sooner than milder flavors do. This is why many "I" Diet menus include foods such as Mexican dishes, curried chicken salad and baked apples flavored with cinnamon. Also, the more aware you are of the taste of food, the more you'll enjoy it and the more satisfying it will be.

Holidays at Home

In our research at Tufts, we've discovered two important predictors of weight regain after weight loss: 1) how tempted you are by foods that are just lying around, and 2) how much you overeat situationally—at holiday gatherings and other special events. Some people seem to put on all their excess weight during holidays because they don't know how to deal with the general abundance of food and the huge variety of high-calorie temptations all around them.

If you're entertaining at home, plan a menu in which half is made up of low-calorie fruit and vegetable dishes, and don't have more than one starch (plain bread or potatoes, for example) with the entrée. Minimizing variety makes dinner easier to prepare and results in less overeating: a win-win situation. But if you have time to put more work in, add a soup or another vegetable or fruit. This will make the meal that much more interesting.

In my experience, guests are positively relieved to sit down to a good meal that doesn't make them overeat. In our recipe section, you'll find an example of a weight-friendly dinner party menu festive enough for any holiday event.

Eating Out

Many of us get 50% of our meals from restaurants and takeout places, which means choosing from a huge variety of high-calorie foods. Cutting down on restaurant meals is a simple way to diminish their harmful effects without giving up the undeniable pleasure of eating out. If you normally have dinner at a restaurant twice a week, limiting yourself to once a week will cut excess calories in half! If you normally eat breakfast out every day, you can cut that down to two days a week and enjoy those breakfasts all the more because now they feel special.

If you have to eat out all the time, try ordering the same thing whenever you go to a particular place. This is another good way to curtail the wrong kind of variety and make calorie control easier. For example, when I get Chinese takeout for lunch, it's almost always the same meal: chicken with green vegetables and steamed rice. One container is far too much for my calorie needs (an individual lunch container contains about 1,200 calories), but because I eat the same thing every time, it's easy to leave most of the rice and about half the chicken without feeling deprived.

Hunger reinforces your interest in variety, so have a bowl of high-fiber cereal or an apple before heading out for a fancy meal. If you're going to someone's house, offer to bring something—and make sure it's satisfying and tasty. There are lots of "I" Diet recipes that you can prepare and take to parties, and your hostess will never realize you're bringing "diet" food.

On Vacation

If you're like many vacationers, you're not too interested in breakfast when you're away from home. Consider reducing unnecessary variety by having a "regular" meal of just high-fiber cereal and fruit or perhaps eggs and fruit only. (Pack a box of high-fiber cereal in your suitcase.) For lunch and dinner, while you're practicing your better eating habits, allow yourself one good entrée and just a dollop of one or two other high-calorie foods. Fill up your plate with the rich variety of steamed vegetables and fruits that a buffet usually offers, so that you have a full plate that includes but isn't dominated by a few of the high-calorie things you love. Over time, you will probably find it easier to eat a wider variety of calorie-rich foods in smaller portions, but cutting back on high-calorie variety and increasing vegetable variety at first is an easy way to get more control. For snacks, take along some fruit, nuts and Snack Attack Packs (page 248) and ignore the poor-tasting brownies, pretzels and other junk food you find in hotels.

Be picky—*really* picky. If the food isn't so great, don't eat it. Why waste hundreds of calories you can spend later on something really healthy and delicious? Just keep in mind how thrilled you'll be when you get home and weigh the same as (or less than) you did when you left!

CHAPTER 7

The Five Food Instincts

A Crib Sheet

N ow that you've begun to understand your food instincts, you may find yourself becoming impatient to start losing weight. *Let's get on with it already,* you may be saying to yourself. I understand, believe me, but just for a minute think about how your food instincts have worked against you in the past to make weight control an exercise in defeat. Lose weight; put it back on. Lose weight; put it back on. Talk about an uphill struggle!

I hope I've convinced you that it doesn't have to be that way. Using the strategies we've talked about, you *can* move forward. You can make simple changes that will give you greater control over not just what you eat but what you weigh. All you have to do is harness your five natural food instincts. It's not that hard—particularly if you keep reminding yourself about what you can do to change the pattern. To help you out, I've compiled an Instinct Crib Sheet. Why not make a copy and put it on your refrigerator door? Read it every day while you're losing weight.

The Five Food Instincts

HUNGER Confront hunger head-on, every day! Make sure *every* meal and *every* snack makes you feel satisfied and cuts hunger with one or (better still) more of the following compositions:

* High fiber
* High protein/low carb
* High volume
* Mixed high- and low-GI carbs

AVAILABILITY No excuses here! You *can* take charge of your food environment, and you *can* make changes to reduce temptation, overeating and even hunger.

* Keep your kitchen stocked with the ready-to-eat, healthy, satisfying foods that are called for in your menu plan. Throw out the junk.
* Keep eating out to a minimum.
* "Spring-clean" your mind. Control sights and smells to keep temptations at bay.

CALORIE DENSITY You love food in general and rich treats in particular. These simple tricks can help you keep pleasure up and calories down:

* Use the "sandwich" technique with moderate portions of high-calorie foods in the middle of a meal, low-calorie foods high in fiber and protein at the beginning and end.
* Make low-calorie foods more appetizing. Add a little fat or strong flavoring like Parmesan cheese to make them taste better. Keep some indulgences, but cut calories and add fiber to make them healthier.

FAMILIARITY Let's hear it for routines and rituals. With a little direction, this instinct can be turned around to help you create healthy food preferences.

* Eat at regular times so your body will learn not to expect food at other times. This will increase enjoyment and reduce temptation.
* Learn to get greater enjoyment from healthy, satisfying foods by eating them when you're hungry!
* Reduce cravings by carefully following your food plan and using our proactive craving stoppers.

VARIETY By influencing what you eat without being aware of it, this instinct can help or hinder weight control, depending on what you put in your kitchen and on your plate.

* Keep a low variety of unhealthy foods. This reduces how many calories you eat.
* Keep a high variety of healthy foods. This *good* variety reduces calories and increases satisfaction.
* Use the 50% Variety Rule (make sure at least 50% of foods in each meal and snack are low in calories and high in fiber or protein).

PART II

THE PROGRAM

CHAPTER 8

Ready, Set, Go

Stepping Toward Success—
For Now and Forever

Now that you understand that the "I" Diet really is a different, better and *easier* way to lose weight, you're ready to go on your last diet ever. Following the program carefully is important for success. And in order to do that, you need to be prepared both practically and mentally. The practical part speaks for itself—it just means stocking your kitchen with good things to eat. But what does it mean to be mentally prepared? Well, that depends on how much work you expect to do in relation to the benefit you hope to get. For example, if you won a free dinner at the best restaurant in town, you would probably be delighted with your prize and use it at the first opportunity. But if you were offered a free dinner in return for mowing somebody's lawn all summer, you would probably feel that it was just too much work for such a small reward and say "No, thank you." Even more important than the work/benefit ratio, though, is the issue of how long it will take to see the benefit.

Is It Worth It?

The relatively new field of behavior economics explains how, in all spheres of life, we overvalue benefits we get today and undervalue benefits we get later. The fundamental tug-of-war between having what we want today and planning for future rewards because of our good behavior pervades our whole life; this explains why we choose to spend $50 a month on morning coffee rather than putting the $50 in a retirement account. When it comes to dieting, the conflict is between enjoying that slice of chocolate cake today and the pleasure derived from being thinner and feeling better in the future. We want both. But since we *can* have the cake now (and eat it, too), the cake often wins.

Why do we act this way? Probably because living well in the present had great survival value in our earliest history. Being sensible about the future is worth it only when there's a future to be sensible for, and there was no incentive to eat well in order to stay healthy for 80 or even 50 years when the average life span was much shorter than that. In fact, the smart thing to do back then was to have another meal whenever one could be found, so that some extra fat could be stored up to help cope with lean times. This overriding survival mechanism is one of the reasons you might have trouble remembering that you've succeeded in losing 10 pounds—and really do want to keep them off—when you're offered some leftover pizza at work. Again, it has nothing to do with weakness. It's just that being sensible means something very different today.

Changes Ahead

By following the "I" Diet menu plan carefully without substitutions, you not only get less hungry but also experience less temptation since you're making fewer of your own decisions about food—decisions that tend to favor eating now rather than waiting. Even so, you still have to be prepared to resist challenges. If you're ready to say yes to each of the following questions, you're getting set to move ahead to Stage I of the plan.

✳ Are you willing to eat three meals and two snacks every day even if you normally eat fewer meals and/or skip snacks?

fiction: You always "hit the wall" soon after starting a diet.
fact: You don't have to.

As you lose weight, your calorie needs decrease because your body requires less energy and your metabolic rate drops to adjust to this new circumstance. Your weight stabilizes temporarily and you might think you've "hit the wall." In our program at Tufts, however, the "wall" doesn't show up for many months after weight loss begins. And getting past it is simply a matter of weighing yourself daily so you get to see the progress you make every week. If you're backsliding and eating more than you should, returning to the "I" menus and following them very carefully is all it will take to get weight loss going again.

✳ Are you willing to commit yourself to learning to like new foods?

✳ Are you willing to forgo casual snacking and eat no food other than what's on the menu, in the appropriate amounts?

✳ Are you willing to get rid of junk food in your home and replace it with more satisfying food that will help your weight loss?

✳ Are you willing to go shopping weekly so you always have the good, healthy foods you need on hand?

All the Right Reasons

Knowing *why* you want to lose weight is important. Are you genuinely overweight? Do you feel heavy and lack energy? Have you outgrown all your clothes and worry that if you don't lose weight now, you never will? These are all good reasons for wanting to drop some pounds. Poor reasons include succumbing to your partner's nagging or thinking you should shed five pounds before a vacation even though you know you'll put them right back on before you even get home.

Once you know you have good strong motivation, you need to come up with some powerful ways to reward yourself. I'm not really talking about rewards for weight loss after it happens (although that's a good idea, too). This is more about incentives for resisting temptation when you feel challenged.

Everyone has a price, so think about what yours might be. Also think in terms of *immediate* gratification (if not right at the moment, then at least within the same day). Be prepared to give yourself something that will make you smile after you manage to resist temptation, and don't give up if your incentive fails

Never forget that you'll be getting healthier by the hour as you lose weight.

you—sometimes it can take a while to find out what your "price" really is. Below are some examples of incentives that may work for you.

✳ *A treat:* a bottle of perfume, theater tickets or a big fat magazine.

✳ *Money:* a sum tucked away toward buying new clothes, a new gold watch or something else you've been dreaming of.

✳ *Downtime:* 20 minutes of relaxation to listen to music, meditate or read a good book.

✳ *A walk:* a leisurely stroll on a beautiful day.

Take a Minute

Whenever I talk to people who have finally, truly, made the decision to lose weight, the first thing I tell them is to slow down. Sounds counterintuitive, but if you don't approach the diet correctly—with all the necessary preparation—you won't get through the first two weeks. And to state the obvious, if you don't get through the first two weeks, you'll never get to Week 3. So let's get you started . . . the right way.

Fiber First

Thinking about what you now eat is important before you start Stage I of the "I" Diet, and the first thing to look at is dietary fiber. If you currently have regular daily servings of high-fiber cereals and whole-grain breads or legumes, as well as vegetables and one or two pieces of fruit a day, you're already eating a diet quite high in fiber and can start right out on the "I" Diet menus. However, if you're eating the typical low-fiber North American diet, a very rapid change to a diet with more fiber can occasionally cause some gastrointestinal discomfort, so I recommend spending a week ramping up your fiber intake before you begin. Look in the diet section of your local supermarket or drugstore for a box of high-fiber bars. Pick out 10 bars with at least 9 grams of fiber and fewer than 160 calories per bar. Also buy 10 pieces of fruit—apples, oranges, pears, plums—and substitute them for less healthy foods that you would otherwise eat. As you follow the plan outlined below, be sure to decrease the amount of other things you eat so you don't gain weight.

Days 1 and 2: Add half a bar in the morning with breakfast and half a bar with dinner.

Days 3 and 4: Keep eating the half-bars morning and night, adding a piece of fruit during the day.

Days 5, 6 and 7: Have one whole bar in the morning and one at night. Add two pieces of fruit during the day.

Weigh Yourself Daily

Some diets tell you to weigh yourself only once a week because, as I pointed out earlier, the weight loss you see on your bathroom scale tells you almost nothing about fat loss. But even though they don't match up well on a day-to-day basis, those weights are still useful at different times for different reasons. The sample chart on page 69 is designed to show you how to keep a record of your weight throughout the eight-week "I" Diet program. The fact is, the more regularly you record your numbers, the easier it will be to stick to your plan.

✳ **Start your weigh-ins several days before beginning your diet.** Most people who know they need to lose weight will avoid stepping on the scale more than once before they start a diet program. They don't want to confront the numbers, but this is a big mistake. If you happen to weigh in after a "good" day, your "baseline" will be artificially low and you won't see the full extent of your progress when you start dieting in earnest. And if you happen to choose a "heavy" day, you may be so miserable that you'll put off starting at all! It's better to accept the facts and take at least three morning weights in a row before you start the "I" Diet so you know what your average pre-diet weight really is. Be sure to weigh yourself in minimal (or no) clothing right after you get up and go to the bathroom (before you have breakfast) so that the numbers you record are less influenced by food and other variable factors. A realistic baseline will allow you to see success sooner.

Also, get a tape measure and measure your waist circumference at the same time that you weigh yourself. If you repeat this measurement every two weeks, you'll get still another good indication of how your body fat is changing.

❋ **Weigh yourself daily in Stage I.** Don't fuss about the daily numbers going up and down a bit. Just keep in mind that it's impossible to lose more than about 3.5 pounds of actual fat a week on any diet. The "I" Diet composition for long-term dieting has been proven to cause weight loss that is close to 100% fat, whereas ketogenic diets (ones that are so low in carbohydrates that your body has to make ketones for brain fuel and also excretes a lot of water) and low-sodium diets cause huge weight loss initially because of water excretion but the same or less fat loss—and, of course, weight will come right back on when the diet is over.

❋ **Weigh yourself at least twice weekly in Stage II, preferably daily.** You can cut down to twice a week now, but daily weights are still best. As weight loss slows down (you will have lost all your surplus water), the easiest way to be sure weight is still coming off is to look for a lower weight every week or to take the average of a week's daily numbers and compare it to that of the previous week.

Because of day-to-day fluctuations and because of that water loss in Stage I, your weight may appear to become stable at the start of Stage II. Not to worry. As long as you stick carefully to the menus, this should be a temporary halt that will not keep fat from continuing to come down. Your weight loss will be gradual, but the plan is designed to help you lose 16 (typical value) and up to 20 pounds during the eight-week program.

Sample Weight Chart

Recording your weight regularly helps you stay on track! Make your own chart so you have a clear picture of how well you're doing on the weight-loss program. First record three consecutive morning weights taken before you begin your diet, then write in the average of these three numbers (your baseline weight) at the top of the chart with five-pound increments below. In the example below, the pre-diet average weight is 142 with daily weights plotted for the first two weeks (Stage I) and average weekly weights shown for the start of the last six weeks (Stage II).

Pre-diet weights: __141__   __143__   __142__

Three-day average ⟶ 142

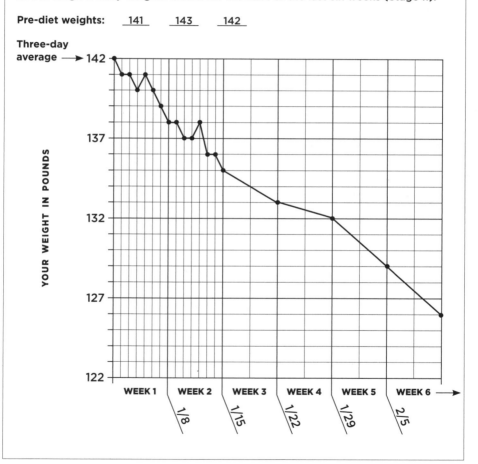

69

Starter Shopping List

Here are the basic items you'll need for the meals in the Stage I menus (with a good head start for Stage II). Take a moment to check out the menus on pages 80–85 for additional ingredients called for in recipes that you want to prepare.

Produce:
Bags of prewashed salad greens; green beans; tomatoes; broccoli; snow peas; packages of baby carrots; celery sticks; cucumbers; onions; garlic; sweet peppers; legumes; button mushrooms; small apples and oranges; grapefruits; pears; strawberries; lemons; plums; prunes; melon chunks; grapes; raisins; dill; crystallized ginger; sunflower seeds

Breads:
A loaf of low-carb bread; 100% coarse whole-wheat bread if you don't get too hungry; low-carb pitas and tortillas

Deli and meats:
Sliced turkey and ham; Canadian bacon; individual portions of plain grilled chicken and fish

Cans and jars:
Soups; beans; low-cal sauce for steak and fish; tomato sauce; low-fat pizza sauce; mustard; peanut butter; unsweetened applesauce; fruit spread; honey; ground cinnamon; ground cloves; low-cal salad dressing; extra-virgin olive oil and good vinegar (e.g., balsamic); caramel sauce

Dairy:
Nonfat or 1% milk; low-fat buttermilk; plain Greek and/or sugar-free low-fat yogurt; sweetened light whipped cream; low-fat sour cream; low-fat mayonnaise; part-skim mozzarella cheese sticks; low-fat cottage cheese and cream cheese; grated Parmesan cheese, preferably imported; non-trans fat tub margarine; eggs and Egg Beaters egg substitute

Cereals and baking:
High-fiber and high-fiber/protein cereals such as Fiber One, Fiber One Honey Clusters, All-Bran Extra Fiber or Trader Joe's High Fiber Cereal; good-quality granola; wheat berries; oat bran; coarse bran; stone-ground whole-wheat flour; white bread flour; baking powder; baking soda; dark brown sugar; sugar substitute (if you use it)

Snacks and drinks:
Peanuts and pecans (no sugary coatings); mineral water or seltzer; diet soda; coffee/tea

Frozen foods:
Vegetables (no sauce); raspberries; grilled chicken or fish steaks (no breading); veggie burgers; sugar-free ice cream

Chocolate:
Bittersweet chocolate; Dutch-process cocoa for "I" Diet Hot or Cold Chocolate, Droste brand if possible

Shop for Stage I

Getting smart about supermarket shopping is crucial for weight control. Yes, some diets just have you eat lean meats, veggies and the odd grape here and there, so you don't have to measure portions or fuss about whether to buy product X or Y. But you can't stick with those programs, because they don't satisfy all your food instincts. To be *sustainable,* a diet has to include the foods your body needs and wants: different carbs, grains, dairy, some treats . . . the whole gamut.

So here's the challenge. The average suburban supermarket contains something like 30,000 to 40,000 products, many of them unhealthy enticements, but buried in that mass of terrible stuff are the 20 or so items that you need to eat in order to lose weight more easily. How do you find them? It's easy! Just make a really good shopping list and check out our Savvy Shopper Supermarket Directory (Appendix E) so you know which specific products are helpful for weight control and where to find them. When you have some time to browse, a field trip will help you locate different items so you'll know where to find them again and will be all set.

On the facing page is a basic shopping list. Go through the menus for Stage I and pick out what you want to eat, then make an *exact* list of everything you will need. The first shopping trip will cost more than later ones, because many of these items will last for the whole program. Don't go on an empty stomach and do take a coffee into the store with you in case you get tempted—you can sniff it as you go up and down the aisles to keep enticing smells out of your head.

Are You Ready?

I hope you won't let your past weight-loss failures stop you from giving this more effective, more sustainable diet your wholehearted commitment. That said, do be honest with yourself. You're the only one who knows if you're *really* ready. Again, you need your doctor's assurance that you're in good health. Also, it's best to start when you have no unusually stressful events coming up and a little slack in the system so you have some downtime every day and get enough sleep.

Below is a final set of questions for you to answer before you begin the "I" Diet program.

1. Keeping in mind that dieting will take some work at first, is this a good time to change your life? **yes** ❏ **no** ❏

2. Are you sure about your motivation? **yes** ❏ **no** ❏

Write two things that will help you through the next two weeks with joy and enthusiasm:

_____

_____

3. What reward will you give yourself when you resist the temptation to break your diet? _____

4. Have you done your shopping for at least a week of Stage I meals and snacks? **yes** ❏ **no** ❏

5. Have you recorded at least three days of pre-diet baseline weights on your chart? **yes** ❏ **no** ❏

When you've answered each question positively, you're ready to begin!

CHAPTER 9

Stage I
The Two-Week "Getting Started" Diet

The "I" Diet menu plan is easy. This may not be apparent on Day 1 or Day 2, because it all may feel a little unfamiliar. But if you like to cook, the recipes are simple—I promise you. Also, the Simply Good menus are great for those days when you just want to grab something from the store or your kitchen shelf. And there are separate menus for vegetarians, divided the same way. If you go vegetarian, I recommend opting for snacks made with milk or cheese to be certain you get enough protein. (Vegetarian menus tend to have lower amounts.) For all the menus, you can save work by eating the same foods two or even three days running!

You'll see that we give you the first three days of menus. When you've gone through all three days, just go back to the beginning and start over—you'll cycle through the menus almost four times before completing the two weeks of Stage I. And, as I said, you can repeat meals to save work.

This variety-reducing schedule is designed to give you an extra dose of hunger suppression right off the bat. Be sure to eat at regular times and include a low-cal drink (or water) with each meal and snack. And let me repeat: Don't tweak the menus—they are designed for success and changes typically add calories and hunger.

Choose Your Plan

The basic menus provide about 1,200 calories a day and are usually the right way to start if you weigh between 120 and 160 pounds. If your starting weight is above 160, this may be too few calories for you to begin with and you risk getting so hungry that you'll be tempted to cheat. See the suggestions below for ways to modify the basic menus in order to increase calories.

✳ If you weigh between 160 and 200 pounds, I recommend starting with a 1,600-calorie daily menu by making the following changes:

Breakfast. Add one extra slice of low-carb toast on a no-cereal or no-egg day, or one tablespoon of granola to cereal.

Lunch. Add one extra slice of meat or tofu to salad and sandwich lunches. Or add extra vegetables and a slice of low-carb bread to soup lunches and turn your bread into a sandwich.

Dinner. Increase the size of the entrée by a third. For example, a 4-ounce portion becomes a 5.3-ounce portion.

Extra. Add a healthy 100-calorie bonus food and be sure to eat it *with* your meal. See Appendix D for a list of foods that you can enjoy as free-choice treats.

✳ If you weigh between 200 and 240 pounds, start with an 1,800-calorie menu by making these changes:

Breakfast. Add one extra slice of low-carb toast on a no-cereal or no-egg day, or 2 tablespoons of granola to cereal.

Lunch. Double the amount of lean meat, tofu and bread with salad and sandwich lunches. For soup lunches, add one extra slice of lean meat, an egg or tofu, some salad and another slice of bread to make one and a half sandwiches.

Dinner. Increase the size of the entrée by 50%. For example, a 4-ounce portion becomes a 6-ounce portion.

Extra. Add a healthy 100-calorie bonus food and be sure to eat it *with* your meal. See Appendix D for a list of foods that you can enjoy as free-choice treats.

This Is My Schedule and I'm Sticking with It!

While you're on the "I" Diet, promise yourself that you'll stick with a regular schedule of meals and snacks unless a tree falls on your house or you win the lottery. You should eat three meals every day and either one or two snacks. Each menu is designed for two snacks, which is helpful for avoiding hunger. If you don't get hungry and want to cut down to one snack, just add those foods to the other snack or a meal. And remember to have a low-calorie drink with each meal and snack. This helps you feel full and also helps to regularize your eating habits.

Breakfast: _____ A.M.

Morning snack: _____ A.M.

Lunch: _____ P.M.

Afternoon snack: _____ P.M.

Dinner: _____ P.M.

Just in case:

Look over the emergency meal suggestions in Appendix G so you always have something that's okay to eat if you get too busy to follow your plan. Write your emergency meals in here for reference:

Breakfast: _____

_____

_____

Lunch: _____

_____

_____

Dinner and dessert: _____

_____

_____

Snacks: _____

_____

"Free" Foods

Not much is "free" in Stage I of the "I" Diet. I encourage you to stick closely to the menus as you start the important job of getting your food instincts to work for you. Try to eat *at least* the recommended portions of vegetables and high-fiber cereals to maintain fullness and *not more* than the recommended portions of other foods to keep those calories from creeping up. But if you feel truly unsatisfied on any day during this stage, you can have more of any of the following:

✷ Extra-fiber cereal with 1% milk or an extra "I" Diet cereal dessert (page 236). Both are terrific hunger stoppers and especially useful for meat menus, which tend to have less fiber than the vegetarian ones.

✷ Free Fiber Baggies: A half cup of high-fiber cereal plus 2 teaspoons of any flavor of your choice (chocolate chips, raisins, walnuts, whatever you like) is a great free food for any time you are hungry.

✷ Cooked green vegetables with half a teaspoon of margarine or low-fat sour cream and fresh lemon juice per extra serving.

✷ An extra salad with a little oil and vinegar or a nonfat dressing.

✷ Fresh and dried herbs and spices with menu dishes. All kinds—the more, the better.

✷ Water and no-cal drinks such as soda, mineral water, Refreshing Limonata (page 250), Fennel Infusion (page 251).

✷ Black coffee and plain tea.

✷ A little low-fat milk for coffee and tea on the menu.

✷ No-cal sugar substitutes and sugar-free gelatin desserts (if you use artificial sweeteners).

> ### A Double-Edged Sword
>
> Not only is alcohol loaded with calories, but its intoxicating effects encourage you to let down your guard when it comes to your food choices. For the first two weeks of your diet, you're asked to forgo alcohol altogether. In Stage II, you'll have a daily 100-calorie allowance that can include alcohol, but remember—even a little can impair your judgment. My advice: Less is more!

Substitutions

Use your head when it comes to menu substitutions. "I" Diet menus are scientifically structured to offer meals that are helpful for weight loss, so it's important to keep substitutions to a bare minimum. Be sure to use *similar* foods and watch portion sizes very carefully.

✳ *Bread.* If hunger isn't a problem, you can substitute 100% whole-wheat bread for the low-carb breads recommended in Stage I, but watch your calories. Whole-wheat slices tend to run about twice as high as low-carb (usually 60 to 70 calories per slice).

✳ *Desserts or carbs?* "I" Diet desserts are sweet-tasting, fiber-rich choices that help to reduce cravings. If you prefer, you can add one of the following 100-calorie carbohydrates to your entrée instead:

> 2 Potato Skins (page 226)
> ½ cup cooked 100% whole-wheat pasta
> One slice low-carb bread, lightly buttered,
>   or a low-carb wrap or pita bread
> ⅓ cup Three-Bean Salad (page 183) or
>   Wheat Berry Salad (page 180)

✳ *Fruit.* Any non-starchy fruit (i.e., no bananas), raw or cooked without sugar or added fruit juice.

✳ *Sandwiches and salads.* Any one of the following can be substituted in lunchtime meals:

> 2 ounces grilled skinless chicken breast
> 2 slices (2 ounces) turkey, ham or leanest roast beef
> 1 hard-boiled egg
> ⅓ cup solid water-packed tuna
> 1½ slices low-fat cheese or ⅔ slice regular cheese
> 2 one-inch cubes grilled tofu

✳ *Margarine.* Use butter if you prefer.

✳ *Nuts.* Have any nuts you like in amounts equivalent to those in the menus. One tablespoon equals about 14 peanuts, 4 pecan or walnut halves, or 8 cashews.

ıles. Any non-starchy cooked or salad vegetable (no potatoes).

❋ *Non-dairy drink.* Unsweetened Almond Breeze instead of milk, if you prefer.

❋ *Salad dressings.* Half as much regular dressing instead of low-cal dressing is fine. Different oils and vinegars (balsamic, fig, etc.) add great variety.

❋ *Emergency meals.* Check Appendix G for good instant meals to keep your diet on track when life gets in the way of your diet.

Take a Supplement

Supplements are a valuable insurance policy during weight loss, helping to prevent deficiencies when your total food intake is reduced. I suggest a one-a-day multivitamin and 500 milligrams of calcium (taken at a different time of day from your multivitamin since calcium competes with other minerals for absorption), plus fish oil with 200 to 300 milligrams DHA.

To Sweeten or Not to Sweeten?

Scientific studies give conflicting results about artificial sweeteners and weight control. I personally think of artificial sweeteners as a useful way to wean yourself off sugar. They allow you to enjoy sweet tastes without calories, and this means that over time they're easier to give up because your brain will come to realize that the sweet taste doesn't bring any nutrients with it. However, one study did suggest a link between worsened mood and the use of an artificial sweetener in people with depression, so whether to use them or not should be an individual decision.

The "I" Diet menus use commercial products that come with or without sweeteners depending on the brand, so you can buy either kind. There are also a few "I" Diet recipes whose ingredients include an artificial sweetener, but you can substitute a teaspoon of honey or sugar for just a few extra calories. In Stage III, you'll be encouraged to reduce both artificial sweeteners and the real thing, because then you'll be ready for the more natural whole-food diet that will more easily sustain a healthy weight.

Looking Ahead

The "I" Diet is a healthy program, and I expect you will experience few or no problems or side effects. But if you should ever get that I-really-have-to-eat-something-right-now feeling on the diet, here's what I suggest:

✻ **Recognize that this is probably not real hunger.** Most likely, it's your food triggers acting up. Try having a cup of tea or brushing your teeth, and reread Chapter 5 for help in reducing cravings and temptation. Also, spend a couple of minutes each morning thinking about your food plan—what you will eat and when. This way, you'll stay on schedule and know when it's *not* okay to eat.

✻ **Be sure to have a low-calorie drink with each meal and snack.** Don't let this slide. It makes a big difference.

✻ **Rearrange your eating schedule if necessary.** If you feel hungry at a particular time of day, try to eat more at that time. If you get too hungry around lunchtime, have breakfast an hour later than usual, even if you have to take it to work with you. If you're not hungry in the morning but feel unsatisfied in the late afternoon, you can switch the morning and afternoon snacks—morning snacks tend to be bigger.

✻ **Choose higher-fiber options.** For example, an "I" Diet cereal dessert (page 236) is a high-fiber substitution for a fruit-based dessert. You might also try adding some of the "free" foods listed on page 76.

And if you really can't handle it, consider moving on to the next-higher calorie level (see page 74). What you must *not* do is have something that's not on your menu. Stick with the program!

Is High Fiber Making You Feel Low?

In our studies at Tufts, most of our volunteers are pleasantly surprised by how easily they adapt to the high-fiber menus that help weight loss. Still, some bloating or diarrhea can occur as you adjust to higher fiber levels. If this happens, try eating a bit less of the cooked vegetables, legumes and high-fiber cereals. You can also take a week off and follow the plan for ramping up your fiber intake on page 67.

Constipation, a rare occurrence, can usually be resolved by drinking at least eight ounces of water or low-cal fluids with every meal and snack.

With Meat

	SIMPLY GOOD	HOME COOKING
Continental Breakfast	2 slices low-carb toast* with 2 teaspoons low-fat cream cheese, peanut butter or fruit spread ½ grapefruit Coffee/tea or water	2 slices "I" Diet Soda Bread (page 160) or low-carb toast* with 2 teaspoons low-fat cream cheese, peanut butter or fruit spread ⅓ cup Homemade Cinnamon Applesauce (page 140) with ¼ cup 2% plain Greek yogurt or ½ grapefruit Coffee/tea or water
Mid-Morning Snack	"I" Diet Hot or Cold Chocolate (page 253) **or** 1 apple and 4 pecan halves Water, diet soda or coffee/tea	
Lunch	Salad Plate: 2–3 cups salad greens and non-starchy veggies, ⅓ cup legumes, 2 slices (2 ounces) turkey breast, 1 teaspoon bacon bits or sunflower seeds, 2 tablespoons low-cal dressing *Optional:* 1 sugar-free gelatin dessert Water, diet soda or coffee/tea	Crispy Taco Pinto Bean Salad (page 181) **or** Thai Chicken Salad with Warm Peanut Sauce (page 177) *Optional:* 1 sugar-free gelatin dessert Water, diet soda or coffee/tea
Afternoon Snack	2 part-skim mozzarella cheese sticks Water, diet soda or coffee/tea	
Dinner	4 ounces plain grilled fish or shellfish with 2 tablespoons low-cal sauce 1½ cups cooked green beans (no sauce) 1 sliced tomato with drizzle of olive oil and vinegar or 1 teaspoon low-cal dressing *Optional:* small baked sweet potato with 1 teaspoon low-fat sour cream instead of dessert	Cajun Cod (page 206) **or** Baked Salmon with Lemon-Dill Sauce (page 203) 1½ cups green beans with ½ teaspoon tub margarine Tomato Salad (page 172) *Optional:* small baked sweet potato with 1 teaspoon low-fat sour cream instead of dessert
Dessert	Chocolate-Tipped Strawberries and Cream (page 246) **or** Ice Cream Sundae (page 236) Water, diet soda or coffee/tea	

*Asterisks mark items that vary a lot in composition and size. Check the Savvy Shopper

Vegetarian

SIMPLY GOOD	HOME COOKING
2 slices low-carb toast* with 2 teaspoons low-fat cream cheese, peanut butter or fruit spread	2 slices "I" Diet Soda Bread (page 160) or low-carb toast* with 2 teaspoons low-fat cream cheese, peanut butter or fruit spread
½ grapefruit	⅓ cup Homemade Cinnamon Applesauce (page 140) with ¼ cup 2% plain Greek yogurt or ½ grapefruit
Coffee/tea or water	Coffee/tea or water

"I" Diet Hot or Cold Chocolate (page 253)
or
6 ounces sugar-free, low-fat yogurt and 4 pecan halves
Water, diet soda or coffee/tea

Salad Plate: 2–3 cups salad greens and non-starchy veggies, ⅓ cup legumes, 1 hard-boiled egg, 1 teaspoon sunflower seeds, 2 tablespoons low-cal dressing	Vegetarian Taco Pinto Bean Salad (page 181)
1 sugar-free gelatin dessert	**or**
Water, diet soda or coffee/tea	Bibb Salad with Mushrooms and Shaved Parmesan (page 170)
	Optional: 1 sugar-free gelatin dessert
	Water, diet soda or coffee/tea

2 part-skim mozzarella cheese sticks
Water, diet soda or coffee/tea

1 veggie burger or 2 meat-free hot dogs with 1 low-carb roll* on the side, mustard and ketchup	Steamed Tofu and Mixed Vegetables with Warm Peanut Sauce (page 207)
2 cups mixed garden salad with drizzle of olive oil and vinegar or 2 teaspoons low-cal dressing	**or**
	Vegetarian Home Run Hot Dogs (page 193)
	Side salad with 2 teaspoons Tarragon Dressing (page 172)
	Optional: low-carb roll* instead of dessert

Chocolate-Tipped Strawberries and Cream (page 246)
or
Ice Cream Sundae (page 236)
Water, diet soda or coffee/tea

directory (Appendix E) for help in choosing suitable products for your diet.

With Meat

	SIMPLY GOOD	HOME COOKING
Cereal and Fruit Breakfast	1/3 cup or more high-fiber cereal* with 2 tablespoons granola and 1/2 cup nonfat or 1% milk 1/2 cup sliced strawberries Coffee/tea or water	1/3 cup or more high-fiber cereal* with 2 tablespoons granola and 1/2 cup nonfat or 1% milk 4 Spicy Prunes (page 141) or 1/2 cup sliced strawberries Coffee/tea or water
Mid-Morning Snack	1 apple and 1 tablespoon peanuts Water, diet soda or coffee/tea	
Lunch	Soup and Sandwich: 1 cup broth-based vegetable soup*; 1 ham sandwich made with 2 slices low-carb bread*, 2 slices (2 ounces) ham, optional 1 slice fat-free cheese, 1 teaspoon low-cal mayo, mustard, lettuce, tomato, onion, hot peppers (as desired) 1/4 cup frozen grapes Water, diet soda or coffee/tea	Hummus and Veggie Plate with Spicy Sesame Cracker Chips (page 182) 1/4 cup frozen grapes Water, diet soda or coffee/tea
Afternoon Snack	"I" Diet Hot or Cold Chocolate (page 253) **or** 1/2 cup low-fat cottage cheese and 2 celery sticks Water, diet soda or coffee/tea	
Dinner	4 ounces cooked lean steak with 2 tablespoons low-cal sauce 1 1/2 cups steamed broccoli (no sauce) Side salad with drizzle of olive oil and vinegar or 2 teaspoons low-cal dressing *Optional:* 1 small low-carb pita bread* instead of dessert	Florentine Steak (page 190) 1 1/2 cups steamed broccoli with 1 teaspoon low-fat sour cream and fresh lemon juice Side salad with drizzle of olive oil and vinegar or 2 teaspoons low-cal dressing *Optional:* 1/2 cup cooked whole-wheat pasta* instead of dessert
Dessert	1 fresh pear with 1 teaspoon warm caramel sauce **or** Ginger-Pecan Crunch (page 237) Water, diet soda or coffee/tea	

Asterisks mark items that vary a lot in composition and size. Check the Savvy Shopper

Vegetarian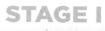

SIMPLY GOOD	HOME COOKING
⅓ cup or more high-fiber cereal* with 2 tablespoons granola and ½ cup nonfat or 1% milk	⅓ cup or more high-fiber cereal* with 2 tablespoons granola and ½ cup nonfat or 1% milk
½ cup sliced strawberries	4 Spicy Prunes (page 141) or ½ cup sliced strawberries
Coffee/tea or water	Coffee/tea or water

1 part-skim mozzarella cheese stick and 2 celery sticks
Water, diet soda or coffee/tea

Soup and Sandwich: 1 cup broth-based vegetable soup*; 1 cheese sandwich made with 2 slices low-carb bread*, 1 slice low-fat cheese, 2 teaspoons low-cal dressing, lettuce, tomato, mustard, hot peppers (as desired)	Hummus and Veggie Plate with Spicy Sesame Cracker Chips (page 182)
	¼ cup frozen grapes
¼ cup frozen grapes	Water, diet soda or coffee/tea
Water, diet soda or coffee/tea	

"I" Diet Hot or Cold Chocolate (page 253)
or
½ cup low-fat cottage cheese and 2 celery sticks
Water, diet soda or coffee/tea

Easy Bean-and-Cheese Burritos (page 269)	Broiled Tofu (page 208)
Side salad with drizzle of olive oil and vinegar or 2 teaspoons low-cal dressing	1½ cups steamed broccoli with 1 teaspoon low-fat sour cream and fresh lemon juice
	Side salad with drizzle of olive oil and vinegar or 2 teaspoons low-cal dressing
	Optional: ½ cup Boiled Barley* (page 217) instead of dessert

1 fresh pear with 1 teaspoon warm caramel sauce
or
Ginger-Pecan Crunch (page 237)
Water, diet soda or coffee/tea

directory (Appendix E) for help in choosing suitable products for your diet.

With Meat

	SIMPLY GOOD	HOME COOKING
Cooked Breakfast	1 egg fried/boiled/poached and 1 slice low-carb toast* with 1 teaspoon tub margarine ½ cup melon chunks Coffee/tea or water	Bacon and Eggs Breakfast (page 137) **or** Vegetable "Frittata" (page 136) ½ cup Plum Compote (page 141) or melon chunks Coffee/tea or water
Mid-Morning Snack	6 ounces sugar-free, low-fat yogurt with 4 pecan halves Water, diet soda or coffee/tea	
Lunch	1 cup thick non-creamy soup such as lentil or beef and barley 1 small orange and 1 tablespoon peanuts Water, diet soda or coffee/tea	Beef and Barley Soup (page 154) **or** Lentil Vegetable Soup (page 149) 1 small orange and 1 tablespoon peanuts Water, diet soda or coffee/tea
Afternoon Snack	Strawberry-Blueberry Smoothie (page 270) **or** ½ cup low-fat cottage cheese and 2 celery sticks Water, diet soda or coffee/tea	
Dinner	4 ounces grilled skinless chicken breast with ¼ cup tomato sauce and 1 tablespoon grated Parmesan 1½ cups steamed mixed veggies (no sauce) Side salad with Rosemary-Thyme Dressing (page 262) *Optional:* low-carb pita bread* instead of dessert	Chicken Parm (page 198) 1½ cups steamed snow peas with ½ teaspoon tub margarine Side salad with drizzle of olive oil and vinegar or 2 teaspoons low-cal dressing *Optional:* ½ cup Boiled Barley* (page 217) instead of dessert
Dessert	Almost Apple Cobbler (page 245) **or** Chocolate-Raspberry Parfait (page 237) Water, diet soda or coffee/tea	

Asterisks mark items that vary a lot in composition and size. Check the Savvy Shopper

Vegetarian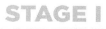

SIMPLY GOOD	HOME COOKING
1 egg fried/boiled/poached and 1 slice low-carb toast* with 1 teaspoon tub margarine ½ cup melon chunks Coffee/tea or water	Vegetable "Frittata" (page 136) ½ cup Plum Compote (page 141) or melon chunks Coffee/tea or water

6 ounces sugar-free, low-fat yogurt with 4 pecan halves
Water, diet soda or coffee/tea

1 cup thick non-creamy soup such as lentil or minestrone 1 small orange and 1 tablespoon peanuts Water, diet soda or coffee/tea	Mushroom and Barley Soup (page 154) **or** Lentil Vegetable Soup (page 149) 1 small orange and 1 tablespoon peanuts Water, diet soda or coffee/tea

Strawberry-Blueberry Smoothie (page 270)
or
½ cup low-fat cottage cheese and 2 celery sticks
Water, diet soda or coffee/tea

No-Fuss Pizza (page 212) **or** Veggie cheese wrap: 1 low-carb tortilla* filled with ½ cup grilled veggies, ¼ cup bean salad or cooked beans, 2 tablespoons low-fat Alfredo sauce Side salad with Rosemary-Thyme Dressing (page 262)	Stuffed Green Peppers (page 216) **or** Barbecue Vegetable Pizza (page 211) Side salad with drizzle of olive oil and vinegar or 2 teaspoons low-cal dressing

Almost Apple Cobbler (page 245)
or
Chocolate-Raspberry Parfait (page 237)
Water, diet soda or coffee/tea

directory (Appendix E) for help in choosing suitable products for your diet.

The "I" Diet has one more great advantage that you need to know about now. *It's easy to get back to it if you fall off the wagon.* Let's say you went to a friend's wedding, lost it and ate everything in sight. Just put yourself back on fiber the next day (half a cup of Fiber One with each meal) and it will be easy to start dieting again. I'm not recommending a casual attitude about going on and off your diet, but if it happens, it's empowering to know that there's an easy way to snap right back again.

Besides, things are about to get easier and more fun. There's a daily bonus of 100 calories, which you can spend on sweet treats or a glass of wine, or save up for some pizza and ice cream. You'll also be able to mix-and-match your meals and snacks if that works better for you, and you'll notice that the variety of food you're eating becomes much more interesting. Think of Stage II as the preamble to the rest of your life . . .

CHAPTER 10

Stage II
The Six-Week "Keeping It Going" Diet

W elcome to the next stage of your "I" Diet plan. This is where weight loss gets fun. (Lots more choices!) Before too long, you should start to see amazing changes in your body's shape and proportions. Tracking our Tufts volunteers' success in this stage of the program is very exciting. The changes are visible and dramatic, reminding me of those unfinished Michelangelo statues that show well-defined, muscular torsos pulling themselves effortlessly out of blocks of marble.

Of course, your new body won't emerge overnight. It takes a while to whittle down body fat. Weigh yourself daily and calculate weekly averages. (Any water you may have lost in Stage I could be normalizing now.) Focus instead on following the menus. Every good meal puts another brick in the wall you're building toward permanent weight loss, even if the scale doesn't show it right away.

fiction: It's harder to lose weight if you're over 40.
fact: No, it isn't.

Although our energy requirements decrease with age, weight loss does *not* get harder. At Tufts, we've found that the people who lose the most weight are somewhat older, whereas college students and recent graduates have the most trouble dropping pounds. True, the average person gains about 40 pounds between the ages of 20 and 50, so calorie intake has to be balanced with energy expended, but older people successfully lose weight once they set their minds to it. This may be because they're more patient than younger people or because their maturity works to good advantage when it comes to sticking with their weight-loss strategies. Whatever the reason, being older clearly is not a lifelong sentence to being overweight.

What's New in Stage II

In some ways, Stage II is more of the same: more good meals guaranteed to suppress hunger and more healthy snacks to keep your weight coming down. You will still find Simply Good and Home Cooking menus with both meat and vegetarian options, but there are some important differences designed to help keep you feeling happy, full and energetic.

✳ **More delicious variety.** Stage II offers a much wider variety of foods to choose from. This might seem like more work, but after the first week it gets easy. Plus it's more fun! One evening, you might be in the mood for Mexican food; the next, a Chinese dinner might hit the spot. No problem. We've also added some classic American favorites as well as Italian and Indian entrées. You don't have to add all the new variety if you're satisfied with less. Keeping Stage I meals is fine, too. And the more you enjoy eating at home, the less tempted you'll be to (over)eat at restaurants.

✳ **Daily treats.** Now you can have a 100-calorie free-choice treat every single day if you want to. Or you can save up this 100-calorie treat allowance for several days, lump all the extra calories together and have a small 400-calorie chocolate sundae on Day 4 if you think you can to resist the

Motivation Check

Take a minute to remind yourself why you're doing this. Review your reasons and your incentives—the nice things you give yourself when you don't give in to temptation. If your incentives didn't prove up to the challenges you faced in Stage I, plan some better ones for Stage II.

My reasons for losing weight:

1. _____

2. _____

3. _____

When I resist eating larger portions or things that are not on the menu, I'll reward myself by:

1. _____

2. _____

3. _____

Great Motivations

- To look better.
- To feel better.
- To have more energy.
- To get your blood pressure and cholesterol back to normal.

Great Incentives

- Book a massage.
- Take a break. Relax, call a friend, do something fun outdoors.
- Buy that book you've been wanting to read.

temptation to have another helping. This 100-calorie bonus is there to incorporate into your meal plan as you wish as long as you don't eat *more,* or you can choose to skip it if you're trying to be super careful.

✳ **A new seven-day menu plan.** Instead of repeating the menus every three days as in Stage I, you'll repeat them after each week. This makes it easier to enjoy healthy foods, because you're eating them in a regular pattern that satisfies your instinct for both familiarity and variety.

✳ **A mix-and-match option.** If sticking with the menus is just impossible for you (say, because of travel or other lifestyle issues), you can now mix-and-match your meals and snacks. See the list starting on page 106.

Calorie Check

Are you where you want to be in terms of calories? If you lost two to five pounds in Stage I, congratulations! You're doing fine. The diet is working exactly as it should. Stay on the same calorie level as in Stage I and follow the same advice for modifying the basic menus if you were using the 1,600- or 1,800-calorie plan (page 74).

Did you lose six pounds or more? If so, super congratulations! The diet is really working for you. Now, though, you might move to the next higher-calorie plan if you were hungry in Stage I.

Did you lose one pound or less? You may have inadvertently eaten more than the specified calories. Even "good" calories add up! Try to stick to the portion sizes specified, and don't "embellish" the recipes or meals until your weight loss is firmly established. If you were on one of the higher-calorie plans, you can also consider moving to the next lower one.

Your Treat or Mine?

Everyone is different when it comes to controlling treats. Some people find that having a few bites makes them lose control. In this case, the only real solution is to give up the worst offenders altogether and focus on getting enjoyment from healthier foods. Other people find that by using good strategies they can enjoy most or even all of their favorite foods without overeating them. The suggestions below will help ensure that the treats you do eat are not only controllable but a good learning experience for the future.

✳ **Never eat your treat by itself.** Bonus foods should be eaten *only with meals*. Chapter 4 explains why this is so important and tells how to use the "sandwich" technique for increasing enjoyment without losing control.

✳ **Make sensible choices.** The more wisely you use your treat allowance, the easier control will be. Even though we've tested these allowances at Tufts and found that on average they make no difference to weight loss, we did discover something interesting. Some volunteers' taste preferences changed so much with weight loss that they no longer had any desire for sweet treats like chocolate or ice cream; they simply wanted to eat other healthy diet foods that weren't on the menu. And for those volunteers who needed more help to feel full and satisfied, using the 100-calorie allowance on an extra "I" Diet cereal dessert was the perfect choice.

> ### Small, Small, Slow
>
> Keep portions small. Make bites small by cutting food into tiny pieces. And don't rush. You can also close your eyes for intense taste. You won't actually feel fuller, but you'll enjoy your food more—and feel more satisfied with less.

✳ **Know your portion size.** Appendix D gives portion sizes for 100-calorie treat allowances. As long as your choice doesn't make you hungry for more, pick whatever you like. Selections range from a daily glass of wine or a beer to a small baked potato or some miniature chocolates. Just remember to *think control.*

Pizza and Ice Cream!

Can you picture 100 calories of pizza? What it amounts to is about a third of a regular slice (much less for deluxe or extra-cheese). And what about 100 calories of premium ice cream? Less than a quarter-cup! Even if you follow all the rules of careful eating, it would still be pretty hard to turn such tiny portions into satisfying treats. One reasonable option is to save up your daily allowance and then once a week have two slices of not-too-indulgent regular pizza (choose the *smallest* slices from a large pizza) or try a slice of pizza and a half-cup of ice cream (plus a salad with nonfat dressing to fill you up).

Better yet, you'll find ways to make your own hearty pizza in our recipe section (pages 211 and 212), and ice cream can be enjoyed every night without using up your treat allowance if you get used to the sugar-free products and have them as a cereal dessert (page 236). Before you know it, these healthier versions can start to taste delicious. Take this as a sure sign that your familiarity instinct is alive and well—and helping you with the important job of weight loss.

With Meat

	SIMPLY GOOD	HOME COOKING
Special Breakfast	"I" Diet Instant Hot Cereal with Maple Syrup and Blueberries (page 135) Coffee/tea or water	Orange-Crumbed French Toast (page 138) or Bannock Cakes (page 134) Coffee/tea or water
Mid-Morning Snack	1 wedge Laughing Cow cheese spread with 3 sticks celery **or** ½ cup baby carrots with 1 tablespoon ranch dressing Water, diet soda or coffee/tea	
Lunch	Soup and Sandwich: 1 cup broth-based vegetable soup; 1 tuna sandwich made with 2 slices low-carb bread*, ¼ cup water-packed solid tuna, 2 teaspoons low-cal mayo, lettuce, tomato, onion, etc. 1 sugar-free gelatin dessert Water, diet soda or coffee/tea	Easy Tomato, Barley and Basil Soup (page 145) "I" Diet Tuna Salad wrap (page 162) 1 sugar-free gelatin dessert Water, diet soda or coffee/tea
Afternoon Snack	"I" Diet Hot or Cold Chocolate (page 253) **or** 1 apple and 1 tablespoon peanuts (14 individual peanuts) Water, diet soda or coffee/tea	
Dinner	4 ounces grilled skinless chicken breast heaped with ⅓ cup cooked pinto beans, ¼ cup salsa, 1 tablespoon grated Parmesan cheese, 2 teaspoons low-fat sour cream, optional chopped fresh cilantro 1½ cups sliced fresh tomato and cucumber with 1 teaspoon olive oil and fresh lemon juice	Mexican Lettuce Wraps (page 194) **or** Tanzanian Chicken Kebabs (page 195) with Cucumber-Mint Raita (page 174) Side salad of baby greens with drizzle of olive oil and fresh lemon juice
Dessert	Ice Cream Sundae (page 236) **or** ⅔ cup raspberries with 2 tablespoons light whipped cream Water, diet soda or coffee/tea **or** Refreshing Limonata (page 250)	

*Asterisks mark items that vary a lot in composition and size. Check the Savvy Shopper

Vegetarian

SIMPLY GOOD	HOME COOKING
"I" Diet Instant Hot Cereal with Maple Syrup and Blueberries (page 135)	Orange-Crumbed French Toast (page 138) or Bannock Cakes (page 134)
Coffee/tea or water	Coffee/tea or water

½ cup low-fat cottage cheese with ⅓ sweet red pepper
or
2 low-fat mozzarella cheese sticks
Water, diet soda or coffee/tea

Soup and Sandwich: 1 cup broth-based vegetable soup; 1 cheese sandwich made with 2 slices low-carb bread*, 1 slice cheese, 1 teaspoon low-cal mayo, mustard, lettuce, tomato, onion, etc.	Easy Tomato, Barley and Basil Soup (page 145)
	Broiled Tofu sandwich (page 161)
	1 sugar-free gelatin dessert
1 sugar-free gelatin dessert	Water, diet soda or coffee/tea
Water, diet soda or coffee/tea	

"I" Diet Hot or Cold Chocolate (page 253)
or
1 apple and 1 tablespoon peanuts (14 individual peanuts)
Water, diet soda or coffee/tea

Easy Bean-and-Cheese Burritos (page 269)	Mixed Vegetable Curry (page 219)
1½ cups sliced fresh tomato and cucumber with 1 teaspoon olive oil and fresh lemon juice	Moong Dal Stew (page 222) with 1 teaspoon Lemon and Date Chutney (page 223) or mango chutney and 2 tablespoons low-fat plain yogurt
	½ cup Boiled Barley* (page 217) or 1 small low-carb pita bread*

1 cup fresh mango
or
⅔ cup raspberries with 2 tablespoons light whipped cream
Water, diet soda or coffee/tea **or** Refreshing Limonata (page 250)

directory (Appendix E) for help in choosing suitable products for your diet.

With Meat

	SIMPLY GOOD	HOME COOKING
Continental Breakfast	1 cup "complete" high-fiber cereal* with 1/2 cup nonfat or 1% milk 1/2 cup sliced strawberries Coffee/tea or water	1/3 cup high-fiber cereal* with 2 tablespoons granola, 2 pecan halves and 1/2 cup nonfat or 1% milk 4 Spicy Prunes (page 141) or 1/2 cup sliced strawberries Coffee/tea or water
Mid-Morning Snack	2 part-skim mozzarella cheese sticks **or** 1 small high-protein, high-fiber snack bar** and 1 plum or kiwi Water, diet soda or coffee/tea	
Lunch	Asian Salad Plate: 2–3 cups salad greens and non-starchy veggies, 2 slices (2 ounces) chicken breast, 1/3 cup legumes, 1 tablespoon mandarin orange segments, 1 teaspoon sesame seeds, 2 tablespoons low-cal Asian-style dressing Water, diet soda or coffee/tea	"I" Diet Chicken Salad wrap (page 161) **or** Indian Kebab Wrap (page 165) 2–3 palm hearts Water, diet soda or coffee/tea
Afternoon Snack	Snack Attack Pack (page 248) **or** "I" Diet Cereal Dessert (page 236) Water, diet soda or coffee/tea	
Dinner	Veggie burger served on a low-carb roll*, lettuce, tomato, onion, 1 teaspoon low-fat mayo, relish, ketchup 1 1/2 cups broccoli (no sauce) with 1 teaspoon low-fat sour cream and fresh lemon juice Side salad of crispy romaine with 2 teaspoons low-fat blue cheese dressing	The Ultimate "I" Burger (page 264) **or** Belgian-Style Beef Stew (page 266) Iceberg Wedges with Blue Cheese (page 169) 1 1/2 cups steamed broccoli with 1 teaspoon low-fat sour cream and fresh lemon juice
Dessert	Almost Apple Cobbler (page 245) **or** Orange Flan (page 241) Water, diet soda or coffee/tea **or** Fennel Infusion (page 251)	

*Asterisks mark items that vary a lot in composition and size. Check the Savvy Shopper
**Small high-protein, high-fiber snack bars contain 80 to 100 calories.

SIMPLY GOOD	HOME COOKING
1 cup "complete" high-fiber cereal* with 1/2 cup nonfat or 1% milk	1/3 cup high-fiber cereal* with 2 tablespoons granola, 2 pecan halves and 1/2 cup nonfat or 1% milk
1/2 cup sliced strawberries	4 Spicy Prunes (page 141) or 1/2 cup sliced strawberries
Coffee/tea or water	Coffee/tea or water

2 part-skim mozzarella cheese sticks

or

1 small high-protein, high-fiber snack bar** and 1 plum or kiwi

Water, diet soda or coffee/tea

Asian Salad Plate: 2–3 cups salad greens and non-starchy veggies, 1 hard-boiled egg, 1/3 cup legumes, 1 tablespoon mandarin orange segments, 1 teaspoon sesame seeds, 2 tablespoons low-cal Asian-style dressing	Vegetarian Chicken Salad wrap (page 161) **or** Leftover curry (page 219) in a small low-carb pita bread with side salad of romaine
Water, diet soda or coffee/tea	2–3 palm hearts
	Water, diet soda or coffee/tea

6 ounces sugar-free, low-fat yogurt with 4 pecan halves

or

1/2 cup low-fat cottage cheese

Water, diet soda or coffee/tea

Veggie burger served on a low-carb roll* with lettuce, tomato, onion, 1 teaspoon low-fat mayo, relish, ketchup	Vegetarian Burger Delight (page 189)
	Iceberg Wedges with Blue Cheese (page 169)
1 1/2 cups broccoli (no sauce) with 1 teaspoon low-fat sour cream and fresh lemon juice	1 1/2 cups steamed broccoli or snow peas with 1 teaspoon low-fat sour cream and fresh lemon juice
Side salad of crispy romaine with 2 teaspoons low-fat blue cheese dressing	

Almost Apple Cobbler (page 245)

or

Orange Flan (page 241)

Water, diet soda or coffee/tea **or** Fennel Infusion (page 251)

directory (Appendix E) for help in choosing suitable products for your diet.
Check the Savvy Shopper directory for suitable brands.

With Meat

	SIMPLY GOOD	HOME COOKING
Continental Breakfast	2 slices low-carb bread* with 2 teaspoons low-fat cream cheese, peanut butter or fruit spread ½ cup melon chunks or ½ grapefruit Coffee/tea or water	2 slices low-carb bread* or "I" Diet Soda Bread (page 160) with 2 teaspoons low-fat cream cheese, peanut butter or fruit spread ¼ cup nonfat plain Greek yogurt with ½ cup sliced strawberries or ½ grapefruit Coffee/tea or water
Mid-Morning Snack	"I" Diet Hot or Cold Chocolate (page 253) **or** 1 cup grapes and 4 pecan halves Water, diet soda or coffee/tea	
Lunch	Picnic Plate: 1 sliced apple and 1" cube (1 ounce) extra-sharp 50% reduced-fat cheddar cheese 6 ounces sugar-free, low-fat yogurt sprinkled with 3 tablespoons or more high-fiber cereal* Water, diet soda or coffee/tea	Hummus and Veggie Plate with Spicy Sesame Cracker Chips (page 182) Masala Tea (page 252) and/or water, diet soda or coffee/tea
Afternoon Snack	1 small high-protein, high-fiber bar** and ⅓ sweet red pepper **or** Strawberry-Blueberry Smoothie (page 270) Water, diet soda or coffee/tea	
Dinner	4 ounces plain grilled fish with 2 tablespoons low-cal sauce 1½ cups green beans (no sauce) Side salad of baby spinach with drizzle of olive oil, balsamic vinegar and 2 teaspoons dried cranberries	Cajun Cod (page 206) **or** Baked Salmon with Lemon-Dill Sauce (page 203) 1½ cups steamed asparagus or 1 cup A Perfect Ratatouille (page 228) Side salad of baby spinach with drizzle of olive oil, balsamic vinegar and 2 teaspoons dried cranberries
Dessert	Ginger-Pecan Crunch (page 237) **or** Indian Barley Pudding (page 242) Water, diet soda or coffee/tea	

Asterisks mark items that vary a lot in composition and size. Check the Savvy Shopper
**Small high-protein, high-fiber snack bars contain 80 to 100 calories.*

SIMPLY GOOD	HOME COOKING
2 slices low-carb bread* with 2 teaspoons low-fat cream cheese, peanut butter or fruit spread	2 slices low-carb bread* or "I" Diet Soda Bread (page 160) with 2 teaspoons low-fat cream cheese, peanut butter or fruit spread
1/2 cup melon chunks or 1/2 grapefruit	1/4 cup nonfat plain Greek yogurt with 1/2 cup sliced strawberries or 1/2 grapefruit
Coffee/tea or water	Coffee/tea or water

"I" Diet Hot or Cold Chocolate (page 253)

or

1 cup grapes and 4 pecan halves

Water, diet soda or coffee/tea

Picnic Plate: 1 sliced apple and 1" cube (1 ounce) extra-sharp 50% reduced-fat cheddar cheese	Thai Salad with Warm Peanut Sauce (page 177)
	or
6 ounces sugar-free, low-fat yogurt sprinkled with 3 tablespoons or more high-fiber cereal*	Hummus and Veggie Plate with Spicy Sesame Cracker Chips (page 182)
Water, diet soda or coffee/tea	Masala Tea (page 252) and/or water, diet soda or coffee/tea

1 small high-protein, high-fiber bar** and 1/3 sweet red pepper

or

Strawberry-Blueberry Smoothie (page 270)

Water, diet soda or coffee/tea

2 veggie hot dogs with a low-carb roll* on the side, ketchup and mustard	2-egg omelet prepared with 1/2 teaspoon tub margarine
or	1/2 cup Wheat Berry Salad (page 180)
2 veggie hot dogs and 1/2 cup baked beans	**or**
Side salad of baby spinach with drizzle of olive oil, balsamic vinegar and 2 teaspoons dried cranberries	Vegetarian Home Run Hot Dogs (page 193)
	Side salad of baby spinach with drizzle of olive oil, balsamic vinegar and 2 teaspoons dried cranberries

Ginger-Pecan Crunch (page 237) **or** Indian Barley Pudding (page 242)

Water, diet soda or coffee/tea

directory (Appendix E) for help in choosing suitable products for your diet.
Check the Savvy Shopper directory for suitable brands.

With Meat

	SIMPLY GOOD	HOME COOKING
Cooked Breakfast	1 egg fried/boiled/poached and 1 slice low-carb toast* with 1 teaspoon tub margarine ½ cup melon chunks Coffee/tea or water	Bacon and Eggs Breakfast (page 137) **or** Vegetable "Frittata" (page 136) ½ cup Plum Compote (page 141) or melon chunks Coffee/tea or water
Mid-Morning Snack	Snack Attack Pack (page 248) **or** 1 apple and 3 dried black mission figs Water, diet soda or coffee/tea	
Lunch	Soup and Sandwich: 1 cup French onion soup (no cheese); 1 roast beef sandwich made with 2 slices low-carb bread*, 2 slices (2 ounces) roast beef with no visible fat, 1 teaspoon mustard, lettuce, tomato, sliced onion, etc. 1 sugar-free gelatin dessert Water, diet soda or coffee/tea	Costa Rican Black Bean Soup (page 148) Side salad with 1 tablespoon grated cheese and 2 teaspoons low-cal dressing 1 sugar-free gelatin dessert Water, diet soda or coffee/tea
Afternoon Snack	"I" Diet Hot or Cold Chocolate (page 253) **or** ½ cup low-fat cottage cheese with ⅓ sweet pepper Water, diet soda or coffee/tea	
Dinner	4 ounces grilled skinless chicken breast with 2 tablespoons low-cal sweet-and-sour sauce 1 cup Chinese-style veggies Mixed garden side salad with drizzle of olive oil and vinegar	Hoisin Pork (page 192) with Asian Coleslaw (page 175) Mixed garden side salad with Rosemary-Thyme Dressing (page 262)
Dessert	Chocolate Cereal Dessert (page 236) **or** 1 ripe pear with 1 teaspoon warm caramel sauce Water, diet soda or coffee/tea	

Asterisks mark items that vary a lot in composition and size. Check the Savvy Shopper

SIMPLY GOOD	HOME COOKING
1 egg fried/boiled/poached and 1 slice low-carb toast* with 1 teaspoon tub margarine	Vegetable "Frittata" (page 136)
½ cup melon chunks	½ cup Plum Compote (page 141) or melon chunks
Coffee/tea or water	Coffee/tea or water

Snack Attack Pack (page 248)
or
1 apple and 3 dried black mission figs
Water, diet soda or coffee/tea

1½ cups thick soup such as lentil or minestrone with 1 tablespoon grated cheese topping	Costa Rican Black Bean Soup (page 148)
Side salad with 1 tablespoon grated cheese and 2 teaspoons low-calorie dressing	Side salad with 1 tablespoon grated cheese and 2 teaspoons low-cal dressing
1 sugar-free gelatin dessert	1 sugar-free gelatin dessert
Water, diet soda or coffee/tea	Water, diet soda or coffee/tea

"I" Diet Hot or Cold Chocolate (page 253)
or
½ cup low-fat cottage cheese with ½ sweet pepper
Water, diet soda or coffee/tea

1 cup cucumber slices with 1 tablespoon low-cal dressing	Mushroom and Barley Risotto (page 218)
1 grilled cheese sandwich made with 2 slices low-carb bread* and 1" cube (1 ounce) 50% fat-reduced sharp cheddar	Watercress and Orange Salad with Parmesan Toasts and Hummus (page 171) **or**
½ cup baked beans	Spicy Tofu and Mixed Vegetable Stir-Fry (page 206)

Chocolate Cereal Dessert (page 236)
or
1 ripe pear with 1 teaspoon warm caramel sauce
Water, diet soda or coffee/tea

directory (Appendix E) for help in choosing suitable products for your diet.

With Meat

SIMPLY GOOD	HOME COOKING

Hot Cereal Breakfast

"I" Diet Instant Hot Cereal with Raisins, Pecans and Cinnamon (page 135)

Coffee/tea or water

Irish Oatmeal (page 133)

Coffee/tea or water

Mid-Morning Snack

"I" Diet Hot or Cold Chocolate (page 253)
or
6 ounces sugar-free, low-fat yogurt with 1 teaspoon dried fruit
Water, diet soda or coffee/tea

Lunch

Ham and Cheese Salad Plate:
2–3 cups salad greens and non-starchy veggies, 1/3 cup legumes, 2 slices (2 ounces) ham, 2 tablespoons feta cheese, 2 tablespoons low-cal dressing

1/4 cup frozen grapes

Water, diet soda or coffee/tea

Apple, Walnut and Blue Cheese Salad (page 168)
or
Bibb Salad with Mushrooms and Shaved Parmesan (page 170)

1 slice "I" Diet Soda Bread (page 160) or low-carb toast*

Water, diet soda or coffee/tea

Afternoon Snack

1 small high-protein, high-fiber bar** and 1/2 orange
or
1/2 cup low-fat cottage cheese with 1/4 cup baby carrots
Water, diet soda or coffee/tea

Dinner

No-Fuss Pizza (page 211)
or
Cheese-and-veggie wrap: 1 low-carb tortilla* filled with warmed 1/2 cup grilled veggies, 1/4 cup legumes or bean salad, 2 tablespoons low-cal Alfredo sauce

1 large tomato, sliced, with chopped fresh basil and drizzle of olive oil and balsamic vinegar

John's Pasta Supper (page 213)
or
Italian Meatballs (page 262)

Florentine Braised Kale (page 227)

Tomato Salad (page 172)

Dessert

Chocolate-Raspberry Parfait (page 237)
or
Chocolate-Tipped Strawberries and Cream (page 246)
Water, diet soda or coffee/tea

*Asterisks mark items that vary a lot in composition and size. Check the Savvy Shopper
**Small high-protein, high-fiber snack bars contain 80 to 100 calories.

SIMPLY GOOD	HOME COOKING

"I" Diet Instant Hot Cereal with Raisins, Pecans and Cinnamon (page 135)

Coffee/tea or water

Irish Oatmeal (page 133)

Coffee/tea or water

"I" Diet Hot or Cold Chocolate (page 253)
or
6 ounces sugar-free, low-fat yogurt with 1 teaspoon dried fruit
Water, diet soda or coffee/tea

Cheese Salad Plate: 2–3 cups salad greens and non-starchy veggies, 1/2 cup legumes, 1 slice cheese, 1 teaspoon sunflower seeds, 2 tablespoons low-cal dressing

1/4 cup frozen grapes

Water, diet soda or coffee/tea

Mexican Black Beans with Chips, Salsa and Sour Cream (page 265)

or

Bibb Salad with Mushrooms and Shaved Parmesan (page 170)

1 slice "I" Diet Soda Bread (page 160) or low-carb toast*

Water, diet soda or coffee/tea

---

1 small high-protein, high-fiber bar** and 1/2 orange
or
1/2 cup low-fat cottage cheese with 1/4 cup baby carrots
Water, diet soda or coffee/tea

No-Fuss Pizza (page 212)

or

Cheese-and-veggie wrap: 1 low-carb tortilla* filled with 1/2 cup warmed grilled veggies, 1/4 cup legumes or bean salad, 2 tablespoons low-cal Alfredo sauce

1 large tomato, sliced, with chopped fresh basil and drizzle of olive oil and balsamic vinegar

Barbecue Vegetable Pizza (page 212)

or

Stuffed Green Peppers (page 216) or Afghan Stuffed Peppers (page 268)

Tomato Salad (page 172)

Chocolate-Raspberry Parfait (page 237)
or
Chocolate-Tipped Strawberries and Cream (page 246)
Water, diet soda or coffee/tea

---

*directory (Appendix E) for help in choosing suitable products for your diet.
Check the Savvy Shopper directory for suitable brands.*

With Meat

	SIMPLY GOOD	HOME COOKING
Continental Breakfast	1 cup "complete" high-fiber cereal* with 1/2 cup nonfat or 1% milk 1/2 orange Coffee/tea or water	1/3 cup high-fiber cereal* with 2 tablespoons granola, 2 teaspoons raisins and 1/2 cup nonfat or 1% milk 1/2 orange Coffee/tea or water
Mid-Morning Snack		"I" Diet Hot or Cold Chocolate (page 253) **or** 1/2 cup low-fat cottage cheese with 3 celery sticks Water, diet soda or coffee/tea
Lunch	Chicken Caesar wrap: 1 small low-carb tortilla* filled with 2 slices (2 ounces) chicken, 1 tablespoon low-cal Caesar dressing, 1 tablespoon grated Parmesan cheese, chopped lettuce Side salad with 2 teaspoons low-cal dressing 1 sugar-free gelatin dessert Water, diet soda or coffee/tea	Thai Chicken Salad with Warm Peanut Sauce (page 177) **or** Crispy Taco Pinto Bean Salad (page 181) 1 sugar-free gelatin dessert Water, diet soda or coffee/tea
Afternoon Snack		Snack Attack Pack (page 248) **or** "I" Diet Cereal Dessert (page 236) Water, diet soda or coffee/tea
Dinner	3 ounces grilled salmon on a toasted low-carb roll* with 1 teaspoon low-fat mayo, fresh lemon juice, lettuce, tomato 1 1/2 cups cooked snow peas (no sauce)	Perfect Grill shrimp or chicken with Creamy Mustard Sauce (page 199) 1 1/2 cups grilled mixed veggies Side salad with drizzle of olive oil and vinegar
Dessert		1 cup sugar-free fresh fruit salad **or** Baked Apples with Figs (page 243) Water, diet soda or coffee/tea

*Asterisks mark items that vary a lot in composition and size. Check the Savvy Shopper

Vegetarian

SIMPLY GOOD	HOME COOKING
1 cup "complete" high-fiber cereal* with 1/2 cup nonfat or 1% milk	1/3 cup high-fiber cereal* with 2 tablespoons granola, 2 teaspoons raisins and 1/2 cup nonfat or 1% milk
1/2 orange	1/2 orange
Coffee/tea or water	Coffee/tea or water

"I" Diet Hot or Cold Chocolate (page 253)
or
1/2 cup low-fat cottage cheese with 3 celery sticks
Water, diet soda or coffee/tea

Cannellini Caesar wrap: 1 small low-carb tortilla* filled with 1/4 cup cooked cannellini beans, 1 tablespoon low-cal Caesar dressing, 2 tablespoons grated Parmesan cheese, chopped lettuce	West African Bean Cakes with Spicy Dip and Green Salad (page 224)
	or
	Thai Salad with Warm Peanut Sauce (page 177)
Side salad with 2 teaspoons low-cal dressing	1 sugar-free gelatin dessert
1 sugar-free gelatin dessert	Water, diet soda or coffee/tea
Water, diet soda or coffee/tea	

Snack Attack Pack (page 248)
or
"I" Diet Cereal Dessert (page 236)
Water, diet soda or coffee/tea

2-egg omelet prepared with 1/2 teaspoon tub margarine	Hoisin Tofu (page 210)
1 slice lightly buttered low-carb toast*	1 1/2 cups grilled mixed veggies
1 1/2 cups mixed garden salad with 1 tablespoon low-cal dressing	Side salad with drizzle of olive oil and vinegar

1 cup sugar-free fresh fruit salad
or
Baked Apples with Figs (page 243)
Water, diet soda or coffee/tea

directory (Appendix E) for help in choosing suitable products for your diet.

With Meat

	SIMPLY GOOD	HOME COOKING
Continental Breakfast	2 slices low-carb bread* with 2 teaspoons low-fat cream cheese, peanut butter or fruit spread ½ cup fresh pineapple chunks Coffee/tea or water	2 slices low-carb bread* or "I" Diet Soda Bread (page 160) with 2 teaspoons low-fat cream cheese, peanut butter or fruit spread ½ cup Homemade Cinnamon Applesauce (page 140) or fresh pineapple chunks Coffee/tea or water
Mid-Morning Snack	2 part-skim mozzarella cheese sticks and ⅓ sweet red pepper Water, diet soda or coffee/tea	
Lunch	Soup and Salad: 1 cup hearty soup* such as lentil or minestrone; side salad with 1 teaspoon sunflower seeds and 2 teaspoons low-cal dressing 1 apple Water, diet soda or coffee/tea	Spicy Stew, North African Style (page 155) 1 apple Water, diet soda or coffee/tea
Afternoon Snack	"I" Diet Hot or Cold Chocolate (page 253) **or** 6 ounces sugar-free, low-fat yogurt with 2 pecan halves Water, diet soda or coffee/tea	
Dinner	4 ounces grilled skinless chicken breast with 2 tablespoons low-fat Alfredo sauce 1 cup cooked green peas (no sauce) Mixed garden side salad with 2 teaspoons low-cal dressing	"Sallat" of Field Greens and Herbs (page 167) Arista Chicken (page 197) **or** Veal Scaloppine in Creamy Mushroom Sauce (page 191) Summer Squash with Butter and Sage (page 231)
Dessert	Chocolate Cereal Dessert (page 236) **or** Chocolate Bread Pudding (page 240) Water, diet soda or coffee/tea	

*Asterisks mark items that vary a lot in composition and size. Check the Savvy Shopper
**Small high-protein, high-fiber snack bars contain 80 to 100 calories.

SIMPLY GOOD	HOME COOKING
2 slices low-carb bread* with 2 teaspoons low-fat cream cheese, peanut butter or fruit spread	2 slices low-carb bread* or "I" Diet Soda Bread (page 160) with 2 teaspoons low-fat cream cheese, peanut butter or fruit spread
1/2 cup fresh pineapple chunks	1/2 cup Homemade Cinnamon Applesauce (page 140) or fresh pineapple chunks
Coffee/tea or water	Coffee/tea or water

2 part-skim mozzarella cheese sticks and 1/3 sweet red pepper
Water, diet soda or coffee/tea

Soup and Salad: 1 cup hearty soup* such as lentil or black bean; side salad with 1 teaspoon sunflower seeds and 2 teaspoons low-cal dressing	Spicy Stew, North African Style (page 155)
	1 apple
1 apple	Water, diet soda or coffee/tea
Water, diet soda or coffee/tea	

"I" Diet Hot or Cold Chocolate (page 253)
or
1 small high-protein, high-fiber bar** and 1/2 orange
Water, diet soda or coffee/tea

1 cup cooked whole-wheat pasta with 1/2 cup tomato sauce and 2 tablespoons grated Parmesan cheese	"Sallat" of Field Greens and Herbs (page 167)
	Tomato and Broccoli Lasagna (page 215)
2 cups mixed garden side salad with 1 tablespoon low-cal dressing	Summer Squash with Butter and Sage (page 231)

Chocolate Bread Pudding (page 240)
or
4 ounces 2% plain Greek yogurt with 1/4 cup fresh fruit and 2 pecan halves
Water, diet soda or coffee/tea

directory (Appendix E) for help in choosing suitable products for your diet.
Check the Savvy Shopper directory for suitable brands.

Mix-and-Match Food Lists

The menu plan for Stage II was designed to guarantee that you get a wide variety of calorie-controlled foods, and following this plan should result in steady weight loss. If you prefer, however, you can mix-and-match different meals and snacks from the lists below, choosing three meals and two snacks that you prefer each day. If you go this way, be sure to have at least two high-fiber (HF) choices every day; if you opt for vegetarian, choose a higher-protein (HP) daily snack (see page 111). (Asterisks mark items that vary a lot in composition and size. Check the Savvy Shopper directory in Appendix E for help in choosing suitable products for your diet.)

Breakfasts

(choose 1 per day)

Simple Breakfasts

✻ ⅓ cup or more high-fiber cereal* with 2 tablespoons granola and ½ cup nonfat or 1% milk; ½ cup fresh fruit, such as blueberries (HF)

✻ 1 cup "complete" high-fiber cereal* with ½ cup nonfat or 1% milk; ½ cup fresh fruit, such as sliced strawberries (HF)

✻ "I" Diet Instant Hot Cereal with either maple syrup and blueberries (page 135) or raisins, pecans and cinnamon (page 135) (HF)

✻ Everyday Continental Breakfast: 2 slices low-carb bread* with 2 teaspoons low-fat cream cheese, peanut butter or fruit spread; ½ cup fresh fruit or ½ grapefruit (HF)

✻ 1 egg fried/boiled/poached and 1 slice low-carb toast* with 1 teaspoon tub margarine; ½ cup fresh fruit, such as melon chunks

Special Breakfasts

✻ Orange-Crumbed French Toast (page 138)

✻ Irish Oatmeal (page 133)

✻ Vegetable "Frittata" (page 136); ½ cup fresh fruit or sugar-free fruit sauce such as Spicy Prunes (page 141)

✻ Bacon and Eggs Breakfast (page 137); ½ cup fresh fruit, such as melon chunks, or Plum Compote (page 141)

❋ Special Continental Breakfast: 2 slices "I" Diet Soda Bread (page 160) with 2 teaspoons low-fat cream cheese, peanut butter or fruit spread; ½ cup fresh fruit, such as Homemade Cinnamon Applesauce (page 140) (HF)

Lunch and Dinner

(choose 1 each per day)

Simple Soup, Sandwich and Salad Options

❋ Soup and Sandwich: 1 cup broth-based vegetable soup; 1 sandwich made with 2 slices low-carb bread* and ¼ cup water-packed solid tuna or 1 slice cheese or 2 ounces roast beef or turkey, 2 teaspoons low-fat mayo, lettuce, tomato, onion, etc.

❋ Ham and Cheese Salad Plate: 2 to 3 cups salad greens and non-starchy veggies, ⅓ cup legumes, 2 slices (2 ounces) ham, 2 tablespoons feta cheese and 2 tablespoons low-cal dressing

❋ Cheese Salad Plate: 2 to 3 cups salad greens and non-starchy veggies, ½ cup legumes, 1 slice cheese, 1 teaspoon sunflower seeds and 2 tablespoons low-cal dressing

❋ Asian Salad Plate: 2 to 3 cups salad greens and non-starchy veggies, 2 slices (2 ounces) chicken breast or 1 hard-boiled egg, ⅓ cup legumes, 1 tablespoon mandarin orange segments, 1 teaspoon sesame seeds and 2 tablespoons low-cal Asian-style dressing

❋ Picnic Plate: 1 apple, 1-inch cube (1 ounce) 50% reduced-fat extra-sharp cheddar cheese and 6 ounces sugar-free, low-fat yogurt sprinkled with 3 tablespoons or more high-fiber cereal*

❋ Soup and Salad: 1 cup hearty soup* such as lentil or minestrone; side salad with 1 tablespoon grated cheese or 1 teaspoon sunflower seeds and 2 teaspoons low-cal dressing; 1 apple

Homemade Soup, Sandwich and Salad Options

❋ Costa Rican Black Bean Soup (page 148); side salad with 1 tablespoon grated cheese and 2 teaspoons low-cal dressing

❋ Mexican Black Beans with Chips, Salsa and Sour Cream (page 265)

❋ Easy Tomato, Barley and Basil Soup (page 145); "I" Diet Tuna Salad wrap (page 162) or Broiled Tofu sandwich (page 161)

✳ Spicy Stew, North African Style (page 155); 1 apple

✳ "I" Diet Chicken Salad wrap (page 161); side salad with 2 teaspoons low-cal dressing

✳ "I" Diet Vegetarian Chicken Salad wrap (page 161); side salad with 2 teaspoons low-cal dressing

✳ Chicken Caesar wrap: 1 small low-carb tortilla* filled with 2 slices (2 ounces) chicken, 1 tablespoon low-cal Caesar dressing, 1 table-spoon grated Parmesan cheese and chopped lettuce; side salad with 2 teaspoons low-cal dressing

✳ Cannellini Caesar wrap: 1 small low-carb tortilla* filled with ¼ cup cooked cannellini beans, 1 table-spoon low-cal Caesar dressing, 2 tablespoons grated Parmesan cheese, chopped lettuce; side salad with 2 teaspoons low-cal dressing

✳ Grilled cheese sandwich: 2 slices low-carb bread* and 1-inch cube (1 ounce) 50% reduced-fat sharp cheddar cheese (sliced thin for grilling); ½ cup baked beans

✳ Leftover curry (page 219) or Tanzanian Chicken Kebabs (page 195) in a small low-carb pita bread* with low-fat plain yogurt, chutney and 2 to 3 palm hearts

✳ Hummus and Veggie Plate with Spicy Sesame Cracker Chips (page 182)

✳ Thai Chicken Salad with Warm Peanut Sauce (page 177)

✳ Apple, Walnut and Blue Cheese Salad (page 168); 1 slice "I" Diet Soda Bread (page 160) or low-carb toast*

✳ Bibb Salad with Grilled Mushrooms and Shaved Parmesan (page 170); 1 slice "I" Diet Soda Bread (page 160) or low-carb toast*

✳ West African Bean Cakes with Spicy Dip and Green Salad (page 224)

✳ Crispy Taco Pinto Bean Salad (page 181)

Simple Dinners

✳ Grilled skinless chicken breast (4 ounces) heaped with ⅓ cup cooked pinto beans, ¼ cup salsa, 1 tablespoon grated Parmesan cheese, 2 teaspoons low-fat sour cream and optional chopped fresh cilantro; 1½ cups sliced fresh tomato and cucumber with 1 teaspoon olive oil and fresh lemon juice

✳ Bean-and-cheese burrito: 1 low-carb tortilla* filled with ¼ cup pinto beans, ½ cup grilled veggies, 2 tablespoons salsa, 2 tablespoons grated Parmesan cheese, 2 teaspoons low-fat sour cream and optional chopped fresh cilantro; 1½ cups sliced fresh tomato and cucumber with 1 teaspoon olive oil and fresh lemon juice

✳ Plain grilled white fish (4 ounces) with 2 tablespoons low-cal sauce; 1½ cups green beans (no sauce); side salad of baby spinach with drizzle of olive oil, balsamic vinegar and 2 teaspoons dried cranberries

✳ 2 chicken or veggie hot dogs on a low-carb roll* with ketchup and mustard; side salad of baby spinach with drizzle of olive oil, balsamic vinegar and 2 teaspoons dried cranberries

✳ 2 chicken or veggie hot dogs; ½ cup baked beans; side salad of baby spinach with drizzle of olive oil, balsamic vinegar and 2 teaspoons dried cranberries

✳ Grilled chicken breast (4 ounces) with 2 tablespoons low-cal sweet-and-sour sauce; 1 cup Chinese-style veggies; mixed garden side salad with drizzle of olive oil and vinegar

✳ No-Fuss Pizza (page 211); 1 large tomato, sliced, with chopped fresh basil and drizzle of olive oil and balsamic vinegar

✳ Cheese-and-veggie wrap: 1 low-carb tortilla* filled with ½ cup warmed grilled veggies, ¼ cup legumes or bean salad and 2 tablespoons low-cal Alfredo sauce; one large tomato, sliced, with chopped fresh basil and drizzle of olive oil and balsamic vinegar

✳ Grilled salmon (3 ounces) on a toasted low-carb roll* with 1 teaspoon low-fat mayo, fresh lemon juice, lettuce and tomato; 1½ cups cooked snow peas (no sauce); mixed garden side salad with 2 teaspoons low-cal dressing

✳ Grilled skinless chicken breast (4 ounces) with 2 tablespoons low-fat Alfredo sauce; 1 cup cooked green peas (no sauce); side salad of crispy romaine lettuce with 2 teaspoons low-cal dressing

✳ Whole-wheat pasta (1 cup) with ½ cup tomato sauce and 2 tablespoons grated Parmesan cheese; 2 cups mixed garden salad with 1 tablespoon low-cal dressing

✳ Two-egg omelet prepared with ½ teaspoon tub margarine; 1 slice lightly buttered low-carb toast*; 1½ cups mixed garden salad with 1 tablespoon low-cal dressing

Home-Cooked Dinners

✳ Mexican Lettuce Wraps (page 194); side salad of baby greens with drizzle of olive oil and fresh lemon juice

✳ Tanzanian Chicken Kebabs (page 195) with Cucumber-Mint Raita (page 174); side salad of baby greens with drizzle of olive oil and fresh lemon juice

✳ Mixed Vegetable Curry (page 219); Moong Dal Stew (page 222) with 1 teaspoon Lemon and Date Chutney (page 223) or mango chutney and 2 tablespons low-fat yogurt; ½ cup Boiled Barley* (page 217)

✳ The Ultimate "I" Burger (page 264) or Vegetarian Burger Delight (page 189) served on a low-carb roll* with lettuce, tomato, onion, 1 teaspoon low-fat mayo, relish and ketchup; 1½ cups steamed broccoli with 1 teaspoon low-fat sour cream and fresh lemon juice

✳ Cajun Cod (page 206) or Baked Salmon with Lemon-Dill Sauce (page 203); 1½ cups steamed asparagus or 1 cup A Perfect Ratatouille (page 228); side salad of baby spinach with drizzle of olive oil, balsamic vinegar and 2 teaspoons dried cranberries

✳ Two-egg omelet prepared with ½ teaspoon tub margarine; ½ cup Wheat Berry Salad (page 180); side salad with 2 teaspoons low-cal dressing

✳ Home Run Hot Dogs (page 193) and side salad of baby spinach with drizzle of olive oil, balsamic vinegar and 2 teaspoons dried cranberries

✳ Hoisin Pork (page 192) with Asian Coleslaw (page 175); mixed garden side salad with drizzle of olive oil and vinegar

✳ Mushroom and Barley Risotto (page 218); Watercress and Orange Salad with Parmesan Toasts and Hummus (page 171)

✳ Spicy Tofu and Mixed Vegetable Stir-Fry (page 206)

✳ John's Pasta Supper (page 213); garden side salad with 2 teaspoons low-cal dressing

✴ Northern Italian Lasagna (page 214); Florentine Braised Kale (page 227); Tomato Salad (page 172)

✴ Barbecue Vegetable Pizza (page 212); Tomato Salad (page 172)

✴ Stuffed Green Peppers (page 216); Tomato Salad (page 172)

✴ Perfect Grill shrimp or chicken with Creamy Mustard Sauce (page 199); 1½ cups grilled mixed veggies; side salad with drizzle of olive oil and vinegar

✴ Arista Chicken (page 197); Summer Squash with Butter and Sage (page 231); "Sallat" of Field Greens and Herbs (page 167)

✴ Veal Scaloppine in Creamy Mushroom Sauce (page 191); Summer Squash with Butter and Sage (page 231); "Sallat" of Field Greens and Herbs (page 167)

✴ Hoisin Tofu (page 210); 1½ cups grilled mixed veggies; side salad with drizzle of olive oil and vinegar

✴ Tomato and Broccoli Lasagna (page 215); Summer Squash with Butter and Sage (page 231); side salad of romaine lettuce with Tarragon Dressing (page 172)

✴ The Ultimate "I" Burger (page 264); Iceberg Wedge with Blue Cheese (page 169); steamed broccoli

✴ Italian Meatballs (page 262); Florentine Braised Kale (page 227); Tomato Salad (page 172)

✴ Belgian-Style Beef Stew (page 266); Iceberg Wedge with Blue Cheese (page 169); steamed broccoli

Snacks

(2 per day)

✴ 1 Snack Attack Pack (page 248) (HF)

✴ 1 apple, 1 cup grapes or 1 orange; 1 tablespoon nuts or 3 dried black mission figs

✴ 2 part-skim mozzarella cheese sticks (HP)

✴ 1 part-skim mozzarella cheese stick; ⅓ sweet red pepper or ¼ cup baby carrots

✴ 1 small high-protein, high-fiber snack bar*; 1 plum, 1 kiwi, ½ orange or ⅓ sweet red pepper (HP)

✴ 6 ounces sugar-free, low-fat yogurt or 4 ounces 2% plain Greek yogurt; 4 pecan halves or 1 tablespoon dried fruit (HP)

* ½ cup low-fat cottage cheese; ⅓ sweet pepper, ¼ cup baby carrots or 3 celery sticks (HP)

* "I" Diet Hot or Cold Chocolate (page 253)

* Any "I" Diet cereal dessert selection (see below) (HF)

* Strawberry-Blueberry Smoothie (page 270)

Carbs

(choose 1 per day for dinner instead of dessert, if preferred)

* 2 Potato Skins (page 226)

* ½ cup whole-wheat pasta or Boiled Barley* (page 217)

* 1 low-carb wrap or 1 slice low-carb bread or toast*

* ⅓ cup cooked legumes, such as Tuscan Beans with Rosemary and Olive Oil (page 233), or Wheat Berry Salad (page 180)

Desserts

(choose 1 dessert to have with dinner or 1 carb selection per day)

* Ice Cream Sundae (page 236) (HF)

* Chocolate Cereal Dessert (page 236) (HF)

* Ginger-Pecan Crunch (page 237) (HF)

* Chocolate-Raspberry Parfait (page 237) (HF)

* Chocolate Bread Pudding (page 240)

* Chocolate Pudding II (page 239) (HP)

* 1 cup fresh mango

* 1 ripe pear with 1 teaspoon warm caramel sauce

* 1 cup unsweetened fresh fruit salad

* ⅔ cup raspberries with 2 tablespoons light whipped cream

* 4 ounces 2% plain Greek yogurt; ½ cup fresh fruit (HP)

* Orange Flan (page 241)

* Indian Barley Pudding (page 242)

* Baked Apples with Figs (page 243)

* Almost Apple Cobbler (page 245)

* Chocolate-Tipped Strawberries and Cream (page 246)

* Rhubarb Yogurt (page 249)

CHAPTER 11

Stage III
Your Personal Maintenance Plan

O kay, you've done a great job. You've lost weight, and now the trick is to figure out a reliable way to *keep* it lost. This absolutely does not have to be hard, but making it work requires a different approach because now the emphasis is a bit less on hunger control and more on finding your own balance for treats and pleasures.

In this chapter, you'll learn to think about a weight maintenance program that meets your individual needs. You'll find out how to assess your new calorie requirements and choose a suitable plan for controlling your daily calorie intake. You'll also learn how to put together your own food plan. And last but not least, you'll discover the best ways to keep your weight down when you're at a restaurant or on vacation. The guidelines are simple, but the results can be spectacular!

The New, Smaller You

There is less of you now. It probably feels great to be able to wear clothes in sizes you haven't been able to get into for a while, but what this means is that your body needs fewer calories than it did before you lost weight. Let's use an easy example: If you lost 10% of your weight, it would make sense that you would now need about 10% fewer calories. But before you lost weight, you were likely gaining weight and consuming more calories than you needed, so you have to take this into account.

(Some studies indicate that metabolism drops a bit more than weight when you diet, also reducing calorie needs.) In short, you now need to eat about 15% fewer calories every day than you did before. In other words, if you weighed 200 pounds at the start and were consuming 2,500 calories a day, you've shed 10% of your body weight if you got down to 180 pounds. You now need 15% fewer calories a day, which comes to 375 fewer calories, or 2,125 calories daily to maintain your weight.

This probably sounds more confusing than it really is. All you have to do to get started here is turn to Appendix B, where you can find a table that gives estimated calorie requirements after weight loss for people of different heights, weights and activity levels.

Successful Calorie Control

In the end, it all comes down to eating fewer calories in ways that allow you to feel fully satisfied. What's important now is learning how to make that happen without feeling frustrated, hungry or deprived. I have a friend who says, "You know the best way to lose weight? Keep your mouth shut." Sure, I tell him, I've heard it all before. But just see how long that works! There are, however, three different approaches to successful calorie control. They can all work, so just decide which one appeals to you the most and get started.

fiction: Women have a much easier time with weight control than men do.
fact: Not true!

First of all, women tend to be smaller than men and have to eat fewer calories to stay slim in our world of huge portions. As if that's not enough, a woman's cyclical fluctuations right through menopause cause variations in hunger and water retention, making it even more difficult than usual to gauge day-to-day weight change. And what about premenstrual hunger and the postmenopausal weight gain that plagues some women? On top of all this, statistics show that the average woman will gain a surprising 19 pounds in the first three years of marriage!

Fortunately, all of these add-on challenges can be met by following the "I" Diet carefully and working out individual maintenance plans for weight control.

✳ **No-Count Calorie Control.** This is the easiest plan in terms of what you have to do to keep track of your food. Simply make a what-I'm-not-allowed-to-eat list, focusing on the high-calorie foods that you find particularly hard to resist. Be sure to make whole groups of tempting foods off limits. These might include "white" carbohydrates like flour and sugar as well as fried foods, beverages with calories, foods with saturated fat like cream, butter and cheese, and candy except maybe for one kind you can eat in small amounts. And don't forget about portion sizes of allowed foods! By monitoring your weight, you can shorten or lengthen your list of restrictions to keep calories in balance.

You might also consider becoming a vegetarian or vegan, if this appeals to you. This can be a very healthy way to eat, provided you take a multivitamin. And by cutting out whole classes of things you might overeat, you can cut back on calories more easily.

✳ **Consistent Calorie Control.** This plan is for people who have a pretty good handle on controlling temptations but need more structure than just a list of what's not allowed. What you do is include lots of the satisfying foods

The Exercise Equation

Although exercise does little to speed up weight loss, it can be a big help in keeping your weight under control once you've lost it. Why? Because it burns some of those calories you no longer need, allowing you to make smaller changes in what you eat. Also, exercise is great for building confidence and reducing stress; some research even suggests that it improves the symptoms of depression. Just 15 or 30 minutes a day can make a positive difference. Climb stairs. Walk when you don't have to drive. Keep some free weights at home and learn how to use them. Every little bit counts when it comes to weight control, so try to work exercise into your life as often as you can.

you ate in Stages I and II in a structured personalized food plan. Start out by making a 7- or 14-day menu plan for eating the healthy foods you like that add up to the number of calories you need each day (see Appendix B). Lots of people prefer this method because it teaches them what they can eat without gaining weight and without counting calories every day. After a while, you won't have to follow your menus so carefully because you will have worked out what and how much you can eat to keep your weight where you want it. This plan doesn't let you indulge in lots of extras, so it may not be the one for you if you go to restaurants three or four times a week.

* **Dynamic Calorie Control.** So what if you do eat out a lot or want to feel free to enjoy temptations more often? You might be what psychologists call a "disinhibited eater"—somebody who really loves food, is exposed to good food often and has trouble keeping it all under control. This plan gives you a lower daily target for everyday calorie intake, so that the extra calories you get when you eat in restaurants balance out with the fewer calories on your menu and by the end of the week you've eaten just the number of calories you're shooting for. You should keep track of the calories you take in most days for this to work. The best way to do this is to use the handheld device called a personal

The right balance is the name of the game if you choose the Dynamic Calorie Control plan.

digital assistant (PDA) with calorie-counting software loaded into it. There are also free web calorie-counting programs like www.mypyramid.gov and www.fitday.com that let you type in your calories.

Hitting the Target

If you choose to use Consistent Calorie Control, your daily calorie target equals your estimated calorie needs after weight loss, which you can find in Appendix B. This is the number you'll be aiming for when you devise your personal eating plan.

Daily calorie target after weight loss: _____

To use the Dynamic Calorie Control plan, start with a daily calorie target that's lower than your estimated calorie needs so you bank calories for days when you plan to have a nice meal at a restaurant—what we can call a "small splurge." Don't count regular meals out when you intend to stick to your calorie target—just those fancy meals that are harder to control. To get to your target, subtract 5% from your estimated daily calorie needs after weight loss for each day of the week when you plan to eat out. For example, if your estimated daily calorie need is 2,000 calories and you plan to eat two nice meals out, your calorie target for other days will be 90%, or 1,800 calories a day. If you eat out three times a week, your target will be 1,700, and so on.

Daily calorie target after weight loss: _____

Next, calculate your target calories for each meal and snack, perhaps following the meal-by-meal breakdown shown below. But if you know you like one meal bigger and another meal smaller, that's okay. Just put in different percentages that add up to the same total:

CALORIES

Weight maintenance breakfast (20%) _____

Weight maintenance lunch (25%) _____

Weight maintenance dinner (25%) _____

Weight maintenance healthy snacks (10%) _____

Free choices (everything else) (20%) _____

Staying On Top of It

NO-COUNT CALORIE CONTROL

Choose this plan if . . .   *Counting calories and planning aren't your thing.*

Average calories   Average calorie needs per week should

Are there day-to-day variations in calories?   Daily calorie intake is not planned. Calories are kept down as a consequence of limited food choices.

Do you make a meal-by-meal menu plan?   No menu plan required; just follow your lists of allowed and off-limits foods.

What do you include in your regular meals and snacks?   Anything on your "allowed" list. (You choose which foods to restrict!)

Can you have treats?   Treats are not part of your daily plan.

What about eating in restaurants?   Stick with your allowed food selections, whether you're eating out or not.

How do you handle holidays and vacations?   Not factored into regular eating plans. If you go off your

Is weight tracking necessary?   Record your weight weekly as a reality check on how your

CONSISTENT CALORIE CONTROL	DYNAMIC CALORIE CONTROL
You've been weight-challenged for years and are willing to follow a plan but want it to include treats.	*You can't or won't give up eating out regularly.*

be the same for all eating styles.

Calorie intake changes little from day to day.	Daily calorie intake is higher on more indulgent days and lower on regular days. Highs and lows balance out to make a good average during each week.
You design an individual menu that's enjoyable and practical to follow.	You can keep track of calorie intake with a web program or personal digital assistant (PDA); a personally designed menu can help get you started.
Regular meals and snacks provide your average daily calorie requirements. These meals and snacks emphasize mostly "I" Diet foods and other natural food choices.	Regular meals and snacks have fewer calories than your average requirement and emphasize mostly "I" Diet foods.
Plan ahead to include daily free-choice foods in your regular meals. Don't eat casually.	Treats are fine on days when you eat out.
If you eat out, carefully count calories.	You may eat out on a regular basis. Some of your restaurant meals may have more calories than you need, so it's important to eat less at other times.

plan, use Stage II menus to recover: one day for each "small splurge"; two for bigger splurges.

balance act is doing. Food plans and allowed variety can be revised until weight is stable.

Go Natural

Now that you've reached Stage III, I'd like to encourage you to go as natural and pure as you can, cutting down on additives including artificial sweeteners and refined carbs such as sugar and white flour. During weight loss, it's useful to get all the help you can from artificial sweeteners, because you were probably used to a sweet diet and were combating hunger as well as changing what you ate. Now you're moving on to the rest of your life, and in my experience the more natural and additive-free you go, the easier it will be to keep weight off. Since these chemicals don't provide calories, you'll probably find them quite easy to give up, and when you do, the natural taste of things like fresh fruits will take over and give you all the sweet flavor you need.

As with any change in a dietary routine, it will take a little while to adjust, but time is the treatment and that means all you need is a little patience to see you through.

Your Own Menu Plan

Creating a personalized food plan takes a little work, but the payoff is well worth the time invested if you want to keep your weight under control. You'll definitely need your own menu plan if you intend to use Consistent Calorie Control, and one is useful if not essential for Dynamic Calorie Control. If you don't want to do this right now, you can always come back to it. You'll find suggestions for weight-healthy maintenance meals in Appendix F.

Your menu plan, specifying meals and snacks for each day of the week, really needs to work for you and the life you lead. If you don't have time to cook, write in mostly easy-to-prepare store-bought foods. Our volunteers at Tufts often take several weeks and go through several drafts before they come up with menus that are both enjoyable and easy to follow. If you find yourself cheating, go back to the drawing board. This doesn't mean you're failing; it's just that your plan needs tweaking. Here's what to do:

❋ **Keep it simple.** You can always "embellish" your menu over time, but bear in mind that it's easier to follow through with a simpler plan.

✳ **Write in any meals you buy or eat out.** If you're using Dynamic Calorie Control, specify regular meals (when you want to eat only those calories allowed by your calorie target) and those not so carefully monitored for calories—your "small splurges."

✳ **Write in regular meals and snacks.** It's good to eat three meals every day; regular snacks are also good if you get hungry. The sample breakfasts, lunches, dinners and snacks in Appendix F show calculated portion sizes for different calorie amounts. Treats are described below.

These regular meals and snacks should contain the same healthy foods as in "I" Diet meals, plus additional whole-grain foods that were not great for weight loss but are fine now that you're maintaining weight, including oatmeal, other whole-grain hot cereals and whole-wheat bread made with either finely ground flour or whole-grain kernels. If, based on your experience in Stages I and II, you feel that one type of eating (e.g., high-fiber, low-GI or high-protein) is better than others for keeping you satisfied, you can choose more meals emphasizing that combination. However, since satisfying hunger is less challenging now that you're eating more foods in total, the big focus here is on establishing routines so you can enjoy them without letting them get out of control.

Make sure you write in a no-cal (water or diet soda) or low-cal (e.g., coffee with 1% milk) beverage with every meal and snack. Having a drink every time you eat means you won't need anything at other times and your mouth will learn not to expect continuous flavor experiences.

✳ **Add free choices.** You will remember that we saved 20% of your calorie requirements after weight loss for

Small Splurges

Nice restaurant meals can include a few delicious extras in reasonable amounts, but aim for pleasure *plus* mostly weight-healthy foods. If you plan on splurging a little on a night out, skip your free choice during the day and have a cereal dessert (page 236) or an apple before you leave home. And if you experience the "second-meal effect" that makes you hungrier the next day, get back on track with a big bowl of high-fiber cereal for breakfast. If you're still unsatisfied, have some extra fiber with lunch, too, and avoid further indulgences that feed a negative cycle of hunger and overeating. You can also go back to Stage II for a day or so to counter the effects of a splurge that turned out to be bigger than you planned.

Make the Most of Your Free Choices

When it comes to "spending" the 20% of the daily calorie requirements that you've saved for free choices, just look at all the good things you can have:

- Any food in amounts greater than on your menu plan
- Any food not similar to "I" Diet items
- All spreads other than small amounts with meals (e.g., extra margarine, cream cheese, peanut butter, jam, jelly, honey)
- Cream and sugar in coffee or tea; whipped cream with anything
- All "mindless eating," such as "tastes," kid leftovers and bites of food grabbed here and there
- Alcohol—wine, beer, cocktails, etc.
- Milk as a drink; sweetened yogurt; flavored and full-fat milks for more than occasional use
- White-bread pizza

- White bread; bagels that are not 100% whole wheat; potatoes (including French fries), bananas and other "white" starches
- Full-fat cheeses other than grated Parmesan and blue cheese for flavoring entrées
- Desserts, cookies, muffins, cakes, brownies
- All chocolate and candy
- Smoothies, slushes; whole-milk lattes; other creamy or frozen drinks
- Sodas, sweetened iced tea, juice drinks (½ cup juice is okay if part of your menu plan)
- Salty snacks; nuts in excess of small amounts for Stage II snacks

free-choice allowances. This might sound like a lot, but most people eat much more. Also, free choices comprise a larger group of foods that are not intended to be exclusively indulgent treats. This is because people usually find it easier to keep count when everything that isn't a good "I" Diet food is counted as a free choice. On days when you're not having a "small splurge" meal, you can add your free-choice calories in any combination to any meal, e.g., a dessert with dinner, or chips with a lunch sandwich, or a bit of each. On days when you have a special meal, your free-choice calories are included as part of the meal. Some of these free choices are things you probably took for granted before, but planning for them carefully now will help you avoid slipping back into old overeating habits and let you enjoy things that would otherwise be hard to know what to do with. Calling less satisfying but common foods like potatoes and white bread "free choices" also helps you focus on whether you really like them. If you do, go ahead and enjoy them to the max. If not, save those calories for something better! Remember that anything you can't eat responsibly should not be eaten regularly and instead saved for very occasional times like holidays.

Here's what my own free-choice plan looks like: My daily calorie target is 1,600 calories, which means I'm allowed 320 calories daily for free choices. Typically, I have one glass of wine (100 calories), two squares of dark or milk chocolate (80 calories), one extra tablespoon of peanut butter with breakfast toast (90 calories) and plenty of milk in coffee and tea. Occasionally, I have things like chocolate cake, French fries, a white bagel or baked potato, and on those days I cut back on my regular free choices.

✳ **Add a daily "satiety booster."** One thing it's hard to get enough of in any weight-control plan is fiber. Even the extra vegetables and whole grains in your menu plan may not provide enough when calories are fairly low. That's why I'm adding a daily "free" "I" Diet cereal dessert (page 236) or Snack Attack Pack (page 248) to your plan. You don't *have* to eat this, but I encourage you to think of it as your daily weight-control "medicine" and enjoy the fact that it doesn't count as a free choice—you can have it in addition to your calorie target provided you don't gain weight.

Test-Drive Your Menu Plan

We all overeat at one time or another, so test-driving and revising your personal menu plan is always a good idea. Weigh yourself weekly. After the first week and again after the first month, you can review your weight and your plan. Did your weight stay where it should? If not, were you sticking with your calorie-control plan? If you found yourself reluctant to follow through on some days and gained weight, what could you change to make the plan easier? Perhaps you tried Dynamic Calorie Control and found yourself overeating, in which case moving on to Consistent Calorie Control at least for now will probably help. If you gained weight even though you think you followed the plan exactly, lower your calorie target by 100 or 200 calories a day, eat out less often, cut back on treats and add more high-fiber dishes to your diet. Keep this up until your weight stays within two pounds of your end-of-diet weight. You can find a plan that works for you, no matter what season it is, how old you are or what else is going on in your life.

Away from Home

Now that you've been successful in losing weight, here are some tips for eating at restaurants and on vacation during weight maintenance.

Eating Out

In general, it's a good idea to eat a limited variety of meals at places you know and to watch portion sizes carefully. Stick to the items in your menu plan as often as possible, and plan ahead by checking out available information on the web. Our Restaurant Survival Guide (Appendix H) gives examples of meals with a reasonable composition and calorie content according to restaurant reports.

- Try to include a light soup or appetizer salad with light dressing *and* a steamed vegetable to get more fullness on fewer calories. Say no to French onion soup with gobs of melted cheese and old-fashioned corn chowder made with cream and potatoes.
- Take advantage of half-portion options, or ask the server to split an entrée and give you half to take home. Be picky and request changes!
- Limit yourself to one alcoholic drink, and then keep seltzer in your glass to avoid refills.
- Banish the bread basket or at least keep it across the table from you.
- Have dessert only if someone is willing to share it with you.

Vacations

Vacations are tricky because you're eating out all the time. Each meal and snack counts, so don't let one indulgence lead to another.

- Limit the damage by packing a tasty, weight-healthy picnic for the journey: sandwiches made with coarse whole-grain bread, fruit, cut-up veggies and water.
- Avoid all those soggy breakfast pastries and dry bagels. Take along some premeasured individual breakfasts of high-fiber cereal mixed with three tablespoons of mixed nuts and dried fruit (you can add milk and fresh fruit).
- Try to make your meals healthy for weight maintenance by choosing salads, light dressings, plain grilled meat and fruit. Save your calories for those times when there's something on the menu that you can't resist.
- Keep fresh fruit and water in your room. Take along a few Snack Attack Packs (page 248).
- Liquid calories don't reduce hunger. Try to stick with one alcoholic drink a day, at a time you can really enjoy it, and avoid sodas, juice drinks and other forms of "liquid poison."

A Final Word

B ack in the 1950s and '60s, most people in North America and Europe did very little exercise and ate what we would now consider a diet designed for weight gain: white bread, meat loaf, white pasta, pies, full-fat milk. Yet few people were overweight. What happened?

Nutrition scientists don't have all the answers, but we do know that we've lost the cultural norms that once helped to regulate what and how much we ate. When foods like soda, butter, cheese and meat were more expensive (relative to income), people naturally ate smaller portions. When dinner was always served at the same time, often beginning with soup, people filled up faster and ate less. When dessert meant an apple and a small cookie, ice cream and pies signified "special occasion."

But times change, and we must change along with them. That's why weight control is, like so many other things that matter, a journey of self-discovery—one in which you will learn more about yourself as well as the world around you. As you figure out how to satisfy your instinctive needs so that you feel well-fed and safe while also getting thin and healthy, you're ahead of the game. And when you understand how controlling the signals that control your food instincts can continue to help you keep the weight off, you can stay at the top of the game no matter the food "customs" of the people around you.

Permanent weight control doesn't have to be hard. It just requires a willingness to learn how to work *with* your food instincts rather than against them. I hope I've helped you get to a place on your weight-loss journey that makes this commitment possible for you.

Happy travels!

PART III

THE RECIPES

Recipe Notes

All of the easy-to-make recipes on the pages that follow are scientifically formulated to work with—rather than against—your food instincts and keep you satisfied and hunger-free. My theory is that if food isn't good enough to share, it isn't good enough to recommend to dieters. These recipes are so good that I often use them when cooking for my friends and family, whether anyone is dieting or not.

Here's why the recipes will help your diet:

✻ Each recipe includes one or more of the "I" Diet hunger-suppressing formulas: a high-protein/low-carbohydrate combination, a mixture of high- and low-GI carbohydrates, high volume and high fiber.

✻ When it comes to fiber, I often combine several kinds in the same recipe to provide the different metabolic benefits of each. Remember, the more fiber variety, the more enjoyable a high-fiber diet becomes.

✻ I also favor rich, full flavors and chewy textures, all kinds of spices and herbs, and the strongest kinds of cheese and chocolate so you get complex, delicious and satisfying flavors without too many calories.

✻ You'll find many familiar tastes in these recipes.

✻ Because these dishes slow digestion, they should help your cravings disappear over time.

✻ High-calorie flavors are concentrated on the outside of dishes, not buried inside; this way, you don't absorb calories without appreciating the taste.

A few of the recipes use ingredients that may not be found in your supermarket. If you have a natural food store nearby, chances are you'll find them there. Online ordering is also an option. For Indian recipes, check www.indianblend.com. If you have a farmers' market in your area, you can get the best produce and support local farms at the same time. I often substitute vegetables in recipes to take advantage of whatever my local farm has to offer in season—this is a great way to increase the variety of flavors you get from healthy foods!

Portion Sizes

The "I" Diet recognizes that both the composition and portion size of what you eat are important for successful weight loss. The portion sizes given in these recipes are for the 1,200-calorie menus. Turn to page 90 to figure out portion sizes for higher-calorie plans.

Vegetarian Options: Ⓥ Ⓥ

Many people are turning to vegetarian meals for health, and there are lots of vegetarian recipes throughout this section. Recipes that call for no meat, poultry or fish are marked Ⓥ (a "V" inside a gray circle) above the recipe name. Those that can be turned into vegetarian options are marked Ⓥ (a "V" on a white background). (For the purposes of this book, I've included eggs and dairy in my vegetarian recipes.)

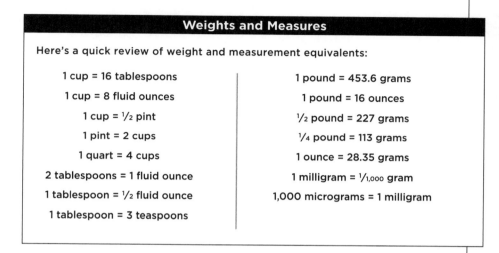

Weights and Measures

Here's a quick review of weight and measurement equivalents:

1 cup = 16 tablespoons	1 pound = 453.6 grams
1 cup = 8 fluid ounces	1 pound = 16 ounces
1 cup = 1/2 pint	1/2 pound = 227 grams
1 pint = 2 cups	1/4 pound = 113 grams
1 quart = 4 cups	1 ounce = 28.35 grams
2 tablespoons = 1 fluid ounce	1 milligram = 1/1,000 gram
1 tablespoon = 1/2 fluid ounce	1,000 micrograms = 1 milligram
1 tablespoon = 3 teaspoons	

Going Green

There are lots of ways to save cooking time and energy. Many cereals and legumes cook in a fraction of the time if you soak them beforehand. And by cooking enough for two or more meals, you save the energy needed to cook another whole meal.

Sugar Substitutes

A few of the recipes include sugar substitute as an optional ingredient. If you're trying to stay chemical-free, you can omit the sugar substitute for a less sweet taste. Or, if you prefer, add a little sugar; just keep in mind that this will add calories to the dish.

Butter and Eggs

The nutritional information given for any recipe calling for margarine is based on the use of tub margarine, but feel free to substitute butter as long as you keep in mind that it's higher in saturated fat. Also, two egg whites can be substituted for each quarter-cup of Egg Beaters listed in the ingredients.

A Note About Water Loss During Cooking

The water content of foods in the "I" Diet is important. Water helps keep food moist and vegetables crisp and flavorful while lowering calories in soups, meat sauces and cooked desserts without having to cut additional fat. Be careful not to reduce the water in the recipes, since less water in a cooked dish would increase the calories per cup. This means you would end up eating more calories than you think despite measuring everything carefully. For these reasons, "I" Diet recipes often ask you to use a pan with a lid. Please be sure to use pans with lids that fit well.

Baking Times

Things like the temperature of a food before it goes in the oven, the size of the baking dish and the accuracy of your oven thermostat make baking times variable. Just keep checking for doneness, following the tips in each recipe for great success every time.

Websites for Free Nutritional Information and Calculations

Nutrient Contents of Different Foods and Meals

www.nal.usda.gov/fnic/foodcomp/search/ (for basic foods, the primary source)

www.calorie-count.com (for restaurants and basic foods)

Free Menu Calculators

www.dailyplate.com

www.calorieking.com

Breakfasts

YOU'VE HEARD IT BEFORE and you'll hear it again: Breakfast is a really important meal. Each good, sustaining meal makes it easier to eat responsibly at the next one, so treat every morning as an opportunity to kick off your day in grand style.

Irish Oatmeal Ⓥ

Bannock Cakes

"I" Diet Instant Hot Cereals Ⓥ

Hot Cereal with Maple Syrup and Blueberries
Hot Cereal with Raisins, Pecans and Cinnamon
Another Hot Cereal

Vegetable "Frittata" Ⓥ

Bacon and Eggs Breakfast

Orange-Crumbed French Toast Ⓥ

Chocolate Pecan Breakfast Bars Ⓥ

Homemade Cinnamon Applesauce Ⓥ

Spicy Prunes Ⓥ

Plum Compote Ⓥ

Great German Rolls Ⓥ

Ⓥ

Irish Oatmeal

Makes four scant 1-cup servings

IF YOU LOVE HOT CEREAL, this Irish oatmeal recipe is the best. With its perfect "I" Diet composition, there is nothing more satisfying. Make a batch on the weekend and serve up quick hot portions during the week. The Bannock Cakes variation is incredibly good in its own right—a truly special Sunday breakfast.

133

For oatmeal:

1 cup Irish (steel-cut) oatmeal

4 cups water

1 cup coarse wheat bran

For each serving of 1 cup cooked oatmeal:

1 tablespoon slivered toasted almonds

2 teaspoons raisins

¼ cup nonfat or 1% milk

Sugar substitute, as desired

Nutritional information per scant 1-cup serving with toppings:

Calories 263

Protein 7.5 grams

Total fat 6.2 grams

Saturated fat 0.5 gram

Total carbohydrates 44.2 grams

Dietary fiber 12.8 grams

1. Place the oatmeal and water in a pot and bring to a boil, then reduce the heat to low and let simmer, covered, for about 20 minutes. The oat grains should be cooked through but retain some bite. Not all of the liquid will be absorbed.

2. Add the wheat bran, stir well and simmer, covered, for 2 minutes longer, or until the mixture is nice and thick.

3. Serve with almonds, raisins and milk, and sweeten to taste. Leftover oatmeal can be stored in the refrigerator for up to 4 days; it will thicken up but can be reheated before use.

Bannock Cakes

Makes one serving

Measure out a scant 1 cup of cooked Irish Oatmeal (fresh or refrigerated) per serving, shape into a cylinder and cut into ½-inch slices. In a nonstick skillet, fry the slices in 1 teaspoon butter or margarine over medium heat until lightly browned, about 3 minutes per side. Serve with ¼ cup blueberries and 2 teaspoons real maple syrup (with some sugar substitute for a sweeter flavor if desired).

Nutritional information per serving with toppings:

Calories 270

Protein 6.3 grams

Total fat 6.3 grams

Saturated fat 0.6 gram

Total carbohydrates 50.9 grams

Dietary fiber 12.9 grams

(V)

"I" Diet Instant Hot Cereals

WHAT IF YOU LOVE HOT CEREAL but don't have time to make Irish Oatmeal? The three hot cereals here really do taste good and are very easy to prepare. Unlike most other kinds, made with thin slices of grains or even powdered grains that are quickly digested, they'll keep you hunger-free for hours.

Hot Cereal with Maple Syrup and Blueberries

Makes one serving

¹/₄ cup quick-cooking oatmeal

¹/₄ cup coarse wheat bran

1 cup nonfat or 1% milk

2 teaspoons maple syrup, for serving

¹/₄ cup blueberries, for serving

> **Nutritional information per serving with toppings:**
>
> **Calories** 255
>
> **Protein** 13.7 grams
>
> **Total fat** 5.1 grams
>
> **Saturated fat** 1.7 grams
>
> **Total carbohydrates** 44.1 grams
>
> **Dietary fiber** 9.0 grams

Place the oatmeal, bran and ⅔ cup of the milk in a microwave-safe bowl. Microwave on high power until the cereal is just boiling, about 1½ minutes; stop it before it begins to boil over. Serve the hot cereal with the maple syrup and the remaining milk and topped with the blueberries.

Hot Cereal with Raisins, Pecans and Cinnamon

Makes one serving

¹/₄ cup quick-cooking oatmeal

¹/₄ cup coarse wheat bran

³/₄ cup nonfat or 1% milk

2 teaspoons raisins, for serving

2 pecan halves, for serving

¹/₄ teaspoon ground cinnamon, for serving

> **Nutritional information per serving with toppings:**
>
> **Calories** 255
>
> **Protein** 13.7 grams
>
> **Total fat** 5.1 grams
>
> **Saturated fat** 1.7 grams
>
> **Total carbohydrates** 44.1 grams
>
> **Dietary fiber** 9.0 grams

Place the oatmeal, bran and ⅔ cup of the milk in a microwave-safe bowl. Microwave on high power until the cereal is just boiling, about 1½ minutes; stop it before it begins to boil over. Serve the hot cereal with the remaining milk and topped with the raisins, pecan halves and cinnamon.

Another Hot Cereal

Makes one serving

1 packet Kashi GOLEAN vanilla-flavored
    instant hot cereal

3 tablespoons coarse wheat bran

2 tablespoons nonfat or 1% milk, for serving

¼ cup blueberries, for serving

> **Nutritional information per serving with topping:**
>
> **Calories** 285
> **Protein** 12.7 grams
> **Total fat** 7.7 grams
> **Saturated fat** 0.7 grams
> **Total carbohydrates** 39.0 grams
> **Dietary fiber** 13.2 grams

Place the instant hot cereal, bran and ⅔ cup of water (or as directed on the package) in a microwave-safe bowl. Microwave on high power until the cereal is just boiling, about 1½ minutes; stop it before it begins to boil over. Serve the hot cereal with the milk and topped with the blueberries.

(V) Vegetable "Frittata"

Makes one serving

WHOLE EGGS ARE A REASONABLE CHOICE if you don't have high cholesterol, but if you need to cut the saturated fat and cholesterol, use a half-cup of Egg Beaters egg substitute when you make the "frittata." In either case—and no matter whether you decide you want to end up with an omelet or a scramble—the result will be a good, solid breakfast.

½ teaspoon tub margarine

1½ cups sliced button mushrooms, or
    1 cup lightly steamed vegetables,
    such as broccoli or spinach

2 eggs, beaten

Salt and freshly ground black pepper

1½ teaspoons ketchup (optional)

> **Nutritional information per serving with ketchup:**
>
> **Calories** 182
> **Protein** 13.6 grams
> **Total fat** 11.4 grams
> **Saturated fat** 5.0 grams
> **Total carbohydrates** 6.7 grams
> **Dietary fiber** 1.7 grams

1. Melt the margarine in a nonstick skillet over high heat. Add the mushrooms, if using, and cook, stirring frequently, until they start to brown, about 4 minutes. If you're using steamed vegetables instead, heat them in the margarine.

2. Add the beaten eggs to the skillet, season with salt and pepper to taste and stir the mixture until the eggs are just set. Serve the "frittata" with ketchup, if desired.

Bacon and Eggs Breakfast

Makes one serving

THERE'S NO NEED TO GIVE UP BACON just because you're dieting. Canadian bacon is a delicious substitute.

> 1 slice (about 1 ounce) Canadian bacon
> 1 teaspoon tub margarine
> ½ cup Egg Beaters egg substitute, or
>   1 egg and 2 egg whites, beaten
> 1 slice low-carbohydrate bread, toasted

Nutritional information per serving:

Calories 206	
Protein 23.2 grams	
Total fat 9.9 grams	
Saturated fat 2.0 grams	
Total carbohydrates 10.3 grams	
Dietary fiber 5.1 grams	

1. Using a nonstick pan if possible, cook the Canadian bacon in a dry pan over medium heat for about 1 minute, turning once. Transfer the Canadian bacon to a plate and cover it with aluminum foil to keep it warm.

2. Melt ½ teaspoon of the margarine in the pan, add the Egg Beaters or egg and egg whites and cook over medium heat until just set, 1 to 2 minutes.

3. Use the remaining ½ teaspoon of margarine to lightly butter the toast.

Variation: For more bacon and less egg, use 3 slices of Canadian bacon and ¼ cup Egg Beaters.

Orange-Crumbed French Toast

Makes two servings of 2 slices each, with toppings

A FAVORITE IN MY HOUSE, orange-scented French toast seems like an indulgent breakfast even though it's extremely diet-healthy. In Stage III, it can be made with regular whole-wheat bread, but in Stage I or Stage II use either low-carbohydrate supermarket bread or our satisfying "I" Diet Soda Bread. For kids and the non-dieting adults in your household, just throw some white bread into the mixture.

⅓ cup Egg Beaters egg substitute
¼ cup nonfat or 1% milk
4 slices low-carbohydrate bread, or
    4 thin slices "I" Diet Soda Bread
    (page 160)
2 teaspoons tub margarine
Grated zest of 2 small oranges
1½ tablespoons confectioners' sugar
4 teaspoons pure maple syrup
    (Grade B tastes richer), or 4 tablespoons
    sugar-free pancake syrup, for serving
⅔ cup blueberries or sliced strawberries, for serving

> **Nutritional information per 2-slice serving with toppings:**
>
> **Calories** 293
> **Protein** 12.0 grams
> **Total fat** 8.2 grams
> **Saturated fat** 0.5 gram
> **Total carbohydrates** 45.8 grams
> **Dietary fiber** 11.2 grams

1. Beat the Egg Beaters and milk together in a shallow bowl, then dip the slices of bread in the mixture, turning them to coat evenly.

2. Heat the margarine in a skillet over low heat and cook the French toast until lightly browned on both sides, 3 to 4 minutes per side. Transfer the French toast to a serving dish.

3. As the French toast cooks, mix together the grated orange zest and confectioners' sugar; it will look a bit like sand.

4. Sprinkle the orange sugar over the French toast and serve each slice with 1 teaspoon of the maple syrup or 1 tablespoon of the sugar-free pancake syrup and a quarter of the berries. (You don't need much syrup to make this sweet; the orange sugar does most of this on its own.)

Chocolate Pecan Breakfast Bars

Makes four bars

CEREAL MANUFACTURERS are putting an increasing number of breakfast bars on the market, but I personally find these bars less filling than the original cereal products. (That's probably because their fiber content has been bumped up with finely processed fiber preparations.) The home-prepared breakfast bars made from this recipe satisfy on all accounts, including taste, and cost much less.

1 square (about 10 grams) bittersweet chocolate
2 teaspoons tub margarine
⅓ cup Marshmallow Fluff
8 pecan halves
1⅓ cups high-fiber cereal such as Fiber One
    or All-Bran Extra Fiber
Cooking oil spray

> **Nutritional information per bar:**
> **Calories** 113
> **Protein** 2.3 grams
> **Total fat** 5.0 grams
> **Saturated fat** 0.9 gram
> **Total carbohydrates** 24.4 grams
> **Dietary fiber** 9.9 grams

1. Place the chocolate and margarine in a microwave-safe container and melt in the microwave on high power, about 20 seconds.

2. Add the Marshmallow Fluff and microwave briefly until melted.

3. Crush the pecans into small pieces, then lightly smash the cereal (putting it in a plastic bag and using a rolling pin works well). Mix the pecans and cereal together with the melted chocolate mixture. Stir well so all of the cereal is covered. Lightly spray a baking dish with cooking oil, then pat the cereal mixture into an approximately 4 by 6-inch rectangle and let cool before cutting into 4 bars. Store the bars wrapped in plastic.

Homemade Cinnamon Applesauce

Makes eleven ½-cup servings

APPLES ARE ON MY LIST of best diet foods because of their low-calorie and high-fiber content, portability and versatility. This made-from-scratch applesauce is a great example of a perfect apple recipe: a good breakfast if you don't like starting the day with raw fruit, or a fine comforting dessert, or a side dish for a pork tenderloin. When you leave the skins on and add lots of cinnamon, you get a more substantial applesauce with some interesting texture that's particularly good for satiety. Cortland apples are ideal because they cook down so well, but they're only available from September through about January. In other months, you can use almost any crisp apples, such as Pink Lady or Rome. When you use these firm apples, the slices will soften but remain intact after they're cooked.

7 large apples (about 3 pounds total)
2 tablespoons dark brown sugar
Sugar substitute equivalent to ¼ cup sugar (optional)
2 tablespoons raisins
3 teaspoons ground cinnamon

Nutritional information per ½-cup serving:

Calories 83
Protein 0.4 gram
Total fat 0.3 gram
Saturated fat 0 grams
Total carbohydrates 22.0 grams
Dietary fiber 3.6 grams

1. Quarter the apples and core but don't peel them. Cut each quarter into 4 or 5 slices.

2. Place the apples and 1 cup of water in a large pot and bring to a boil. Let the apples simmer, covered, until nicely soft, 10 to 15 minutes.

3. Stir in the brown sugar, sugar substitute, if using, raisins and cinnamon and add a little more water if the applesauce seems too dry. Taste for sweetness, adding more brown sugar or sugar substitute if needed. The applesauce can be divided into half-cup portions and frozen. To thaw and warm, microwave on high power for about 1½ minutes.

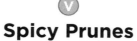

Spicy Prunes

Makes eleven servings of 4 prunes each

DRIED PLUMS, BETTER KNOWN AS PRUNES, don't actually have as much fiber as most of us think—only about half a gram per fruit. But they're good "diet" foods nonetheless, since they're rich, chewy and satisfying. This no-cook recipe isn't just for breakfast—it's also a terrific dessert.

Grated zest of 1 orange,
    or 1 teaspoon orange extract
½ teaspoon ground cinnamon
⅛ teaspoon ground cloves
2 tablespoons honey
Sugar substitute equivalent to ¼ cup sugar (optional)
1 package (about 10 ounces) prunes

Nutritional information per 4-prune serving:	
Calories 79	
Protein 0.7 gram	
Total fat 0 grams	
Saturated fat 0 grams	
Total carbohydrates 14.0 grams	
Dietary fiber 1.6 grams	

1. Heat 2 cups of water nearly to boiling in a saucepan and add the orange zest, cinnamon, cloves, honey and sugar substitute, if using.

2. Place the prunes in a heatproof bowl and pour the spiced liquid over them. Let cool completely, cover the bowl well and let the prunes steep in the refrigerator until they're soft, 1 to 2 days. Serve cold or at room temperature.

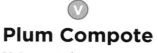

Plum Compote

Makes eight ½-cup servings

THIS RECIPE TURNS those unpromising bullet-hard black plums from the supermarket into a tasty, juicy dish. I like to cook up a batch and freeze individual servings for a quick and easy breakfast fruit or a satisfying snack during the day.

2 pounds hard black plums (about 7 large plums)
1 tablespoon sugar
2 to 3 tablespoons sugar substitute (optional)

Rinse the plums, then quarter them and remove the pits. Place the plums and ¾ cup of water in a pot over low heat and bring to a simmer. Cover the pot and let the plums simmer until they're cooked but still firm and bathed in a rich red sauce, about 30 minutes. Stir in the sugar and sugar substitute, if using, and serve or freeze.

Nutritional information per ½-cup serving:

Calories 58

Protein 0.8 gram

Total fat 0.4 gram

Saturated fat 0 grams

Total carbohydrates 14.5 grams

Dietary fiber 1.6 grams

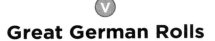

Great German Rolls

Makes twenty-four rolls

DENSE, CHEWY AND UTTERLY DELICIOUS, these rolls that I developed after tasting similar ones in Munich years ago are well worth the time it takes to make them. Try them for breakfast with honey and yogurt or use them for sandwiches filled with a slice of cheese or lean roast beef, horseradish sauce, lettuce, tomato and a thin slice of onion.

½ cup wheat berries
3 cups stone-ground 100% whole-wheat flour
2 cups white bread flour
2 cups coarse wheat bran
3 teaspoons dried instant yeast
1½ teaspoons salt
3 tablespoons wheat gluten (optional)
A little less than 3 cups warm water
1 teaspoon molasses
¼ cup flax seeds
⅓ cup sunflower seeds

Nutritional information per roll:

Calories 133

Protein 5.3 grams

Total fat 2.1 grams

Saturated fat 0.2 gram

Total carbohydrates 26.2 grams

Fiber 4.9 grams

1. Simmer the wheat berries in plenty of water until cooked and just starting to break open, about 45 minutes. Drain and rinse in cold water.

2. Meanwhile, place the whole-wheat and white bread flours, bran, yeast and salt in a large bowl or stand mixer fitted with a bread hook and start to mix. Add the wheat gluten, if using; it isn't necessary but does add protein and makes the rolls rise more.

3. Warm a scant 3 cups of water in a microwave to body temperature, about 1 minute on high power. Add the molasses and stir until dissolved, then pour most of the molasses mixture into the flour mixture, reserving a little. Mix the dough, adding more water as needed to make a soft but not sticky dough. Knead the dough for 5 minutes if you're using a machine or for 10 minutes by hand. Then cover the dough and let it rise until doubled in size, about 1 hour.

4. Mix the cooked wheat berries into the risen dough and knead again for 2 minutes. You can do this directly in the mixer if you're using one. Cut the dough into 24 equal pieces. Knead each one to make it round, then brush a little water on the top and bottom.

5. Spread out the flax seeds and sunflower seeds in separate shallow bowls. Press the top of each roll in the flax seeds. Then press the bottom in the sunflower seeds. The sunflower seeds don't have to cover the entire bottom of each roll; a light covering is fine.

6. Lightly grease a nonstick 10 by 14 by 2-inch baking dish. Arrange the rolls snugly in the center of the baking dish, making 4 rows of 6 rolls. Cover the dish and let the rolls rise until they've doubled in size, about 30 minutes. The rolls will fill the baking dish and be packed tightly together.

7. Preheat the oven to 400°F.

8. Place the rolls in the oven and immediately reduce the temperature to 350°F. Bake the rolls until the tops and bottoms are lightly browned and a skewer inserted in the middle of one roll comes out clean, 35 to 45 minutes. A few seeds will fall off as the rolls bake, but that's fine.

9. When cool, the rolls can be separated and frozen. To reheat, simply pop them in the microwave for about 40 seconds on high power.

Soups

SOUP IS ONE OF THE GREAT DIET FOODS, particularly when it's chunky—you'll feel satisfied quickly and hunger pangs won't return for hours. You can buy soup in cans (as long as you stick with broth-based vegetable soups); however, our homemade soups are very easy to make and transform a sandwich lunch into something out of the ordinary. If you make a batch of soup at the start of your diet, you can freeze individual servings and have them available in the days ahead.

Easy Tomato, Barley
and Basil Soup Ⓥ

Gazpacho Ⓥ

Carrot and Ginger Soup Ⓥ

Costa Rican Black Bean Soup Ⓥ

Lentil Vegetable Soup Ⓥ

Rich Chili Soup Ⓥ

Tuscan Minestrone

Pork and Lemongrass Soup

Beef and Barley Soup Ⓥ

Spicy Stew,
North African Style Ⓥ

Potage of Lamb and
Winter Squash

(V)

Easy Tomato, Barley and Basil Soup

Makes 7 cups

DON'T LET THE CANNED TOMATOES FOOL YOU. This soup is wonderfully satisfying and fresh-tasting enough to serve to company.

1 tablespoon extra-virgin olive oil
1 large onion, finely chopped
1 large clove garlic, finely chopped
1 can (28 ounces) whole tomatoes,
    preferably imported Italian
1 quart low-sodium chicken or vegetable broth
1/4 cup hulled barley
1/3 cup finely chopped fresh basil leaves
1/4 teaspoon freshly ground black pepper
Salt
Grated Parmesan cheese, preferably imported,
    for serving

Nutritional information per 1-cup serving:
Calories 99
Protein 5.7 grams
Total fat 5.7 grams
Saturated fat 0.7 gram
Total carbohydrates 39.0 grams
Dietary fiber 2.0 grams

1. Place the olive oil in a large saucepan over low heat. Add the onion and garlic and cook until lightly browned, 10 to 15 minutes, stirring occasionally.

2. Meanwhile, place the tomatoes in a blender or food processor and puree until partially smooth.

3. Add the tomatoes, broth and barley to the pan with the onion. Cover and let simmer until the barley is just cooked, about 30 minutes.

4. Add the basil and pepper to the soup and season with salt to taste.

5. Serve each bowl of soup with 1/2 teaspoon Parmesan cheese sprinkled on top.

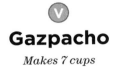

Gazpacho

Makes 7 cups

CHILLED GAZPACHO is a refreshing diet treat at the end of summer when local tomatoes are plentiful. This recipe is my particular favorite because of the perfect balance of fresh flavors. Also, since the vegetables are roughly chopped, you'll end up feeling more satisfied.

2 pounds ripe tomatoes
1 cup chopped English cucumber with skin
1 cup chopped red bell pepper
1 cup chopped green bell pepper
1/2 cup chopped red onion
1 clove garlic
1/2 cup chopped peeled carrots
1 tablespoon extra-virgin olive oil
2 tablespoons cider vinegar
2 tablespoons fresh lime juice
2 1/2 cups tomato juice
1/2 teaspoon paprika
1/8 teaspoon cayenne pepper
2 teaspoons salt
1/4 teaspoon freshly ground black pepper

> **Nutritional information per 1-cup serving:**
> **Calories** 75
> **Protein** 2.4 grams
> **Total fat** 2.3 grams
> **Saturated fat** 0.4 gram
> **Total carbohydrates** 12.7 grams
> **Dietary fiber** 2.3 grams

1. Prepare the tomatoes: Pierce the tomato skins, then place the tomatoes in boiling water for about half a minute until the skins loosen. Drain the tomatoes and rinse them in cold water. Peel the skins from the tomatoes before roughly chopping all the inner flesh (don't bother to remove the seeds). Place the tomatoes in a food processor and puree until smooth. Transfer to a bowl.

2. Prepare the remaining vegetables: Working in batches, grind the cucumber, bell peppers, onion, garlic and carrots in the food processor until very small pieces are formed. (Don't overprocess—you don't want to end up with a liquid.) Transfer each batch to the bowl.

3. Add the olive oil, vinegar, lime juice, tomato juice, paprika, cayenne pepper, salt and pepper to the tomato puree and chopped vegetables in the bowl; mix well. Chill for at least 2 hours before serving.

(V)

Carrot and Ginger Soup

Makes 7 cups

THIS DELICIOUS, FOOLPROOF SOUP goes well with sandwiches. It freezes well, too. Ginger seems to have the same hunger-suppressing properties found in hot peppers, so it's a great addition to any diet recipe!

1 tablespoon tub margarine
1 tablespoon canola or peanut oil
1 large or 2 small onions, coarsely chopped
1 clove garlic, coarsely chopped
2 pounds carrots, coarsely chopped
1 piece (1$\frac{1}{2}$ inches long and
   1 inch in diameter) fresh ginger,
   peeled and finely chopped
4 cups low-sodium chicken or vegetable broth
$\frac{1}{2}$ teaspoon salt
$\frac{1}{2}$ teaspoon freshly ground black pepper
$\frac{3}{8}$ cup orange juice

> **Nutritional information per 1-cup serving:**
>
> **Calories** 81
> **Protein** 1.5 grams
> **Total fat** 1.8 grams
> **Saturated fat** 0.3 gram
> **Total carbohydrates** 15.9 grams
> **Dietary fiber** 3.6 grams

1. Heat the margarine and oil in a large saucepan over low heat. Add the onion and garlic and cook until softened but not at all browned, about 10 minutes.

2. Add the carrots, ginger, broth, salt and pepper to the onions and let simmer, covered, until the carrots are tender, about 30 minutes.

3. Using a food processor or blender and working in batches, blend the soup until velvety. Add the orange juice and taste for seasoning, adding more salt and/or pepper as needed.

ⓥ Costa Rican Black Bean Soup

Makes 10 cups

THE TRADITIONAL COSTA RICAN DISH called *sopa negra* contains black beans, cilantro and whatever other good things are available. My friend Ellen Richstone shared this recipe with me after a trip to Costa Rica. It's easily prepared if you have a blender and makes a great stand-alone lunch with a slice of "I" Diet Soda Bread (page 160) and a piece of fruit for dessert. Freeze the soup in individual portions for easy meals on a moment's notice.

1 pound dried black beans, or
    6 cups canned black beans
    (about four 15-ounce cans; see Notes)
2 tablespoons corn or canola oil
1 medium-size onion, finely chopped
½ red bell pepper, finely chopped
1 clove garlic, chopped
⅓ cup finely chopped fresh cilantro
2 teaspoons salt (optional; see Notes)
1 teaspoon freshly ground black pepper
1¼ cups canned diced tomatoes
Tabasco sauce
1 teaspoon low-fat sour cream per serving (optional),
    for garnish
1 teaspoon finely chopped scallion per serving (optional),
    for garnish

Nutritional information per 1-cup serving with garnishes:

Calories 197	
Protein 10.2 grams	
Total fat 3.9 grams	
Saturated fat 0.7 gram	
Total carbohydrates 35.0 grams	
Dietary fiber 7.8 grams	

1. If using dried beans, soak them overnight in water to cover. Drain the beans and bring to a boil in about 8 cups of water, then reduce the heat and let simmer, covered, until just softened, about 1 hour. Set aside 3 cups of the bean-cooking liquid.

2. Place the oil in a large saucepan over medium heat. Add the onion, bell pepper and garlic and cook until starting to brown, about 5 minutes.

3. Add 3 cups of the black beans and the cilantro, salt, if using, and black pepper and cook for a couple of minutes.

4. Using a blender, puree the bean mixture until it's semi-smooth and then return it to the pan. Add the remaining black beans, the reserved bean-cooking liquid and the tomatoes and let simmer, covered, until the flavors develop, about 10 minutes.

5. Season the soup with Tabasco sauce to taste and garnish with sour cream and/or scallion, if desired.

NOTES If you use canned beans, drain them, reserving the liquid. Add enough low-sodium chicken broth for a total of 3 cups of liquid and use this in place of the bean-cooking liquid.

Add the salt if you cook the beans from scratch or use unsalted canned beans. If you use canned beans with salt, taste for seasoning after adding the cilantro and pepper in Step 3 and add salt as needed.

(V)
Lentil Vegetable Soup

Makes about 7 cups

NOTHING COULD BE HEALTHIER than this thick, richly flavored soup. Created by Judy Bart Kancigor, the author of *Cooking Jewish,* it's almost a meal all by itself.

1 cup lentils, picked over, rinsed and drained
1 can (15 ounces) diced tomatoes, undrained
1/2 cup chopped onion
1/2 cup thinly sliced celery
1/2 cup thinly sliced carrots
1 bay leaf
1/2 teaspoon garlic powder
1 teaspoon coarse salt, or more to taste
1/8 teaspoon freshly ground black pepper, or more to taste
4 to 6 cups low-sodium chicken or vegetable broth

Nutritional information per 1-cup serving:

Calories 134

Protein 11.0 grams

Total fat 0.4 gram

Saturated fat 0.1 gram

Total carbohydrates 22.8 grams

Dietary fiber 9.5 grams

Place the lentils, tomatoes, onion, celery, carrots, bay leaf, garlic powder, salt, pepper and 4 cups of broth in a large saucepan and bring to a boil. Reduce the heat and let simmer, covered, stirring occasionally, for about 2 hours. If the soup thickens too much, add 1 to 2 more cups of broth, depending upon how thick you want it to be. Serve hot.

(V)

Rich Chili Soup

Makes 12 cups

FOR THIS FINE, SATISFYING ONE-BOWL MEAL, you start out with several cans and a few extras and end up, just 30 minutes later, with a huge pot of flavorful homemade soup. Serve some bread on the side for non-dieters. If you're cooking just for one, you can cut this recipe in half and still have plenty for a few days.

1 tablespoon canola oil
1 small onion, chopped
1 clove garlic, minced
1 whole skinless, boneless chicken breast
    (about 1¼ pounds)
1 large red bell pepper, cut in ¾-inch squares
1 tablespoon cornstarch
1 quart low-sodium chicken or vegetable broth
1 can (15 ounces) navy beans, preferably with
    no salt added, undrained
1 can (15 ounces) red kidney beans, preferably with no salt added, undrained
1 can (8 ounces) tomato sauce
½ cup unseasoned canned diced tomatoes
½ cup frozen corn kernels
2 to 3 teaspoons chili powder
1 teaspoon dried oregano
1 teaspoon ground cumin
1½ teaspoons salt
½ teaspoon freshly ground black pepper
Freshly squeezed lime juice (optional)

> **Nutritional information per 1-cup serving:**
> **Calories** 163
> **Protein** 16.2 grams
> **Total fat** 3.7 grams
> **Saturated fat** 0.7 gram
> **Total carbohydrates** 16.8 grams
> **Dietary fiber** 7.0 grams

1. Heat the oil in a large pot over medium heat. Add the onion and garlic and cook until lightly browned, about 5 minutes.

2. Meanwhile, rinse the chicken under cold running water, pat it dry with paper towels and remove any visible fat. Cut the breast in half lengthwise, then cut each half crosswise into ¼-inch slices.

3. When the onion is starting to brown nicely, add the sliced chicken and the bell pepper and cook until the chicken turns white, a couple of minutes.

4. Mix the cornstarch with a couple of tablespoons of the broth, then add this mixture to the pot along with the remaining broth, the undrained navy and kidney beans and the tomato sauce, diced tomatoes, corn, chili powder, oregano, cumin, salt and black pepper.

5. Stir the soup occasionally while it comes to a boil, then cover the pot and let simmer until the chicken is cooked through, about 10 minutes.

6. Add the lime juice, if using, and taste for seasoning, adding more salt and/or black pepper as needed. Serve the chili soup hot.

Vegetarian variation: Omit the chicken breast and add 8 ounces of white button mushrooms, sliced. Add them after the onion and garlic have cooked for 5 minutes and cook until lightly browned, about 5 minutes, before adding the bell pepper in Step 3. Use vegetable broth.

> Nutritional information per 1-cup vegetarian serving:
> **Calories** 108
> **Protein** 6.7 grams
> **Total fat** 2.2 grams
> **Saturated fat** 0.2 gram
> **Total carbohydrates** 16.8 grams
> **Dietary fiber** 7.0 grams

Tuscan Minestrone

Makes 15 cups

ON A COLD, WINTRY DAY when you feel like spending some time in the kitchen, making a pot of Tuscan Minestrone is the perfect solution. This recipe makes a generous amount of soup. It freezes well but thickens up a bit when reheated.

1 generous cup dried cannellini beans
1 thick slice (about 3 ounces) imported prosciutto,
    all visible fat removed
Salt and freshly ground black pepper
1/4 cup extra-virgin olive oil
1 large red onion, diced
2 cloves garlic, minced
1 celery rib, chopped
1 large carrot, peeled and chopped
20 sprigs (about 1/2 cup) fresh flat-leaf parsley,
    coarsely chopped
1/2 medium-size savoy cabbage, chopped
    (about 6 cups)
1 cup canned diced tomatoes with their juices
1 bunch kale, chopped (about 6 cups)
5 tablespoons grated Parmesan cheese,
    preferably imported

Nutritional information per 1-cup serving:

Calories 127	
Protein 6.8 grams	
Total fat 4.5 grams	
Saturated fat 1.0 gram	
Total carbohydrates 15.8 grams	
Dietary fiber 5.4 grams	

1. Either soak the cannellini beans overnight in a big bowl of water or, if you start the same day, bring them to a boil in water to cover, turn off the heat and let them stand for an hour while they plump up. Drain.

2. Put the cannellini beans, prosciutto and 10 cups of water in a stockpot with a tight-fitting lid and bring to a simmer. Let simmer, covered, until the beans are soft, 1 to 2 hours (the cooking time is very variable with dried beans; you just have to check them every once in a while).

3. Heat the olive oil in a saucepan over low heat. Add the onion, garlic, celery, carrot and parsley and cook until lightly browned all over, 15 to 20 minutes.

4. When the beans are cooked, remove and finely dice the prosciutto and set it aside. Place about half of the beans in a blender with a little of the cooking liquid and puree to a smooth paste, then add the bean paste to the pot along with the diced prosciutto. Season with salt and pepper to taste.

5. Add the onion mixture to the stockpot along with the savoy cabbage and the tomatoes. Let simmer, covered, until the cabbage is cooked, about 15 minutes.

6. Add the kale and let simmer until it wilts, about 5 minutes. Taste for seasoning, adding more salt and/or pepper as needed. Serve the soup hot with a generous teaspoon of grated Parmesan cheese on top of each serving.

Pork and Lemongrass Soup

Makes 2 cups

THE COMPLEX FLAVORS OF ASIAN SOUPS make many of them terrific diet food. This one, which uses bits of pork and watercress, is a favorite of mine. It takes only a few minutes to prepare.

2 cups chicken broth
1 stalk lemongrass, about 3 inches long
2 white button mushrooms, sliced
2 thin slices peeled fresh ginger
1 ounce pork tenderloin (see Note)
½ cup chopped watercress (can be the stalks left
    over from salad made with the leaves)
Salt and freshly ground black pepper

> Nutritional information per 1-cup serving:
> **Calories** 64
> **Protein** 8.8 grams
> **Total fat** 2.0 grams
> **Saturated fat** 0.6 gram
> **Total carbohydrates** 2.1 grams
> **Dietary fiber** 0.4 gram

1. Place the chicken broth, lemongrass and mushrooms in a saucepan, bring to a simmer and let simmer, covered, until you can smell the lemongrass fragrance, about 15 minutes. Remove and discard the lemongrass.

2. Slice the pork very thinly, add it to the broth and heat until cooked through, about 2 minutes.

3. Add the watercress and let simmer, covered, about 30 seconds. Season the soup with salt and pepper to taste and serve immediately.

NOTE Cut the end off a pork tenderloin if you're planning on cooking one for dinner.

(V)
Beef and Barley Soup

Makes 9 cups

CHOOSE THE LEANEST CUT OF MEAT, throw in lots of vegetables and end up with a complete meal in a bowl. The soup freezes well, too.

2 teaspoons olive oil
1 large onion, finely chopped
3 ribs celery, finely chopped
2 cloves garlic, finely chopped
1/4 cup finely chopped fresh parsley (optional)
1 pound leanest beef with no visible fat, in 1 piece
   (see Note)
1 can (14 ounces) diced tomatoes
1 1/2 cups sliced white button mushrooms
1 1/2 quarts beef or vegetable broth
1 1/2 teaspoons chopped fresh basil, or
   1/2 teaspoon dried basil
1 1/2 teaspoons chopped fresh oregano, or 1/2 teaspoon dried oregano
1/2 teaspoon freshly ground black pepper
1/4 cup hulled barley
3 large carrots, peeled and sliced
1/2 cup something green, such as raw leftover broccoli stalks, thinly sliced
1/2 cup cooked beans (optional), such as canned navy beans, rinsed and drained
Salt

Nutritional information per 1-cup serving, including beans:
Calories 133
Protein 13.8 grams
Total fat 2.8 grams
Saturated fat 0.7 gram
Total carbohydrates 13.4 grams
Dietary fiber 3.2 grams

1. Heat the olive oil in a large saucepan over medium heat. Add the onion, celery, garlic and parsley, if using, and cook until browning nicely, about 5 minutes.

2. Add the meat, tomatoes, mushrooms, broth, basil, oregano, pepper and barley. Bring to a boil, cover the pan and let simmer until the meat breaks apart, about 2 hours.

3. Add the carrots and green vegetable and cook, covered, until tender, about 15 minutes. Add the beans and cook until just heated through, about 5 minutes. Season the soup with salt to taste.

Vegetarian variation: Mushroom barley soup—omit the beef and use vegetable broth. Increase the mushrooms to 3 cups and the barley to ½ cup.

NOTE Ask your butcher for a piece of bottom round to get the leanest cut.

> **Nutritional information per 1-cup vegetarian serving, including beans:**
>
> **Calories** 100
> **Protein** 5.2 grams
> **Total fat** 1.5 grams
> **Saturated fat** 0.2 gram
> **Total carbohydrates** 18.1 grams
> **Dietary fiber** 4.2 grams

(V)

Spicy Stew, North African Style

Makes 7½ cups

THIS TERRIFIC SPICY SOUP leaves you full and satisfied. The lamb adds a rich taste, but the recipe is good without it, if you want to make a meat-free dish. In either case, if you have a big enough pot, double this recipe for a large gathering. Offer couscous on the side for non-dieters.

½ cup dried chickpeas (garbanzo beans),
    soaked overnight and drained
½ pound leanest leg of lamb, cut into ½-inch cubes
½ medium-size onion, finely chopped
½ teaspoon ground turmeric
½ teaspoon salt, or more to taste
¼ teaspoon freshly ground black pepper
¼ teaspoon ground ginger
3 cups beef or vegetable broth
1 cup cubed rutabaga
1 cup sliced carrots
½ of a 6-ounce can tomato paste
1 medium-size zucchini, sliced
½ small cabbage, cut into chunks
½ cup green beans
1 medium-size red bell pepper, finely diced
¼ cup chopped fresh parsley
2 tablespoons raisins
Cayenne pepper

> **Nutritional information per 1½-cup serving:**
>
> **Calories** 219
> **Protein** 14.4 grams
> **Total fat** 4.3 grams
> **Saturated fat** 1.1 grams
> **Total carbohydrates** 32.9 grams
> **Dietary fiber** 9.0 grams

1. Bring the soaked chickpeas, lamb, onion, turmeric, salt, black pepper, ginger and broth to a boil in a large pot. Reduce the heat and let simmer, covered, until the beans are just beginning to soften, 1 to 2 hours.

2. Add the rutabaga and carrots and let simmer, covered, until partially cooked, about 15 minutes.

3. Add the tomato paste, zucchini, cabbage, green beans, bell pepper, parsley and raisins and let simmer until everything is tender, about 15 minutes.

4. Taste for seasoning, adding cayenne pepper to taste and more salt as needed.

Vegetarian variation: Omit the lamb and use vegetable broth. *Makes 7 cups*

Nutritional information per 1½-cup vegetarian serving:

Calories 188

Protein 8.2 grams

Total fat 1.9 grams

Saturated fat 0.2 gram

Total carbohydrates 34.9 grams

Dietary fiber 9.6 grams

Potage of Lamb and Winter Squash

Makes 4¼ cups

ONE OF THE EARLIEST RECORDED RECIPES, potage was a staple food in cultures ranging from ancient Rome to Elizabethan England. Essentially a thick soup or watery casserole (depending on your point of view) with a whole-grain/vegetable base and perhaps a little meat or fish tossed in, it's still a "daily" food in many parts of the world today. It's also a great diet food—the broth and vegetables make you feel full quickly, and the intact grains and meat prolong digestion to slow down the return of hunger.

Potage is simple to make—just throw a few things into a pot and wait an hour. This version uses lamb, which produces a richly flavored dish with a small portion of meat, but you can substitute chicken or beef for a milder taste. The potage freezes well but is thicker the second time around.

2 ounces lean leg of lamb with no visible fat,
    or very lean beef or chicken
1 tablespoon canola or other oil
$\frac{1}{2}$ small onion, chopped
$\frac{1}{2}$ clove garlic, chopped
2 cups low-sodium chicken or vegetable broth
$\frac{1}{2}$ cup sliced white button mushrooms
$\frac{1}{2}$ cup hulled barley
$\frac{1}{2}$ cup chopped fresh parsley
1 cup chopped winter squash, such as butternut
$\frac{1}{2}$ of a 15-ounce can cannellini or other beans,
    rinsed and well drained
    (save the rest for bean salad)
2 teaspoons dried cranberries
$\frac{1}{2}$ teaspoon ground cinnamon
Salt and freshly ground black pepper

> **Nutritional information per 1-cup serving:**
> **Calories** 190
> **Protein** 8.1 grams
> **Total fat** 4.2 grams
> **Saturated fat** 0.6 gram
> **Total carbohydrates** 30.1 grams
> **Dietary fiber** 7.3 grams

1. Cut the lamb into $\frac{1}{2}$-inch cubes. Heat the oil in a saucepan over high heat. Add the lamb, onion and garlic and cook briefly until lightly browned, about 5 minutes.

2. Add the broth, mushrooms, parsley, barley and $\frac{1}{2}$ cup of water and let simmer until the barley is soft, 50 minutes to 1 hour.

3. Add the squash after the barley has cooked for about 30 minutes. When the squash and barley are cooked, add the beans, cranberries and cinnamon and cook until heated through, about 5 minutes. Season with salt and pepper to taste just before serving.

Sandwiches and Wraps

MANY DIETS DON'T INCLUDE SANDWICHES because of the bread, which is often high in carbohydrates. But sandwiches fit into the "I" Diet with ease. Just follow the simple suggestions below.

1. *A sandwich needs company—never eat one by itself.* Every sandwich you eat while you're on the "I" Diet should be accompanied by something bulky to give you the total volume you need to feel satisfied.

Sandwiches with a few more calories, such as our "I" Diet Chicken Salad sandwich (page 161) and Indian Kebab Wrap (page 165), should be accompanied by a side salad and light dressing, which add only a few calories.

Sandwiches like the "I" Diet Tuna Salad sandwich (page 162), The American Classic Sandwich (page 162) and the Italian-Style Panini (page 164) can be paired with either a salad or a broth-based soup.

Pickles are a terrific accompaniment to a sandwich meal, in addition to a salad or soup, provided you don't have high blood pressure (in which case, check the container for the amount of salt). Dill pickles are particularly great because they're strong-flavored and have only about 7 calories per huge spear—plus a gram of fiber as a bonus!

2. *Choose your bread carefully.* The low-carbohydrate bread you can get in regular supermarkets is ideal for sandwiches, or, for the best taste, the homemade "I" Diet Soda Bread on page 160 is a winner. Two slices of low-carb bread or Soda Bread make a sandwich that fits the regular 1,200-calorie "I" Diet menu (three slices for one and a half sandwiches if you're on a higher-calorie plan).

3. *Pick your fillings with equal care.* First, think about spreads. A couple of teaspoons of low-fat salad dressing adds to the taste. Mustard or plain yogurt is also good. After that, pack in as much

salad stuff as you can manage to make a really substantial-looking sandwich—up to a cup of lettuce, cucumber, thinly sliced onion, tomato slices and hot peppers!

Only then is it time to focus on your protein source. Any of these should be fine:

> 2 ounces (slice sizes vary so check the package) turkey,
>   lean ham or roast beef
> 1 hard-boiled egg, sliced
> ¼ cup water-packed solid tuna
> 3 ounces Broiled Tofu (page 208)
> 1 tablespoon crunchy peanut butter
>   and 1 teaspoon fruit spread

If you want a break from high-protein fillings, try a watercress or cucumber sandwich instead. Use two slices of bread, such as our Soda Bread, lightly buttered. Then fill the sandwich with ½ cup or so of watercress or some thin cucumber slices for a delicious and unusual treat.

"I" Diet Soda Bread ⓥ

"I" Diet Chicken or Tofu Salad ⓥ

"I" Diet Tuna Salad

The American Classic Sandwich

The New Yorker

Italian-Style Panini

Indian Kebab Wrap

"I" Diet Soda Bread

Makes 40 thin slices

MANY DIETS TREAT BREAD LIKE POISON. Bad idea. Low-carbohydrate breads (such as Arnold's) are a useful aid to weight loss. The problem is that these breads can be hard to find. The solution is a much tastier homemade bread. This version doesn't have quite as much fiber as low-carb bread, but it doesn't have to—it has wheat berries and a very dense, coarse texture, which also slows digestion. And since it doesn't call for yeast, you just mix up the ingredients and bake!

½ cup wheat berries
3 cups stone-ground whole-wheat flour
2 cups coarse bran (regular red wheat bran, not white wheat bran)
2 cups white bread flour
3 teaspoons baking powder
2 teaspoons baking soda
½ teaspoon salt
3¼ cups low-fat buttermilk, or more as needed

Nutritional information per slice:

Calories 72
Protein 3.2 grams
Total fat 0.5 gram
Saturated fat 0.1 gram
Total carbohydrates 16.4 grams
Dietary fiber 3.8 grams

1. Lightly grease two 9 by 4 by 3-inch loaf tins.

2. Place the wheat berries in a saucepan with plenty of water and let simmer until the grains are plump and some are starting to break open, about 45 minutes. Drain the wheat berries.

3. Preheat the oven to 350°F.

4. Place the whole-wheat flour, bran, white bread flour, baking powder, baking soda and salt in a large bowl and mix well. Add the drained wheat berries and mix again.

5. Add 3¼ cups of buttermilk and stir to mix well to make a stiff dough with no dry flour in it. Because flour is drier at some times of the year, you might have to add ¼ cup or even more buttermilk. Divide the dough in half, place each half in a prepared loaf pan and gently pat it into the pan.

6. Bake the bread until the loaves are lightly browned and have pulled away from the sides of the pan, 45 to 55 minutes. A skewer inserted in the center will come out dry when the bread is done.

7. Let the bread cool completely before slicing. Slices freeze well and can be thawed in a microwave or toasted.

Higher-fiber variation: If you're somebody who gets really hungry, add ¼ cup of corn bran to the dry ingredients for more fiber (one source of corn bran: www.honeyvillegrain.com).

Bread-for-life variation: After weight loss, you can reduce the wheat berries to ⅓ cup if you want. Since you won't need quite so much all-out hunger suppression, the bread can be a bit lighter and still good for preventing weight gain.

(V)

"I" Diet Chicken or Tofu Salad

Makes enough filling for two sandwiches

THIS SANDWICH FILLING has more calories than some of the others here, so pair it with a vegetable salad rather than soup.

3 tablespoons low-fat plain yogurt
1 teaspoon brown sugar
½ teaspoon lemon juice
3 ounces cooked skinless chicken (store-bought or leftover), or 3 ounces Broiled Tofu (page 208)
1 scallion, both white and green parts, thinly sliced
2 tablespoons thinly sliced celery
1 tablespoon raisins

Nutritional information per sandwich (including 2 slices of low-carb bread):

Calories 250
Protein 2.9 grams
Total fat 6.8 grams
Saturated fat 1.3 grams
Total carbohydrates 24.9 grams
Dietary fiber 8.7 grams

1. Mix the yogurt, brown sugar and lemon juice together to make a sauce.

2. Cut the chicken or tofu into ½-inch or smaller cubes, then mix it with the scallion, celery, raisins and yogurt sauce. Serve immediately or refrigerate until ready to use.

"I" Diet Tuna Salad

Makes enough filling for three sandwiches

THIS SANDWICH FILLING IS SO GOOD, you'll want to share it with your friends. Be sure to include the black pepper; it suppresses hunger and makes up for the lack of mayonnaise.

1 can (6 ounces) water-packed solid tuna,
    drained well
1 large or 2 small scallions, both white and green parts,
    finely chopped
3 to 4 tablespoons low-fat plain yogurt
2 teaspoons finely chopped fresh parsley (optional)
⅛ teaspoon salt
¼ teaspoon freshly ground black pepper

Mix the tuna, scallion, yogurt, parsley, if using, salt and pepper together. Taste for seasoning, adding more salt and/or pepper as needed.

Nutritional information per sandwich (including 2 slices of low-carb bread):
Calories 197
Protein 20.6 grams
Total fat 4.8 grams
Saturated fat 0.3 gram
Total carbohydrates 18.4 grams
Dietary fiber 8.7 grams

The American Classic Sandwich

Makes one sandwich

SIMPLY PERFECT.

2 slices low-carbohydrate bread
2 teaspoons low-fat Thousand Island
    dressing or blue cheese dressing
1 ounce (about 1 slice) turkey, or 1 piece
    (1 ounce) grilled skinless chicken breast, sliced
1 tablespoon grated Parmesan cheese,
    preferably imported
1 tablespoon chopped onion
2 thin slices tomato
2 romaine or iceberg lettuce leaves

Nutritional information per sandwich:
Calories 210
Protein 14.9 grams
Total fat 6.6 grams
Saturated fat 1.4 grams
Total carbohydrates 24.4 grams
Dietary fiber 9.5 grams

Toast the bread, then spread it with the dressing. Pile the meat, Parmesan cheese, onion, tomato and lettuce on one slice of toast and top it with the other slice.

The New Yorker

Makes one sandwich

MY FATHER-IN-LAW, DENNIS FLANAGAN, was the consummate New Yorker, proud to say he lived his whole life there, first uptown, then downtown. This robust, tasty sandwich is a diet version of the one he enjoyed every weekend for decades. I offer it here, knowing he would be pleased to be remembered for the treat he created.

1 slice (about 1 ounce) Canadian bacon
½ teaspoon tub margarine
1 large egg
2 slices low-carbohydrate bread
Thinly sliced onion—a couple of slices,
    or more if you like
Plenty of freshly ground black pepper
1 dill pickle spear

Nutritional information per sandwich:

Calories 260
Protein 17.5 grams
Total fat 12.3 grams
Saturated fat 2.4 grams
Total carbohydrates 20.7 grams
Dietary fiber 9.4 grams

1. Cook the Canadian bacon on both sides in a dry pan over medium heat. Remove the Canadian bacon from the pan. Add the margarine and fry the egg over easy until the white is completely set.

2. Meanwhile, lightly toast the bread.

3. Make a sandwich of the Canadian bacon and egg, seasoned with pepper, and top with the onion and the other slice of toast. Serve the sandwich with the dill pickle on the side.

Italian-Style Panini

Makes one sandwich

IMPORTED PROSCIUTTO AND PARMESAN CHEESE make a big difference in this delightful recipe.

2 slices low-carbohydrate bread

1 thin slice imported prosciutto

1 tablespoon grated Parmesan cheese, preferably imported

1 tablespoon finely chopped onion

1 teaspoon store-bought pesto from the deli refrigerator

2 thin slices tomato

¼ cup sautéed sliced mushrooms (optional; see Note)

Balsamic vinegar

Salt and freshly ground black pepper

4 sprigs watercress

> **Nutritional information per sandwich, including mushrooms:**
>
> **Calories** 225
>
> **Protein** 14.3 grams
>
> **Total fat** 10.6 grams
>
> **Saturated fat** 2.4 grams
>
> **Total carbohydrates** 19.8 grams
>
> **Dietary fiber** 9.1 grams

1. Place a slice of bread on a work surface and layer the prosciutto, Parmesan cheese, onion, pesto, tomato and mushrooms, if using, on top. Add a dash of balsamic vinegar and season with salt and pepper to taste.

2. Heat a panini maker and cook the sandwich according to the manufacturer's directions or heat a frying pan and cook the sandwich on both sides until crisply browned, 2 to 4 minutes per side.

3. Open up the sandwich after it's cooked and add the watercress. Serve.

NOTE To sauté the mushrooms, heat ¼ teaspoon margarine (just enough to moisten the bottom of the pan) in a small nonstick skillet over high heat. Add the mushrooms and cook, stirring constantly, until they release their liquid and are nicely browned, 3 to 4 minutes.

Indian Kebab Wrap

Makes one wrap

THIS SANDWICH USES leftover Tanzanian Chicken Kebabs, but it's so good that you may end up making the kebab recipe just to have the ingredients on hand (the kebabs freeze well). A great side for this dish is the Cucumber-Mint Raita (page 174), which takes only a couple of minutes to prepare and adds just a few calories.

2 skewers (8 pieces of chicken total)
   Tanzanian Chicken Kebabs (page 195)
1 low-carbohydrate pita bread or tortilla
2 to 3 tablespoons low-fat plain yogurt or
   leftover dal (page 222)
1 crisp romaine or iceberg lettuce leaf
1 teaspoon Lemon and Date Chutney (page 223)
   or mango chutney (optional)
2 finely shredded fresh mint leaves (optional)

Nutritional information per wrap:	
Calories 252	
Protein 19.4 grams	
Total fat 6.8 grams	
Saturated fat 1.2 grams	
Total carbohydrates 24.6 grams	
Dietary fiber 3.0 grams	

1. Reheat the kebabs in a microwave oven at high power until just warmed through, about 20 seconds; be careful not to overheat the kebabs or they will be tough.

2. Warm the pita bread by placing it on a microwave-safe plate and heating it on high power for about 10 seconds. Pile the chicken, yogurt, lettuce, chutney and mint, if using, in the pita and enjoy.

Salads

BESIDES TASTING GOOD, salads give you bulk along with the vitamins and minerals you need for vitality and strength. Since salads don't usually contain much fiber, I like to team them up with legumes, high-fiber breads or a high-fiber cereal dessert for a feeling of satisfaction at the end of a meal. Measure your salad dressings—that's where you can pile on calories if you're not careful.

"Sallat" of Field Greens and Herbs ⓥ

Apple, Walnut and Blue Cheese Salad ⓥ

Iceberg Wedges with Blue Cheese ⓥ

Bibb Salad with Mushrooms and Shaved Parmesan ⓥ

**Watercress and Orange Salad
with Parmesan Toasts and Hummus** ⓥ

Tomato Salad ⓥ
Tarragon Dressing

Tomato-Cucumber Salad with Greek Dressing ⓥ

Cucumber-Mint Raita ⓥ

Coleslaws ⓥ
Classic Coleslaw
Asian Coleslaw

Crisp Fennel Salad ⓥ

Thai Chicken Salad with Warm Peanut Sauce ⓥ

Curried Chicken Salad on Field Greens ⓥ

Wheat Berry Salads ⓥ
Wheat Berry and Cilantro Salad
Wheat Berry, Raisin and Pine Nut Salad

Crispy Taco Pinto Bean Salad ⓥ

Hummus and Veggie Plate with
Spicy Sesame Cracker Chips Ⓥ

Three-Bean Salad with Fresh Herbs Ⓥ

Thai Tofu Salad Ⓥ

Mixed Fruit with Yogurt Dip Ⓥ

See also Bonus Recipes, pages 261 and 262

Ⓥ

"Sallat" of Field Greens and Herbs

Makes two servings

THE ANCESTORS OF MODERN GREEN SALADS, sallats were popular hundreds of years ago in Europe. This historical recipe, adapted from an English source from the time of Shakespeare, is wonderfully refreshing. It goes well with "I" Diet Tuna Salad (page 162) and is also good with almost any main course. Look for a mix of baby greens, such as red and green leaf lettuce, radicchio, frisée—maybe even dandelion.

4 cups moderately packed
    mixed field greens (mesclun)
½ cup moderately packed arugula or
    watercress, with larger stems removed
¼ cup chopped mixed fresh herbs, such as parsley,
    chives and basil, with smaller amounts of mint,
    chervil and thyme
1½ tablespoons oil, such as canola
2¼ teaspoons cider vinegar or wine vinegar
1 teaspoon sugar
Salt and freshly ground black pepper

> **Nutritional information per serving:**
> **Calories** 123
> **Protein** 2.4 grams
> **Total fat** 10.6 grams
> **Saturated fat** 1.6 grams
> **Total carbohydrates** 6.7 grams
> **Dietary fiber** 3.1 grams

Place the greens, arugula or watercress and herbs in a large bowl and toss to mix. Add the oil and toss to coat, then add the vinegar and sugar and toss again. Season with salt and pepper to taste.

Apple, Walnut and Blue Cheese Salad

Makes two servings

APPLES, WALNUTS AND BLUE CHEESE—they just go together. But most
diets won't let you anywhere near cheese. The secret is choosing a strong-
flavored blue, eating only a small amount and mixing it with other things:
a crisp apple, a soft lettuce, a crunchy stalk of celery.

For the salad:

2 medium-size crisp apples,
    such as Gala or Braeburn
2 tablespoons walnut halves
2 ribs celery
½ head of Bibb lettuce

For the dressing:

1 tablespoon olive oil
1 tablespoon balsamic or cider vinegar
1 teaspoon honey
1½ tablespoons crumbled very strong blue cheese,
    such as Roquefort
2 tablespoons low-fat plain yogurt (optional)
Salt and freshly ground black pepper

> **Nutritional information per serving, including yogurt:**
>
> **Calories** 235
>
> **Protein** 3.9 grams
>
> **Total fat** 13.5 grams
>
> **Saturated fat** 2.7 grams
>
> **Total carbohydrates** 28.6 grams
>
> **Dietary fiber** 5.4 grams

1. Make the salad: Cut the apples into approximately ½-inch cubes. Chop
the walnut halves into medium-size pieces and finely slice the celery. Rinse
the lettuce under cold running water and pat it dry with paper towels.

2. Make the dressing: Place the olive oil, vinegar, honey, blue cheese
and yogurt, if using, in a bowl and stir to mix (the yogurt will make the
dressing creamier). Season with salt and pepper to taste.

3. Add the apples, walnuts and celery to the dressing and toss to mix.
Arrange the lettuce leaves on 2 serving plates, dividing them evenly.
Top with the apple salad and serve immediately.

(V)

Iceberg Wedges with Blue Cheese

Makes four servings

REMEMBER THE GOOD OLD-FASHIONED lettuce and blue cheese wedge, the kind you got in steak houses along with a juicy steak? The restaurant kind will never help your diet, so here's our diet-friendly alternative. The secret is simple: Dilute the dressing with milk. Commercial blue cheese dressing is so thick that you have to use a lot to coat the lettuce. Not the case here!

1 small head of iceberg lettuce
¼ cup low-calorie blue cheese dressing
¼ cup nonfat or 1% milk
2 carrots, peeled and grated
¼ cup finely chopped onion
Handful of cooked chickpeas
    (garbanzo beans; optional)
Chopped fresh parsley (optional), for garnish
2 teaspoons bacon bits (optional), for garnish

Nutritional information per serving with chickpeas and bacon bits:

Calories 55

Protein 1.2 grams

Total fat 3.9 grams

Saturated fat 0.5 gram

Total carbohydrates 4.1 grams

Dietary fiber 0.8 gram

1. Cut the lettuce into quarters and remove and discard the outer leaves. Rinse the lettuce quarters under cold running water and pat dry with paper towels.

2. Mix the blue cheese dressing and milk together.

3. When you're ready to serve, pour the dressing over the lettuce quarters and then garnish them with the carrots and onion and the chickpeas and parsley, if using. Top each serving with ½ teaspoon bacon bits, if desired.

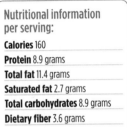

Bibb Salad with Mushrooms and Shaved Parmesan

Makes two servings

THIS SALAD IS EXTRA-SATISFYING because it combines mushrooms and Parmesan cheese. These two foods are packed with the umami flavor that stimulates our fifth class of taste receptors (the other classes are sweet, salty, bitter and sour) to give us the taste that we recognize as savory and meaty.

1 teaspoon tub margarine
8 ounces white button mushrooms, sliced
   (about 3 cups)
4 cups Bibb lettuce, or any
   other greens of your choice
1 tablespoon olive oil
½ teaspoon balsamic vinegar
½ ounce thin Parmesan cheese shavings
Salt and freshly ground black pepper

Nutritional information per serving:

Calories 160
Protein 8.9 grams
Total fat 11.4 grams
Saturated fat 2.7 grams
Total carbohydrates 8.9 grams
Dietary fiber 3.6 grams

1. Melt the margarine in a skillet over high heat. Add the mushrooms and cook until they're lightly browned, about 5 minutes.

2. Rinse the lettuce under cold running water and pat it dry with paper towels. Toss the lettuce with the olive oil, balsamic vinegar and Parmesan cheese. Season the salad with salt and pepper to taste, then mix in the warm cooked mushrooms. Serve immediately.

Watercress and Orange Salad with Parmesan Toasts and Hummus

Makes two servings

SERVE THE WATERCRESS AND ORANGE as a side salad, or pair it with Parmesan toast fingers and hummus for a lovely lunch. Measure out the hummus carefully—it packs a lot of calories and is easy to overeat.

For the salad:

1 small orange
2 teaspoons olive oil
1 teaspoon balsamic vinegar
1 tablespoon orange juice
Salt and freshly ground black pepper
1 scallion, both white and green parts, thinly sliced
1 bunch watercress, tough stems removed (about 2 cups)
2 cups chopped romaine or other mild-tasting greens

For the Parmesan toasts and hummus:

2 slices low-carbohydrate bread
4 teaspoons grated Parmesan cheese, preferably imported
¼ cup hummus

> **Nutritional information per serving:**
>
> **Calories** 212
> **Protein** 8.8 grams
> **Total fat** 10.8 grams
> **Saturated fat** 0.4 gram
> **Total carbohydrates** 22.7 grams
> **Dietary fiber** 8.4 grams

1. Make the salad: Separate the orange into segments, then cut each segment into thirds; reserve 1 tablespoon of the juice to add to the dressing. Mix the olive oil, balsamic vinegar and orange juice together in a salad bowl. Season with salt and pepper to taste, then mix in the scallion, greens and orange pieces.

2. Make the Parmesan toasts: Toast the bread and sprinkle the Parmesan cheese on top. Heat the Parmesan toasts in the microwave on high power until the cheese melts. Cut the toasts into fingers. Serve the salad with the toast fingers and the hummus, for dipping.

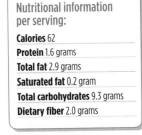

Tomato Salad

Makes one serving

BEST IN SUMMER, when farmers' markets are overflowing with juicy, ripe local tomatoes, but good anytime!

1 large tomato, sliced
1 teaspoon of any dressing, such as
    Tarragon Dressing (recipe follows),
    or a drizzle of extra-virgin olive oil and vinegar
Salt and freshly ground black pepper

Slice the tomato, pour the dressing over it and season with salt and pepper to taste. Serve the salad immediately.

Nutritional information per serving:

Calories 62	
Protein 1.6 grams	
Total fat 2.9 grams	
Saturated fat 0.2 gram	
Total carbohydrates 9.3 grams	
Dietary fiber 2.0 grams	

Variation: Adding a garnish of 1 teaspoon chopped fresh basil gives you herbed tomato salad.

Tarragon Dressing

Makes ¾ cup (12 tablespoons)

This light homemade dressing goes nicely with any salad, but I particularly like it with our Tomato Salad. Also try it as a dipping sauce for crisp green vegetables, such as zucchini and bell peppers.

¼ cup plus 1 tablespoon cider vinegar
¼ cup finely chopped onion
1 tablespoon Dijon mustard
1 tablespoon chopped fresh tarragon,
    or 1 teaspoon dried tarragon
2 teaspoons sugar
1 teaspoon salt
⅛ teaspoon freshly ground black pepper
¼ cup light oil, such as canola or corn
1 teaspoon sugar substitute (optional)

Nutritional information per 1-tablespoon serving:

Calories 47	
Protein 0.1 gram	
Total fat 4.6 grams	
Saturated fat 0.3 gram	
Total carbohydrates 1.7 grams	
Dietary fiber 0.1 gram	

Place the cider vinegar, onion, mustard, tarragon, sugar, salt and pepper in a bowl and stir to mix well. Add the oil whisking constantly until blended. Taste for seasoning, adding more salt and/or pepper and the sugar substitute, if using, as needed. The dressing can be refrigerated, covered, for several days.

Tomato-Cucumber Salad with Greek Dressing

Makes two servings

THIS EASY DISH IS SUITABLE for a quick lunch when you're at home alone or as a side for other main courses. The combination of oregano and lemon makes the classic Greek flavors of tomato and cucumber come to life without the need for feta cheese.

1 cup chopped tomato
1 cup diced cucumber (see Note)
$^1/_4$ cup canned chickpeas (garbanzo beans), well rinsed and drained
1 tablespoon canola oil or olive oil
1 tablespoon lemon juice
1 tablespoon chopped fresh parsley
$^1/_2$ teaspoon dried oregano
Salt and freshly ground black pepper

Nutritional information per serving:
Calories 116
Protein 2.7 grams
Total fat 7.7 grams
Saturated fat 0.8 gram
Total carbohydrates 11.0 grams
Dietary fiber 2.9 grams

Place the tomato, cucumber, chickpeas, oil, lemon juice, parsley and oregano in a bowl and stir to mix. Season with salt and pepper to taste. Serve immediately.

NOTE Try using one of the English (hothouse) cucumbers that come shrink-wrapped in plastic. They're less bitter because they have fewer seeds. Leave the skin on for more fiber.

Ⓥ
Cucumber-Mint Raita

Makes one serving

THIS IS A WONDERFUL SIDE to serve with Tanzanian Chicken Kebabs
(page 195). The baking soda gives the yogurt a milder flavor by helping
to neutralize its acid.

1 cup cucumber slices (see Note)
⅓ cup low-fat plain yogurt
Pinch of baking soda
½ teaspoon finely chopped fresh mint
Salt and freshly ground black pepper

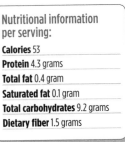

Nutritional information
per serving:

Calories 53	
Protein 4.3 grams	
Total fat 0.4 gram	
Saturated fat 0.1 gram	
Total carbohydrates 9.2 grams	
Dietary fiber 1.5 grams	

Mix the cucumber slices, yogurt, baking soda and
mint together in a bowl. Season with salt and pepper
to taste and refrigerate until ready to use.

NOTE Try using one of the English (hothouse) cucumbers that come
shrink-wrapped in plastic. They're less bitter because they have fewer
seeds. Leave the skin on for more fiber.

Ⓥ
Coleslaws

COLESLAW IS USUALLY AN ABSOLUTE DIET NO-NO—it's loaded with
mayonnaise and way too many calories. With a few simple changes,
as in the two very different recipes here, shredded cabbage becomes
a versatile tasty side dish to go with many lunchtime meals or dinner
entrées. To save work, I usually buy the bags of ready-shredded cabbage.

Although coleslaw is best eaten fresh because it softens with age,
it's still tasty after being stored in the refrigerator for a day or two.
Be sure to keep it covered until you're ready to serve it.

Classic Coleslaw

Makes 4 cups

8 ounces shredded cabbage
   (¹/₂ of a preshredded 1-pound bag)
2 scallions, both white and green parts, finely sliced
1 tablespoon sugar substitute (optional)
1 tablespoon cider vinegar or other vinegar
1 tablespoon low-fat mayonnaise
¹/₃ cup low-fat plain yogurt
¹/₄ teaspoon salt
¹/₄ teaspoon freshly ground black pepper
2 pinches of celery seeds (optional)
2 tablespoons raisins (optional)

> **Nutritional information per 1-cup serving with raisins:**
> **Calories** 65
> **Protein** 2.0 grams
> **Total fat** 3.2 grams
> **Saturated fat** 0.5 gram
> **Total carbohydrates** 8.4 grams
> **Dietary fiber** 1.7 grams

Place the cabbage, scallions, sugar substitute, if using, vinegar, mayonnaise, yogurt, salt, pepper and the celery seeds and raisins, if using, in a large bowl and stir to mix. Taste for seasoning, adding more salt as needed.

Asian Coleslaw

Makes 4 cups

8 ounces shredded cabbage and carrot mix
   (¹/₂ of a preshredded 1-pound bag)
2 tablespoons finely chopped onion
1 tablespoon shredded fresh basil leaves
1 teaspoon shredded fresh mint leaves
2 teaspoons canola or corn oil
1 tablespoon rice vinegar or other vinegar
1 small clove garlic, finely chopped
1 teaspoon sugar
¹/₄ teaspoon salt
¹/₄ teaspoon freshly ground black pepper
2 tablespoons roasted peanuts (optional), crushed

> **Nutritional information per 1-cup serving with peanuts:**
> **Calories** 65
> **Protein** 2.0 grams
> **Total fat** 3.2 grams
> **Saturated fat** 0.5 gram
> **Total carbohydrates** 8.4 grams
> **Dietary fiber** 1.7 grams

Place the cabbage and carrot mix, onion, basil, mint, oil, rice vinegar, garlic, sugar, salt, pepper and peanuts, if using, in a large bowl and toss to mix. Taste for seasoning, adding more salt and/or pepper as needed.

(V)

Crisp Fennel Salad

Makes six servings

THIS LIGHT, ELEGANT SALAD from Sheila Lukins' book *Celebrate!* works as
an appetizer before a special dinner or as a vegetarian lunch on its own,
paired with some bean salad and a slice of "I" Diet Soda Bread (page 160).

2 tablespoons fresh orange juice
1 teaspoon red wine vinegar
1 tablespoon honey
1 tablespoon Dijon mustard
¼ cup extra-virgin olive oil
Salt and freshly ground black pepper
2 cloves garlic, crushed
2 fennel bulbs, trimmed, fronds chopped
4 large red radishes, trimmed and thinly sliced
8 fresh basil leaves, finely sliced
2 large bunches arugula (12 ounces total), rinsed and dried

Nutritional information per serving:
Calories 136
Protein 2.7 grams
Total fat 9.6 grams
Saturated fat 0 grams
Total carbohydrates 11.8 grams
Dietary fiber 3.5 grams

1. Place the orange juice, wine vinegar, honey and mustard in a small bowl
and whisk until smooth. Whisking constantly, add the olive oil in a steady
stream. Continue whisking until the dressing is slightly thickened. Season
with salt and pepper to taste, add the garlic cloves and let rest at room
temperature for at least 1 hour.

2. Meanwhile, cut the fennel bulbs in half lengthwise and remove the
cores and any tough outer pieces. Thinly slice the fennel and place it in
a large bowl. Toss the radish slices with the fennel.

3. Remove the garlic cloves from the dressing, whisk it again and pour it
over the fennel and radishes. (You can dress the fennel and radishes up
to 2 hours before serving and refrigerate.)

4. Shortly before serving, toss the fennel fronds and the basil with the
fennel and radishes.

5. Divide the arugula among 6 salad plates and top with the salad.

ⓥ
Thai Chicken Salad with Warm Peanut Sauce

Makes two servings

ONE OF THE LIKELIEST PLACES to find my colleagues at lunchtime is at the busy Montien, a Thai restaurant across the street from the Tufts downtown Boston medical campus. It's an open secret in Boston that chef and owner Tony Suktheva prepares the best Thai food around, and his skills have received so many good reviews and local awards that they barely fit on the available wall space. Fresh and delicious, Tony's food showcases the many ways that salads and steamed vegetables can make a gourmet dish that's satisfying and healthy.

When I talked to Tony and his co-owner wife about providing an "I" Diet recipe, they amazed me by taking it for granted that Thai food is good for weight control. Thai people have long known that ingredients like fresh ginger and garlic increase satisfaction, something that Western science has only recently figured out.

One of my favorite lunches at Montien is the house salad, which features an abundant selection of vegetables together with a luscious warm peanut sauce. Recognizing that most of us don't have the hours in the kitchen to make this sauce from scratch, Tony has adapted his usually complicated recipe to start with ingredients you can purchase in most big supermarkets. You'll have more peanut sauce than you need for the chicken salad. The sauce is also perfect for steamed tofu and vegetables like cauliflower, broccoli, carrots, zucchini slices and snow peas.

For the peanut sauce:

1/2 cup unsweetened light coconut milk

1/4 cup reduced-fat smooth peanut butter

3 teaspoons sugar

2 teaspoons red curry paste, such as A Taste of Thai

2 teaspoons Asian fish sauce

Nutritional information per serving of salad with 1/4 cup peanut sauce:

Calories 271

Protein 19.8 grams

Total fat 12.3 grams

Saturated fat 5.2 grams

Total carbohydrates 11.3 grams

Dietary fiber 4.6 grams

For the salad:

4 cups chopped iceberg lettuce

3 cups of sliced raw vegetables, such as cucumber, cauliflower florets,
broccoli, green and red bell pepper, mushrooms, carrots and/or
red onion

2 ounces grilled skinless chicken breast, sliced

1 large hard-boiled egg, cut into quarters

1. Make the peanut sauce: Place the coconut milk and peanut butter in a
microwave-safe bowl and heat in a microwave on high power until hot but
not boiling, about 30 seconds, then whisk until well mixed. Add the sugar,
curry paste, fish sauce and 1 tablespoon of water, stir to mix well and
microwave on high power for about 15 seconds. (This makes about 1 cup
of peanut sauce. You can refrigerate the sauce for several days or freeze
individual ¼-cup servings and thaw them in the microwave.)

2. Assemble the salad: Using 2 cups for each serving, make a bed of
lettuce on 2 salad plates. Arrange the vegetables on the lettuce and
top with the chicken and egg quarters. Serve each
plate with ¼ cup of the warm peanut sauce on the
side for dipping or pouring over the salad.

Vegetarian variation: Thai tofu salad—Substitute
2 ounces of sliced Broiled Tofu (page 208) for the
chicken breast.

Nutritional information
per vegetarian serving
with ¼ cup peanut sauce:

Calories 244
Protein 14.1 grams
Total fat 12.0 grams
Saturated fat 5.0 grams
Total carbohydrates 11.4 grams
Dietary fiber 4.6 grams

Ⓥ

Curried Chicken Salad on Field Greens

Makes two servings

THIS RICH, FRAGRANT DISH, a variation on the recipe we use for chicken
salad sandwiches (page 161), is like magic—it makes only four ounces of
chicken go a long way.

½ cup low-fat plain yogurt
1 teaspoon brown sugar
¾ to 1 teaspoon curry powder
½ teaspoon lemon juice
4 ounces cooked skinless, boneless
    chicken breast (store-bought or leftover)
1 scallion, both white and green parts, thinly sliced
2 tablespoons thinly sliced celery
½ cup grapes, cut lengthwise in half
¼ cup small cubes of apple
1 tablespoon raisins
4 to 6 cups field greens
1 teaspoon extra-virgin olive oil
½ teaspoon balsamic vinegar
Salt and freshly ground black pepper

Nutritional information per serving:

Calories 249
Protein 23.2 grams
Total fat 7.9 grams
Saturated fat 1.6 grams
Total carbohydrates 23.1 grams
Dietary fiber 3.8 grams

1. Place the yogurt, brown sugar, curry powder and lemon juice in a medium-size bowl and stir to mix.

2. Cut the chicken into ½-inch or smaller cubes. Add the chicken, scallion, celery, grapes, apple and raisins to the bowl with the yogurt mixture and stir to coat.

3. Place the greens in a large bowl, add the olive oil and balsamic vinegar and toss to coat. Divide the greens between 2 salad plates, spoon the chicken salad on top and season with salt and pepper to taste.

Variation: Classic chicken salad—Omit the curry powder and add 1½ teaspoons chopped fresh tarragon or ½ teaspoon dried tarragon for a classic chicken salad.

Vegetarian variation: Curried tofu salad— Substitute 6 ounces of Broiled Tofu (page 208) for the chicken breast.

Nutritional information per vegetarian serving:

Calories 194
Protein 8.5 grams
Total fat 7.8 grams
Saturated fat 1.0 gram
Total carbohydrates 26.4 grams
Dietary fiber 5.1 grams

Ⓥ
Wheat Berry Salads

WHEAT BERRIES ARE SLOWLY DIGESTED and extremely chewy, which seems to further increase satiety. And they're a snap to cook. I love their taste, but after weight loss you can make these salads with cooked medium-grind bulgur wheat, if you prefer.

Wheat Berry and Cilantro Salad

Makes four ⅓-cup servings

1 cup cooked wheat berries (see opposite)
1 tablespoon olive oil or canola oil
½ tablespoon cider vinegar or wine vinegar
¼ cup finely chopped celery
¼ cup grated carrots
¼ cup finely chopped fresh cilantro
Salt and freshly ground black pepper

Nutritional information per ⅓-cup serving:	
Calories 66	
Protein 1.5 grams	
Total fat 3.3 grams	
Saturated fat 0.5 gram	
Total carbohydrates 8.4 grams	
Dietary fiber 1.5 grams	

Place the wheat berries, oil, vinegar, celery, carrots and cilantro in a bowl and stir to mix well. Season with salt and pepper to taste.

Wheat Berry, Raisin and Pine Nut Salad

Makes four ⅓-cup servings

1 cup cooked wheat berries (see opposite)
1 tablespoon olive oil or canola oil
½ tablespoon cider vinegar or wine vinegar
2 tablespoons raisins
¼ cup chopped fresh parsley
1 tablespoon pine nuts
Salt and freshly ground black pepper

Nutritional information per ⅓-cup serving:	
Calories 88	
Protein 1.9 grams	
Total fat 4.4 grams	
Saturated fat 0.7 gram	
Total carbohydrates 11.5 grams	
Dietary fiber 1.7 grams	

Place the wheat berries, oil, vinegar, raisins, parsley and pine nuts in a bowl and stir to mix well. Season with salt and pepper to taste.

Cooking Wheat Berries

Cover wheat berries with plenty of water and let simmer for 40 to 50 minutes until the berries start to break open. (The precise amount of water doesn't matter.) Or, if you're sufficiently organized, go green: Bring the wheat berries to a boil, turn off the heat and just let them sit for an hour or so before cooking. You'll be cutting the actual cooking time by more than half. Once the wheat berries are done, drain them.

(V)

Crispy Taco Pinto Bean Salad

Makes two servings

SUBSTITUTE CRUNCHY ICEBERG LETTUCE for calorie-laden taco shells and enjoy healthy Mexican food.

5 ounces cooked skinless, boneless chicken breast,
   or 5 ounces Broiled Tofu (page 208), diced
½ cup canned pinto beans, rinsed well and drained
4 cups chopped iceberg or romaine lettuce, plus
   lettuce leaves for serving
1 cup diced fresh tomato
2 scallions, both white and green parts,
   finely chopped
1 tablespoon chopped fresh cilantro
2 tablespoons fat-free Italian dressing
½ to 1 package taco seasoning mix
2 tablespoons nonfat sour cream
1 tablespoon grated Parmesan cheese, preferably imported
Hot sauce (optional)

> **Nutritional information per serving with chicken:**
> **Calories** 292
> **Protein** 31.2 grams
> **Total fat** 5.4 grams
> **Saturated fat** 1.3 grams
> **Total carbohydrates** 30.4 grams
> **Dietary fiber** 7.9 grams

Place the chicken or tofu, pinto beans, lettuce, tomato, scallions, cilantro and Italian dressing in a large bowl and stir to mix. Sprinkle the taco seasoning on top and mix again. Taste for seasoning, adding more taco mix as necessary. Serve the salad immediately on a bed of lettuce, topped with the sour cream, Parmesan cheese and hot sauce, if desired.

V

Hummus and Veggie Plate with Spicy Sesame Cracker Chips

Makes one serving

HUMMUS WITH REGULAR CRACKERS isn't great diet food—it can be just too easy to eat a whole meal's worth of calories without feeling satisfied. But paired with our high-fiber crackers or "I" Diet Soda Bread (page 160) and some good fresh crudités, it's perfect for weight control and makes an easy, satisfying meal.

½ cup baby carrots
2 to 3 ribs celery
½ medium-size green or red bell pepper
¼ cup store-bought hummus of your choice
9 Spicy Sesame Cracker Chips, or 2 slices
    low-carbohydrate bread, toasted

Slice the carrots, celery and bell pepper into crudités. Serve with the hummus and cracker chips or toast.

Nutritional information per serving:	
Calories 309	
Protein 13.0 grams	
Total fat 6.6 grams	
Saturated fat 1.1 grams	
Total carbohydrates 55.1 grams	
Dietary fiber 13.3 grams	

Spicy Sesame Cracker Chips
Makes about eighty-four 1 by 1½-inch crackers

Scientifically designed with several kinds of fiber and with an outer coating of the flavors found in regular chips, these sesame cracker chips taste good alone, with a dip or as part of a meal. (They can even pass as croutons on a salad.) But their real purpose is to satisfy your urge for a salty snack without inducing the more-more-more craving that comes with regular chips.

A single batch of cracker chips will see you through several weeks of weight loss, but plan ahead—you may need to order the corn bran and seasoning powder online.

2 cups coarse wheat bran
$^1/_4$ cup (1 ounce) corn bran (see Notes)
$^3/_4$ cup all-purpose flour
2 tablespoons sesame seeds
1 teaspoon dried instant yeast
1 teaspoon sugar
Scant $^1/_3$ cup (80 grams) tub margarine
2 to 3 teaspoons Cajun- or nacho cheese-flavor
   seasoning powder (see Notes)

> **Nutritional information per cracker chip:**
>
> **Calories** 15
> **Protein** 0.4 gram
> **Total fat** 0.9 gram
> **Saturated fat** 0.1 gram
> **Total carbohydrates** 2.0 grams
> **Dietary fiber** 0.9 gram

1. Preheat the oven to 325°F.

2. Place the wheat bran, corn bran, flour, sesame seeds, yeast and sugar in a bowl and mix them together. Rub in the margarine until the mixture has the texture of coarse meal, add ½ cup of water and knead until the dough is pliable but not sticky, 1 to 2 minutes.

3. Cut the dough into 3 pieces and roll it out as thin as you can, at least ⅛ of an inch thick. Sprinkle the dough well with some of the seasoning powder and cut it into 1 by 1½-inch rectangles. Arrange the rectangles of dough on a baking sheet with the unseasoned side facing up. Sprinkle the unseasoned side with seasoning powder.

4. Bake the cracker chips until crisp and very slightly browned, 20 to 25 minutes. Let the cracker chips cool before storing them in plastic bags.

NOTES One source for corn bran is www.honeyvillegrain.com. Seasoning powders are available from www.spicesetc.com.

(V)

Three-Bean Salad with Fresh Herbs

Makes 5¼ cups

EASY TO PUT TOGETHER, this is a great stand-alone main dish or a suitable dinner carbohydrate. The combination of cilantro and mint gives it a fresh flavor that is very satisfying. The salad will store well in the refrigerator, covered, for a few days.

3 cans (15 ounces each) different beans,
   such as pinto, black or cannellini,
   preferably with no added salt
¼ cup very finely chopped onion
2 tablespoons chopped fresh cilantro
2 teaspoons chopped fresh mint
2 tablespoons canola oil
2 tablespoons cider vinegar or wine vinegar
Salt (about ½ teaspoon if the beans had no salt)
   and freshly ground black pepper

> **Nutritional information per ½-cup serving:**
>
> **Calories** 110
> **Protein** 5.2 grams
> **Total fat** 2.6 grams
> **Saturated fat** 0.2 gram
> **Total carbohydrates** 1.6 grams
> **Dietary fiber** 6.1 grams

1. Rinse all of the beans really well and drain them.

2. Place the onion, cilantro, mint, oil and vinegar in a bowl and stir to mix well. Add the beans and mix again, then season with salt and pepper to taste.

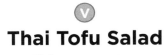

Thai Tofu Salad

Makes two servings

THIS THAI SALAD IS A TERRIFIC WAY to use up leftover broiled tofu at lunch. The cilantro and basil give it a lovely pungency.

For the salad:
4 cups chopped romaine lettuce
½ cup bean sprouts
½ cup thinly sliced cucumber
1 large carrot, shredded
¼ cup chopped fresh basil leaves
2 tablespoons chopped fresh cilantro
4 ounces Broiled Tofu (page 208), sliced
½ cup canned black beans, rinsed and drained
¼ cup frozen green peas, thawed

> **Nutritional information per serving:**
>
> **Calories** 337
> **Protein** 14.5 grams
> **Total fat** 12.8 grams
> **Saturated fat** 1.6 grams
> **Total carbohydrates** 46.0 grams
> **Dietary fiber** 10.6 grams

For the dressing:

1 clove garlic, peeled and crushed

1/3 cup fresh lime juice

2 tablespoons soy sauce

2 tablespoons brown sugar

1 1/2 tablespoons canola oil

1/2 teaspoon finely minced peeled fresh ginger

Salt and freshly ground black pepper

Sugar substitute (optional)

1 tablespoon chopped fresh mint leaves, for garnish

1 teaspoon sesame seeds (optional)

1. Make the salad: Place the lettuce, bean sprouts, cucumber, carrot, basil and cilantro in a large bowl and stir to mix. Arrange the lettuce mixture on 2 plates and top with the tofu slices, black beans and green peas.

2. Make the dressing: Place the garlic, lime juice, soy sauce, brown sugar, oil and ginger in a bowl and whisk to mix. Add salt and pepper to taste and sugar substitute for a sweeter dressing. Pour the dressing over the salads and garnish with the mint and sesame seeds, if using.

Ⓥ

Mixed Fruit with Yogurt Dip

Makes one serving

SOMETIMES NOTHING TASTES BETTER than a lunch of fruit in season. Add a yogurt dip and it's practically decadent.

2 cups sliced or small whole ripe fruit, such as pear, apple, peach, apricot, kiwi, strawberries, grapes, cherries and/or blackberries

1/2 cup sugar-free, low-fat plain yogurt

Rinse the fruit under cold running water and pat dry with paper towels. Serve the fruit nicely arranged on a plate with a bowl of the yogurt for dipping.

Nutritional information per serving:
Calories 225
Protein 7.4 grams
Total fat 1.7 grams
Saturated fat 0.3 gram
Total carbohydrates 50.1 grams
Dietary fiber 7.7 grams

Main Dishes

RARE IS THE PERSON WHO DOESN'T ENJOY a good dinner after a busy day. Scientifically designed to please, our "I" Diet main dishes are packed full of familiar rich flavors with plenty of protein, fiber and volume to leave you satisfied and comfortably full. I serve many of these dishes to non-dieting dinner companions and get rave reviews, so don't feel you have to keep them to yourself!

A Really Good Hamburger

Vegetarian Burger Delight Ⓥ

Florentine Steak

Veal Scaloppine in Creamy Mushroom Sauce

Grilled Pork Tenderloin
Hoisin Pork
BBQ Pork

Home Run Hot Dogs Ⓥ

Mexican Lettuce Wraps Ⓥ

Tanzanian Chicken Kebabs

Arista Chicken

Chicken Parm

Perfect Grill with Creamy Mustard Sauce Ⓥ

Haddock with Tomato-Cumin Sauce

Baked Salmon with Lemon-Dill Sauce

Seafood Stew in Tamarind Broth

Cajun Cod

Spicy Tofu and Mixed Vegetable Stir-Fry ⓥ

A Taste for Tofu ⓥ

Broiled Tofu
Tofu Alfredo
Tofu Parmigiana

Hoisin Tofu ⓥ

Steamed Tofu and Mixed Vegetables with Warm Peanut Sauce ⓥ

No-Fuss Pizza ⓥ

Barbecue Vegetable Pizza ⓥ

John's Pasta Supper

Northern Italian Lasagna ⓥ
"I" Diet Béchamel Sauce

Stuffed Green Peppers ⓥ

Boiled Barley ⓥ

Mushroom and Barley Risotto ⓥ

Keep-Your-Kids-Company "Macaroni and Cheese" ⓥ

Mixed Vegetable Curry ⓥ

Chickpea Masala ⓥ

Moong Dal Stew ⓥ
Lemon and Date Chutney

West African Bean Cakes with Spicy Dip and Green Salad ⓥ

See also Bonus Recipes, pages 262–69

A Really Good Hamburger

Makes four burgers

WHO SAYS YOU HAVE TO GIVE UP HAMBURGERS? Not me! Just eat them at home, where you can control the ingredients (and the portion size). Start with the leanest ground beef, then gather up plenty of flavorful toppings and some low-carb bread rolls. You can eat your hamburger open-face or scoop out the middle of each bun half so you can hold it like a regular burger. If you start the meal with cooked vegetables, you'll fill up and barely miss the French fries.

1 pound extra-lean ground beef
4 low-carbohydrate hamburger buns, middles
    cut out (see Notes)
Plenty of good, healthy toppings per person, such as:
    2 to 3 thin tomato slices
    1 very thin onion slice
    3 to 4 thin dill pickle slices
    1 to 2 crisp lettuce leaves
    1 tablespoon ketchup, low-fat Thousand Island
      dressing or barbecue sauce
    Sautéed sliced mushrooms (see Notes)
    1 tablespoon caramelized onion (page 259)
    1 teaspoon crumbled blue cheese or grated Parmesan cheese,
      preferably imported

Nutritional information per 1-hamburger serving:

Calories 263	
Protein 30.1 grams	
Total fat 8.0 grams	
Saturated fat 2.6 grams	
Total carbohydrates 18.7 grams	
Dietary fiber 3.1 grams	

1. Preheat the grill to high. You can also cook the hamburgers in a frying pan on the stove; there's no need to use any oil.

2. Divide the meat into 4 equal portions and shape each into a patty slightly larger than the buns.

3. When the grill is ready, cook the burgers until well done, 2 to 3 minutes on each side.

4. At the last minute, briefly toast the insides of the buns on the grill or in the frying pan so they're slightly browned.

5. Assemble the burgers, adding the toppings.

NOTES If you can't get low-carb hamburger buns, you can substitute half a 100% whole-wheat roll for each serving.

Cook ½ cup of sliced mushrooms per person over high heat in ¼ teaspoon of tub margarine until lightly browned.

(V)

Vegetarian Burger Delight

Makes eight burgers

TO AVOID THE "TOO STARCHY" TASTE that you get with many homemade vegetarian burgers, give this "I" Diet treat a try. Serve the burgers the conventional way with a roll and ketchup or on their own. Freeze individual burgers for later. You may never go back to meat!

For the burgers:
2 medium-size onions, quartered
1 cup baby carrots
8 ounces white button mushrooms
½ cup grated Parmesan cheese, preferably imported
¼ teaspoon salt
¼ teaspoon freshly ground black pepper
4 teaspoons canola or similar oil

For serving, per burger:
1 low-carbohydrate roll
2 teaspoons ketchup
1 teaspoon relish
As much lettuce and thinly sliced onion as you like

Nutritional information per 1-burger serving, including roll, ketchup and relish:
Calories 193
Protein 9.8 grams
Total fat 7.0 grams
Saturated fat 2.3 grams
Total carbohydrates 27.5 grams
Dietary fiber 6.0 grams

1. Place the onion quarters and carrots in a food processor and run the machine until the mixture is almost smooth. Add the mushrooms and run the machine again until only tiny particles are left. Place the vegetable mixture in a nonstick pan without oil over medium heat and cook until the excess liquid has evaporated, about 10 minutes. You may need to reduce the heat to low and cook the mixture a little longer if it starts to stick before the liquid has evaporated.

2. Add the Parmesan cheese, salt and pepper to the vegetable mixture and stir to mix. Divide the mixture into 8 portions and shape into patties.

3. Heat the oil in a skillet over medium heat. Cook the patties until lightly browned and crisp, about 4 minutes on each side. Be gentle when you turn the patties over—the burgers will not be as solid as regular burgers.

4. Serve the burgers immediately in the rolls, accompanied by ketchup, relish, lettuce and sliced onion, or freeze individually wrapped burgers. You can reheat the frozen burgers in a 400°F oven for about 7 minutes.

Florentine Steak

Makes two 4-ounce servings

FOOD IS OFTEN BEST when simply prepared. The Florentine method of grilling lean steak—with just a little olive oil, crushed garlic, salt and black pepper—is delicious and easy, too.

1 teaspoon extra-virgin olive oil
8 ounces lean tender beefsteak,
    about 1 inch thick
1 clove garlic, peeled and crushed
Salt and freshly ground black pepper

Nutritional information per serving:

Calories 198
Protein 24.5 grams
Total fat 10.3 grams
Saturated fat 3.4 grams
Total carbohydrates 0.6 gram
Dietary fiber 0.1 gram

1. Preheat the grill to high or heat a heavy grill pan over high heat.

2. Spread the olive oil on both sides of the steak. Spread the crushed garlic over the steak and sprinkle it with a little salt and plenty of black pepper.

3. Grill the steak until done to your liking, 2 to 5 minutes per side on high for medium-well to well-done.

Veal Scaloppine in Creamy Mushroom Sauce

Makes four servings

THE THIN SLICES OF VEAL SCALOPPINE go a long way. A two-ounce portion is enough to satisfy, especially in this appetizing recipe. Truffle oil makes the dish special and can be obtained from Italian markets, on the web and in upscale cooking stores like Williams-Sonoma.

About 2 teaspoons olive oil

8 ounces white button mushrooms, sliced (about 3 cups)

8 ounces veal scaloppine (pound them 1/8 inch thin, or ask your butcher to do this)

2 teaspoons all-purpose flour

1/3 cup nonfat or 1% milk

1 tablespoon brandy

1 tablespoon lemon juice

1 teaspoon sugar

Salt and freshly ground black pepper

1 teaspoon black truffle oil (optional)

Chopped fresh parsley (optional), for garnish

> **Nutritional information per serving:**
>
> **Calories** 139
>
> **Protein** 11.0 grams
>
> **Total fat** 7.4 grams
>
> **Saturated fat** 2.2 grams
>
> **Total carbohydrates** 5.7 grams
>
> **Dietary fiber** 0.8 gram

1. Wipe a little olive oil in a saucepan and heat it over high heat. Add the mushrooms and cook, stirring frequently, until browned, about 3 minutes. The mushrooms will release liquid, but this will evaporate before they're nicely browned. Transfer the mushrooms to a bowl and cover with aluminum foil to keep warm.

2. Add 1 teaspoon of olive oil to the saucepan along with the veal and cook until the slices are very lightly browned, 1 to 2 minutes per side, working in batches if necessary. Remove the veal from the pan and reduce the heat to low.

3. Add the remaining 1 teaspoon of olive oil and the flour to the pan and cook until the mixture starts to froth. Then add the milk and brandy and stir to mix well, scraping any brown bits off the bottom of the pan.

4. Add the lemon juice and sugar to the sauce and season with salt and pepper to taste. Stir in the truffle oil, if using.

5. Spoon the mushrooms over the veal and top with the sauce. Serve immediately, topped with parsley, if desired.

Grilled Pork Tenderloin

PORK TENDERLOIN IS VERSATILE, quick to cook . . . and a great diet food. Ounce for ounce, it has no more fat than chicken breast.

Hoisin Pork

Makes three 4-ounce servings

This Chinese-style pork dish is easy to prepare and sure to win accolades from all who try it.

½ cup hoisin sauce
1 tablespoon finely chopped peeled fresh ginger
3 cloves garlic, finely minced
2 tablespoons finely chopped onion
¼ cup dry white wine
1 pork tenderloin, about 12 ounces

> Nutritional information per serving of Hoisin Pork or BBQ Pork:
>
> **Calories** 196
> **Protein** 27.0 grams
> **Total fat** 5.2 grams
> **Saturated fat** 1.6 grams
> **Total carbohydrates** 8.3 grams
> **Dietary fiber** 0.8 gram

1. Mix the hoisin sauce, ginger, garlic, onion and white wine together. Place the pork tenderloin in a baking dish and spoon the hoisin marinade over it. Let the pork marinate in the refrigerator, covered, for 6 to 12 hours.

2. Preheat the grill to medium or preheat the oven to 425°F.

3. Grill the pork, turning once, or bake it until the inside has lost its pink color, about 25 minutes total.

BBQ Pork

Makes three 4-ounce servings

Serve this dish with a big green salad or Southern style with Zesty Baked Beans (page 232) or Black-Eyed Peas (page 234) and a green vegetable such as Healthy Collard Greens (page 228).

1 tablespoon barbecue sauce for the pork, plus more for serving
1 pork tenderloin, about 12 ounces
Salt and freshly ground black pepper
Cooking oil spray

1. Preheat the grill to medium or preheat the oven to 425°F.

2. Spread the barbecue sauce over the pork tenderloin, season it with salt and pepper to taste and spray it with cooking oil spray.

3. Grill the pork, turning once, or bake it until the inside has lost its pink color, about 25 minutes total.

4. Serve the pork sliced, with more barbecue sauce on the side.

Ⓥ

Home Run Hot Dogs

Makes four servings of two hot dogs each

I LOVE THE HOT DOGS you can get from the Italian carts outside Fenway Park in Boston, so I looked for a way to re-create that experience using lower-calorie chicken, turkey or tofu hot dogs. The secret is serving them with lots of onions and sweet peppers. Skip the rolls until you're past active weight loss, or use your 100-calorie free-choice allowance in Stage II for a low-carb bun.

2 large red bell peppers
2 tablespoons canola or peanut oil
2 large onions, sliced
Salt
8 regular-size chicken, turkey or
    tofu hot dogs
8 teaspoons sharp mustard
    (Nathan's is wonderful with this recipe),
    for serving
4 tablespoons ketchup, for serving

Nutritional information per serving:
Calories 189
Protein 16.3 grams
Total fat 16.2 grams
Saturated fat 3.0 grams
Total carbohydrates 21.1 grams
Dietary fiber 4.3 grams

1. Core, quarter and slice the bell peppers.

2. Heat the oil in a heavy-bottomed pot over low heat, then add the bell peppers and onions. Cook over low heat until the onions are soft and lightly golden, 45 minutes or longer, and season with salt to taste.

3. Add the hot dogs to the pot with the peppers and onions, cover the pot and let cook until the hot dogs are heated through, about 5 minutes.

4. Serve the hot dogs with the mustard and ketchup.

(V)

Mexican Lettuce Wraps

Makes twelve wraps; serves four

WHEN YOU'RE IN THE MOOD for Mexican food, here's a way to get your fix with fewer calories. It's okay to let family members who are not on a diet use taco shells rather than the lettuce wraps. Just don't be tempted to nibble!

For the filling:

1 tablespoon olive oil
½ pound ground white meat turkey or extra-lean (90% to 95%) ground beef
1 can (15 ounces) pinto beans, rinsed and drained
1 package taco seasoning mix

For serving:

12 whole iceberg lettuce leaves
½ cup nonfat sour cream
½ cup salsa (see Note)
3 tablespoons grated Parmesan cheese, preferably imported

Nutritional information per 3-wrap serving:

Calories: 270	
Protein: 23.9 grams	
Total fat: 7.3 grams	
Saturated fat: 2.5 grams	
Total carbohydrates 26.9 grams	
Dietary fiber: 7.8 grams	

1. Heat the olive oil in a saucepan over high heat. Add the turkey or beef and cook until browned all over, 3 to 5 minutes.

2. Add the pinto beans, taco seasoning and 1 cup of water. Cover the pan, reduce the heat and let simmer for 10 minutes. Then, if necessary, stir the filling and let it simmer, uncovered, for a few minutes until it thickens.

3. Serve about ¼ cup of the filling wrapped in each lettuce leaf with some sour cream, salsa and a sprinkling of Parmesan cheese.

NOTE You can either use store-bought salsa or make your own: Mix 1 chopped medium-size tomato together with 1 tablespoon of chopped onion and 1 tablespoon of chopped fresh cilantro. Season with salt and freshly ground black pepper to taste.

Vegetarian variation: This recipe can also be made meat-free. Instead of ground turkey or beef, use 8 ounces of firm light tofu cut into small strips. Add 1 teaspoon more olive oil to compensate for the lack of oil in the tofu.

> Nutritional information
> per 3-wrap vegetarian
> serving:
> **Calories** 240
> **Protein** 15.9 grams
> **Total fat** 6.3 grams
> **Saturated fat** 1.0 gram
> **Total carbohydrates** 30.1 grams
> **Dietary fiber** 8.3 grams

Tanzanian Chicken Kebabs

Makes eighteen skewers

ZANZIBAR, TANZANIA, LIES AT THE CROSSROADS of the historical Indian-African-Arab-European trading routes, and its rich, spicy fusion food is pure gastronomic heaven. Bakari Hamdan, former chef of the Matemwe Beach Village guesthouse in Zanzibar, explains that it isn't just the careful balance of freshly ground spices and other ingredients that makes this food so special; cutting meat up small not only makes a little of an expensive food go a long way but allows the spices to permeate for a richer flavor. How lucky that this delicious but simple recipe has the low calories and perfect nutritional balance to make it an honorable weight-loss staple.

Chef Bakari says he hopes you *chakula chema*—Swahili for "enjoy your meal." Serve the *mishkaki*—kebabs—with a large tossed salad and a bowl of cucumber slices mixed with plain yogurt and a little chopped mint and salt. Add some whole-grain rice or chapati on the side for non-dieters, and round out your dinner with sliced ripe tropical fruit, such as mango, and a cup of Masala Tea (page 252) or Kenyan Chai (page 251). Any leftover kebabs can be put to good use when preparing the Indian Kebab Wraps on page 165.

1 pound skinless, boneless chicken breasts
2 tablespoons olive oil
2 tablespoons nonfat plain yogurt
2 tablespoons ground cumin
2 teaspoons very coarsely ground black pepper
   (see Note)
1 piece (1 inch by 1½ inches) fresh ginger,
   peeled and grated
3 to 4 large garlic cloves, peeled and crushed
1 teaspoon salt
18 bamboo skewers

Nutritional information per 3-skewer serving:

Calories 153
Protein 20.1 grams
Total fat 6.2 grams
Saturated fat 1.2 grams
Total carbohydrates 2.9 grams
Dietary fiber 0.5 gram

1. Cut the chicken into very small pieces, approximately 1 inch by ½ inch by ½ inch; you should have about 72 pieces.

2. Place the olive oil, yogurt, cumin, pepper, ginger, garlic and salt in a glass or stainless-steel bowl and stir to mix. Add the chicken and stir until it's well coated. Cover and let marinate in the refrigerator for 2 hours or as long as overnight.

3. Preheat the grill to high and soak the bamboo skewers in water to cover for 30 minutes to keep them from burning.

4. Put about 4 pieces of chicken on each skewer the long way, so they almost touch. Grill the kebabs until just cooked through and nicely browned, about 1 minute per side.

NOTE Grind the pepper on the coarsest setting; if it's too finely ground, the dish will be too spicy.

Arista Chicken

Makes eight servings of about 4 ounces each

IN ITALY, THERE'S A DISH OF ROAST PORK called *arista*. According to legend, Greek bishops visiting Florence for the Ecumenical Council of 1450 exclaimed *"Aristos!"* ("the best" in Greek) after a fine dinner—and the name stuck. In this adaptation of the classic recipe, starting with bone-in chicken breasts helps keep the meat moist during cooking. Before serving the most tender, yummy chicken breasts that ever were, just discard the skin and bones. I serve Arista Chicken fresh and hot with cooked vegetables and Tuscan Beans (page 233) and use leftovers as a fine addition to a green salad.

4 tablespoons chopped fresh rosemary leaves,
  or 4 teaspoons dried rosemary (see Note)
4 large cloves garlic, chopped
2 tablespoons olive oil
1½ teaspoons salt
1½ teaspoons very coarse freshly
  ground black pepper
2 large chicken breasts with skin and
  bones (about 3 pounds total)

> **Nutritional information per 4-ounce serving:**
> **Calories** 180
> **Protein** 26.2 grams
> **Total fat** 4.5 grams
> **Saturated fat** 1.5 grams
> **Total carbohydrates** 8.9 grams
> **Dietary fiber** 3.0 grams

1. Mix the fresh or dried rosemary, garlic, olive oil, salt and pepper together in a small bowl.

2. Using your hands (there is no other way to do this), work most of the rosemary mixture under the skin of the chicken breasts. Rub the remaining rosemary mixture over the skin and bones. Cover the chicken breasts with plastic wrap and refrigerate them for 4 to 10 hours to let the flavors infuse well.

3. Preheat the oven to 375°F.

4. Bake the chicken until the skin is golden brown and the juices run clear when you stick a fork in the thickest part, 1 to 1¼ hours. (An instant-read thermometer should register 165°F when inserted in the thickest part of a breast but not touching the bone.) You can baste the chicken a few times as it bakes, but it will come out fine if you don't.

5. Remove and discard the skin and bones from the chicken before serving.

NOTE To rehydrate dried rosemary, place it in a microwave-safe dish with 1 teaspoon of water and microwave on high power for 10 seconds.

Chicken Parm

Makes four servings

YOU DON'T HAVE TO GO WITHOUT chicken parmigiana on the "I" Diet, and the combination of tomato sauce and cheese is similar enough to pizza to help you through our no-pizza Stage I.

Cooking oil spray
8 ounces white button mushrooms (optional),
    sliced (about 3 cups)
2 skinless, boneless chicken breast halves
    (about 1 pound total)
½ teaspoon salt
1 cup store-bought low-fat pizza sauce
¼ cup grated Parmesan cheese, preferably imported
1 sprig fresh basil, chopped (optional)

Nutritional information per serving with mushrooms:	
Calories 192	
Protein 31.0 grams	
Total fat 3.7 grams	
Saturated fat 1.6 grams	
Total carbohydrates 7.5 grams	
Dietary fiber 1.9 grams	

1. Preheat the oven to 400°F.

2. If you're using mushrooms, spray a frying pan with cooking oil and cook them on high heat, stirring, until lightly browned, about 3 minutes.

3. Place a chicken breast half on a cutting board and, using a sharp knife, make a cut into the thickest part parallel to the cutting board so you "butterfly" the breast to open it out flatter. Repeat with the remaining half chicken breast.

4. Place a piece of aluminum foil on a baking sheet and spray it with cooking oil. Arrange the chicken breasts on the foil, salt them lightly and top them with the mushrooms, if using, and the pizza sauce.

5. Pull the aluminum foil up so that it partially covers the chicken and bake the chicken until it's cooked and the juices run clear when you stick a fork in the thickest part, 30 to 40 minutes.

6. Remove the chicken from the foil and top with the Parmesan cheese (it will melt). Serve the chicken immediately, sprinkled with the chopped basil, if using.

Variation: Mexican chicken (a high-fiber version)— Follow the recipe for Chicken Parm, substituting salsa for the pizza sauce and sprinkling only 2 tablespoons of Parmesan cheese on top after baking. Serve the cooked chicken with ½ cup of nonfat refried beans in place of dessert, sprinkling the remaining 2 tablespoons of Parmesan over the beans along with the chopped green parts of scallions, and perhaps have ¾ teaspoon of fat-free sour cream and fresh salsa on the side for each serving.

Nutritional information per serving with refried beans:
Calories 281
Protein 35.8 grams
Total fat 4.5 grams
Saturated fat 1.9 grams
Total carbohydrates 29.2 grams
Dietary fiber 7.8 grams

(V)

Perfect Grill
with Creamy Mustard Sauce

Makes four servings

EVERY DIETER SHOULD HAVE a simple grilling recipe on hand. This one uses a marinade that works equally well with any meat or tofu. Be sure to choose a lean protein source like shrimp, chicken or tofu; most of the oil isn't absorbed, but it's important to keep an eye on total calories—you don't want them to get too high.

If the weather is too cold or wet to grill on the day you decide to use this recipe, just turn on your oven and bake everything instead.

For the grill:

1 pound peeled and deveined raw shrimp, skinless, boneless chicken breast or firm light tofu

8 cups or more cut-up nonstarchy raw veggies, such as mushrooms, onion and zucchini slices, asparagus spears, quarters of green and red bell pepper and green beans (see Notes)

For the marinade:

½ cup canola oil

¼ cup cider vinegar

Piece of lemon peel (optional)

2 cloves garlic, crushed and peeled

1 teaspoon salt

½ teaspoon freshly ground black pepper

¼ cup chopped fresh herbs, such as basil or parsley, or 1 tablespoon dried rosemary or oregano (see Notes)

For the creamy mustard sauce:

¼ cup low-fat plain yogurt

¼ cup whole-grain mustard

> **Nutritional information per serving of shrimp or chicken with sauce and vegetables:**
>
> **Calories** 294
>
> **Protein** 31.9 grams
>
> **Total fat** 15.0 grams
>
> **Saturated fat** 2.6 grams
>
> **Total carbohydrates** 10.6 grams
>
> **Dietary fiber** 3.9 grams

> **Nutritional information per serving of tofu with sauce and vegetables:**
>
> **Calories** 231
>
> **Protein** 16.8 grams
>
> **Total fat** 16.9 grams
>
> **Saturated fat** 2.4 grams
>
> **Total carbohydrates** 11.6 grams
>
> **Dietary fiber** 4.6 grams

1. Preheat the grill to high or preheat the oven to 450°F.

2. If you're using shrimp or chicken, rinse it under cold running water and pat dry with paper towels. If using tofu, drain it, slice it about ¾ inch thick and let it stand while you prepare the marinade.

3. Prepare the marinade: Mix the oil, cider vinegar, lemon peel, if using, garlic, salt, black pepper and herbs together in a baking dish.

4. Add the shrimp, chicken or sliced tofu and the vegetables to the baking dish. Turn to coat well and let marinate for 5 minutes—longer if you like for chicken (this makes enough marinade for up to 2 pounds if you want to feed more people).

5. Grill or bake the shrimp or chicken until cooked through, 2 to 4 minutes for the shrimp, 15 to 25 minutes for the chicken (to test for doneness, make a cut in the thickest part of the breast; it should have lost almost all of its pinkness when cooked through). Grill or bake tofu for 10 to 14 minutes; grill or bake the vegetables 10 to 15 minutes. Use a perforated metal plate to hold the shrimp or tofu and vegetables on the grill.

6. Make the mustard sauce: Mix the yogurt and mustard together in a small bowl. Serve the sauce on the side.

NOTES If cooking chicken and using dried oregano as the herb, squeezing fresh lemon juice on the chicken as it grills makes a wonderfully fragrant Greek grill.

Two cups of raw vegetables will make about 1½ cups when cooked.

Variation: For a Southern barbecue treat, spread 2 teaspoons of barbecue sauce lightly on the cooked meat and serve with Healthy Collard Greens (page 228) and Black-Eyed Peas (page 234).

Haddock
with Tomato-Cumin Sauce

Makes six servings

LET ME COUNT THE WAYS in which haddock and other white fish are a special diet food. First, they taste great. Second, they're a terrific protein source with one of the lowest calorie counts out there—more satisfying calorie for calorie than other high-protein foods like chicken and beef. And third, they're a good source of the omega-3 fatty acid DHA, which appears to offer protection against the neurological degeneration that can occur in older people. In this adapted recipe, cumin is the magic ingredient; it transforms the haddock from a mild white fish into a tangy taste treat. Thanks go to Diane Forley, former chef and owner of Verbena Restaurant in New York City and author of *The Anatomy of a Dish*.

The tomato-cumin sauce is best made a day in advance and refrigerated overnight to let the flavor develop.

2 tablespoons extra-virgin olive oil

1 medium-size onion, cut in half lengthwise
    and sliced

2 ribs celery, trimmed and cut into thin lengths

³/₄ pound Swiss chard, stems cut into thin
    2-inch lengths, leaves chopped

Salt and freshly ground black pepper

1 tablespoon ground cumin

1 tablespoon cracked coriander seeds

4 cups canned tomatoes with their juice, chopped

2 tablespoons sugar

Pinch of cayenne pepper

4 haddock fillets (about 6 ounces each)

Nutritional information
per serving:

Calories 226

Protein 24.6 grams

Total fat 2.1 grams

Saturated fat 0.3 gram

Total carbohydrates 19.9 grams

Dietary fiber 3.4 grams

1. Heat the olive oil in a large, deep skillet over medium heat. Add the onion, celery and chard stems and season with salt and pepper to taste. Cook, stirring frequently, until the vegetables soften slightly, about 5 minutes. Add the cumin and coriander seeds and cook until fragrant. Add the tomatoes and their juice, the sugar and 3 cups of water and let come to a simmer. Add the chard leaves and cayenne and let simmer until the sauce is flavorful and the oil begins to float to the surface, about 40 minutes. Let the sauce cool, then place it in a bowl and keep it, covered, overnight in the refrigerator.

2. When it's time to cook the fish, put the sauce back in a deep skillet and bring it to a simmer. Season the haddock fillets with salt and pepper to taste and add them to the sauce. Spoon a little of the sauce over the fillets and cook, covered, until the fish is just done, about 5 minutes (test by lifting a fillet out of the sauce and sticking a knife in the center—if it flakes, the fish is done).

3. Spoon the fish and sauce into bowls and serve.

Baked Salmon with Lemon-Dill Sauce

Makes four 4-ounce servings

SOME OILY FISHES, like tuna and swordfish, probably shouldn't be eaten too frequently because of their higher mercury levels. Salmon, however, is safe to eat whenever you want. And it contains plentiful amounts of those healthful omega-3 oils (a hefty 1,457 milligrams per 100 grams, or eight times the daily amount of 180 milligrams believed to reduce neurological symptoms in older people). This salmon dish is also good served plain with lemon wedges—and you'll save 19 calories per serving.

For the salmon:

1 pound salmon fillets

1 tablespoon chopped fresh dill, or 1 teaspoon dried dill

Salt and freshly ground black pepper

For the sauce:

1/2 cup low-fat plain yogurt

2 tablespoons lemon juice

1 teaspoon sugar

3/4 teaspoon chopped fresh dill, or 1/4 teaspoon dried dill

1/8 teaspoon salt

Freshly ground black pepper

Nutritional information per serving with sauce:
Calories 216
Protein 24.0 grams
Total fat 12.7 grams
Saturated fat 0.3 gram
Total carbohydrates 2.5 grams
Dietary fiber 0 grams

1. Prepare the salmon: Preheat the oven to 375°F.

2. Line a roasting pan with aluminum foil and place the salmon on top. Sprinkle the dill over the salmon and season with salt and pepper to taste. Partially pull the foil over the salmon so that about half of the fish is loosely covered.

3. Bake the salmon until it breaks into flakes when pierced in the thickest part with a fork, about 30 minutes.

4. Make the sauce: Place the yogurt, lemon juice, sugar, dill and salt in a small bowl and stir to mix. Season with pepper to taste. Serve the lemon-dill sauce on the side.

Seafood Stew in Tamarind Broth

Makes five servings

THIS IS A PERFECT "I" DIET DISH, with loads of lean seafood protein and healthy fiber-filled vegetables. A true masterpiece, it's from Lynne Aronson and Elizabeth Simon's cookbook *BowlFood*.

2 carrots, peeled and cut into 3-inch lengths
1 pound calabaza or winter squash, peeled,
    seeded and cut into 3 large wedges
2 cups Tamarind Broth
2 tablespoons hoisin sauce
1 pound thick white fish fillets (bass, halibut or
    snapper), cut into 2-ounce pieces
1/2 pound medium-size shrimp, peeled and deveined
1/2 pound squid, cleaned and cut into 1-inch strips
Salt and freshly ground black pepper
3 scallions, both white and green parts, chopped, for garnish
1/2 fresh jalapeño pepper, stemmed and minced, with seeds, for garnish

> **Nutritional information per serving:**
>
> **Calories** 268
> **Protein** 34.7 grams
> **Total fat** 3.9 grams
> **Saturated fat** 0.8 gram
> **Total carbohydrates** 17.7 grams
> **Dietary fiber** 2.4 grams

1. Preheat the oven to 250°F.

2. Bring a medium-size saucepan of salted water to a boil over medium heat. Add the carrots and let simmer until softened, about 5 minutes. Using a slotted spoon, transfer the carrots to a large ovenproof serving bowl and keep warm in the preheated oven.

3. Add the squash to the same pan of boiling water and let simmer until softened, about 5 minutes. Transfer the squash to the bowl with the carrots and keep warm. Discard the cooking water.

4. Combine the Tamarind Broth and hoisin sauce in the saucepan, bring to a boil over medium heat and let simmer for about 3 minutes. Add the fish fillets and simmer until just cooked through, about 3 minutes. Using a slotted spoon, transfer the fish to the bowl with the vegetables.

5. Add the shrimp to the broth mixture and simmer until just cooked through, about 3 minutes. Using a slotted spoon, transfer the shrimp to the bowl with the vegetables.

6. Add the squid to the broth mixture and let simmer until just done, about 3 minutes. Using a slotted spoon, transfer the squid to the bowl with the vegetables.

7. Season the hot cooking liquid with salt and pepper to taste, then strain it over the vegetables and seafood. Sprinkle the scallions and jalapeño on top and serve.

Tamarind Broth
Makes about 3 cups

Any leftover broth makes a fantastic base for Pork and Lemongrass Soup (page 153) diluted with an equal amount of water. If you make the soup this way, there's no need to add the lemongrass. I find the broth delicious without adding any sugar, and this saves you about 20 calories per cup.

4 cups chicken stock
3 scallions, both white and green parts, chopped
¼ cup tamarind concentrate
¼ cup peeled chopped fresh ginger
¼ cup soy sauce
2 tablespoons sugar
4½ teaspoons rice vinegar
1 stalk lemongrass, chopped
1 whole star anise
½ fresh serrano pepper, stemmed, with seeds,
    cut in half and chopped

Nutritional information per cup of broth:	
Calories 84	
Protein 4.6 grams	
Total fat 0.7 gram	
Saturated fat 0 grams	
Total carbohydrates 15.8 grams	
Dietary fiber 0.9 gram	

1. Combine the chicken stock, scallions, tamarind concentrate, ginger, soy sauce, sugar, rice vinegar, lemongrass, star anise and serrano pepper in a stockpot and bring to a boil over medium heat. Reduce the heat to low and let simmer, uncovered, for 30 minutes.

2. Remove the broth from the heat and strain through a fine sieve into a medium-size heatproof bowl. Press on the solids with the back of a spoon to extract as much liquid as possible. Use the broth immediately, or let it cool, transfer it to airtight containers and refrigerate it for up to 1 week or freeze it for up to 1 month.

Cajun Cod

Makes four 4-ounce servings

COD IS JUST TERRIFIC DIET FOOD and easier to find really fresh than some other fishes that get shipped halfway around the world. This tasty dish is ready to bake in no time and is particularly good because it adds the satiety benefit of spices to the already high satiety of fish protein.

1 pound cod, pollock or other white fish fillets
1½ teaspoons Cajun seasoning
Sprinkle of salt
Cooking oil spray (not butter flavor)
Lemon quarters, for serving
Chopped fresh parsley (optional), for serving

Nutritional information per serving:	
Calories 111	
Protein 21.5 grams	
Total fat 2.0 grams	
Saturated fat 0.4 gram	
Total carbohydrates 1.0 gram	
Dietary fiber 0.3 gram	

1. Preheat the oven to 400°F.

2. Rinse the fish under cold running water and pat it dry with paper towels. Sprinkle the Cajun seasoning and salt over the fish, then spray it lightly with the cooking oil spray.

3. Bake the fish until it breaks into flakes when pierced in the thickest part with a fork, about 30 minutes.

4. Serve the fish with lemon quarters and sprinkle chopped parsley on top, if desired.

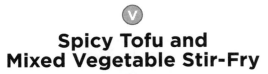

Spicy Tofu and Mixed Vegetable Stir-Fry

Makes three servings

THE STRONG FLAVORINGS of this stir-fry make the tofu seem not just a reasonable substitute for meat but indeed a better alternative. Serve it with low-sodium soy sauce if you'd like, plus some rice for non-dieting family members.

14 ounces firm light tofu
1½ tablespoons dry sherry or rice wine
2½ teaspoons hoisin sauce
2 teaspoons bean paste
½ teaspoon chile paste with garlic (optional)
4 teaspoons canola or corn oil
1 small onion, finely chopped
2 cloves garlic, finely chopped
1 piece (1 inch) fresh ginger, peeled and grated
6 cups mixed vegetables, such as sliced carrots,
     snow peas, sliced green and/or red bell pepper, sliced Chinese cabbage,
     tiny broccoli florets, sliced mushrooms and/or sliced zucchini
6 ounces bean sprouts

> **Nutritional information per 2-cup serving:**
> **Calories** 264
> **Protein** 21.9 grams
> **Total fat** 11.0 grams
> **Saturated fat** 1.5 grams
> **Total carbohydrates** 23.6 grams
> **Dietary fiber** 7.0 grams

1. Drain the tofu in a colander.

2. Place the sherry, hoisin sauce, bean paste and chile paste, if using, in a bowl and stir to mix, then set aside.

3. Slice the drained tofu into thick triangles. Heat 2 teaspoons of the oil in a heavy nonstick pan over high heat and cook the tofu slices, turning once, until both sides are golden brown, about 2 minutes per side. Remove the tofu from the pan and set aside.

4. Heat the remaining 2 teaspoons of oil in a large enameled or nonstick pot over high heat. Add the onion, garlic and ginger and cook for 1 minute. Add ¼ cup of water and the vegetables, cover the pot and let steam for 4 minutes.

5. Add the bean sprouts and let steam for 1 minute longer. Add the reserved sherry mixture and the tofu, stir to coat well, then serve immediately.

A Taste for Tofu

I HAVE TO ADMIT, I didn't used to like tofu—it seemed too bland and generally not my kind of food. And then my editor said, "Sue, get busy and give us a vegetarian line of menus," and so the transformation started. I cooked, tasted, reformulated recipes and tried again. And within a few tries, I found myself no longer missing meat and instead looking forward to my meat-free dinners!

Broiled Tofu

Makes three 4-ounce servings plus leftovers for a sandwich

Broiled tofu is the base for the Tofu Alfredo and Tofu Parmigiana recipes here. It's also great for sandwiches, so make a batch and keep it in the refrigerator.

14 ounces firm light tofu
1/2 teaspoon salt
Freshly ground black pepper
Olive oil spray

1. Preheat the broiler.

2. Drain the tofu in a colander.

3. Cut the tofu into 6 thick slices. Lightly salt and pepper both sides of each slice of tofu, then spray the slices lightly on both sides with olive oil. Broil the tofu slices on each side until lightly browned and a little crisp, about 6 minutes per side.

NOTE Slices of broiled tofu can be refrigerated, covered, for 2 days.

> **Nutritional information per 4-ounce serving of Broiled Tofu:**
> **Calories** 61
> **Protein** 9.4 grams
> **Total fat** 1.9 grams
> **Saturated fat** 0 grams
> **Total carbohydrates** 1.5 grams
> **Dietary fiber** 0 grams

Tofu Alfredo

1/2 teaspoon tub margarine
8 ounces white button mushrooms, sliced (about 3 cups)
1/3 cup store-bought light Alfredo sauce, such as Buitoni
1/4 cup fat-free sour cream
1 tablespoon nonfat or 1% milk
6 thick slices Broiled Tofu
1 teaspoon finely chopped fresh sage (optional), for garnish

1. Melt the margarine in a skillet, add the mushrooms and cook over high heat, stirring, until lightly browned, about 3 minutes. The mushrooms can be cooked ahead and refrigerated, covered, for up to 2 days.

2. Place the Alfredo sauce, sour cream and milk in a saucepan and stir to mix. Heat over low heat until just boiling, about 1 minute.

3. Reheat the tofu slices in a microwave on high power, about 15 seconds per slice, if necessary.

4. Heap the sautéed mushrooms over the tofu slices, pour the Alfredo sauce mixture on top and garnish with the sage, if desired.

Tofu Parmigiana

½ teaspoon tub margarine
8 ounces mushrooms, sliced
   (about 3 cups; optional)
¾ cup tomato sauce
3 tablespoons grated Parmesan
   cheese, preferably imported
6 thick slices Broiled Tofu
1 sprig fresh basil, chopped
   (optional), for garnish

1. If you're using the mushrooms, melt the margarine in a skillet, add the mushrooms and cook over high heat, stirring, until lightly browned, about 3 minutes. The mushrooms can be cooked ahead and refrigerated, covered, for up to 2 days.

2. Heat the tomato sauce in a microwave on high power for about 1 minute, stirring it after 30 seconds so it doesn't boil over.

3. Reheat the tofu slices in the microwave on high power, about 15 seconds per slice, if necessary.

4. Heap the sautéed mushrooms, if using, over the tofu slices, pour the tomato sauce on top and sprinkle with the Parmesan cheese (it will melt). Serve immediately, sprinkled with the fresh basil, if desired.

Nutritional information per 4-ounce serving of Tofu Alfredo or Tofu Parmigiana:

Calories 109	
Protein 13.5 grams	
Total fat 8.7 grams	
Saturated fat 1.2 grams	
Total carbohydrates 3.9 grams	
Dietary fiber 1.3 grams	

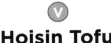

Hoisin Tofu

Makes three 4-ounce servings, plus leftovers for a sandwich

IF YOU STILL HAVE ANY DOUBTS about tofu, try it with an Asian twist.

14 ounces firm light tofu
½ teaspoon salt
Freshly ground black pepper
¼ cup hoisin marinade
    (from Hoisin Pork recipe on page 192)

> **Nutritional information per serving:**
> **Calories** 109
> **Protein** 13.5 grams
> **Total fat** 8.7 grams
> **Saturated fat** 1.2 grams
> **Total carbohydrates** 3.9 grams
> **Dietary fiber** 1.3 grams

1. Preheat the broiler.

2. Drain the tofu in a colander.

3. Cut the tofu into 6 thick slices. Lightly salt and pepper both sides of each slice. Spread the hoisin marinade over the tofu slices and let marinate for 5 minutes.

4. Broil the tofu on each side until lightly browned and a little crisp, about 6 minutes.

Steamed Tofu and Mixed Vegetables with Warm Peanut Sauce

Makes one serving

THIS SIMPLE RECIPE uses the delicious warm peanut sauce that Montien chef Tony Suktheva developed for his signature Thai chicken salad.

2 cups mixed vegetables, such as cauliflower and
    broccoli florets, sliced carrots, green beans,
    baby corn and/or snow peas
¼ pound firm light tofu, cut into slices or triangles
¼ cup warm homemade peanut sauce (page 177)

1. Pour water to a depth of ½ inch in a large steamer pot with a tight-fitting lid (keep the water level well below the bottom of the steamer basket). Bring to a boil, then place the vegetables and tofu loosely in the steamer basket. Steam the vegetables and tofu until the vegetables are just cooked but still a little crisp, about 10 minutes.

2. Drain the steamed vegetables and tofu very thoroughly, then serve it with the warm peanut sauce on the side for dipping.

> **Nutritional information per serving:**
> **Calories** 230
> **Protein** 17.2 grams
> **Total fat** 8.0 grams
> **Saturated fat** 1.3 grams
> **Total carbohydrates** 16.9 grams
> **Dietary fiber** 3.3 grams

No-Fuss Pizza

Makes one individual pizza

SIMPLE—AND SIMPLY DELICIOUS.

> 1 large whole-wheat pita bread, or
>> 2 small low-carbohydrate pita breads
> ⅓ cup pizza sauce
> 1 cup cooked broccoli or sautéed mushrooms
>> (optional, but good to add)
> 2 tablespoons grated Parmesan cheese,
>> preferably imported

1. Toast the pita(s), either whole on a griddle or cut into quarters and placed in an electric toaster.

2. Put the pita(s) on a microwave-safe plate and spoon on pizza sauce and broccoli or mushrooms, if using. Sprinkle the Parmesan cheese on top and microwave briefly on high power until the cheese melts, about 20 seconds.

> **Nutritional information per pizza with broccoli or mushrooms:**
> **Calories** 319
> **Protein** 15.4 grams
> **Total fat** 6.3 grams
> **Saturated fat** 2.5 grams
> **Total carbohydrates** 54.8 grams
> **Dietary fiber** 11.7 grams

(V)
Barbecue Vegetable Pizza

Makes one large pizza; eight slices

IF YOU HAVE TIME to make pizza from scratch, go for it. If not, look in your supermarket for pizza dough or pizza shells made with 100% whole-wheat flour. I like to use a strong Parmesan—less cheese equals fewer calories. And then, if you cook the pizza on a grill, you'll have a treat fit for kings!

1³/₄ cups all-purpose flour
1¹/₂ cups coarse wheat bran
1 package (¹/₄ ounce) active dry yeast
1 teaspoon sugar
1 teaspoon salt
Cooking oil spray
1 cup tomato sauce
¹/₄ cup grated Parmesan cheese, preferably imported
¹/₄ cup finely chopped sweet onion
1 red bell pepper, stemmed, seeded and diced
1 cup steamed broccoli florets or raw mushroom slices
4 slices pepperoni (optional), cut in quarters

> **Nutritional information per 2 slices with pepperoni:**
> **Calories** 361
> **Protein** 16.4 grams
> **Total fat** 5.5 grams
> **Saturated fat** 2.1 grams
> **Total carbohydrates** 70.9 grams
> **Dietary fiber** 14.7 grams

1. Mix together the flour, wheat bran, yeast, sugar and salt.

2. Add enough warm water to make a very soft but not sticky dough; start with 1 cup and add up to ¹/₄ cup more. The dough can be made in a mixer if you have a dough hook.

3. Knead the dough in the mixer for a couple of minutes or for 5 minutes by hand and then pull out the dough to make a large pizza 14 inches in diameter.

4. Spray a pizza stone or baking sheet lightly with cooking oil spray. Place the pizza dough on top, cover it and let it rise for about 30 minutes.

5. Preheat the oven to 425°F.

6. Spoon the tomato sauce, then sprinkle the Parmesan cheese, onion, bell pepper, broccoli or mushrooms, and pepperoni, if using, onto the pizza dough. Bake until cooked through and browning nicely, 15 to 25 minutes.

Variation: Grilled pizza—This is a little more work, but the results are sublime! Preheat the grill to low, then carefully place the rolled-out dough on the grill. Grill until the bottom is lightly browned, 5 to 8 minutes. Turn the pizza crust over carefully and, while the other side is grilling for 5 to 8 minutes, layer the toppings so that they cook while the bottom of the crust is browning. If the toppings are still a little undercooked when the crust is done, broil the top of the pizza for 2 to 3 minutes before serving.

John's Pasta Supper

Makes about 10 cups of sauce

MY HUSBAND'S FAMILY has been handing down this recipe generation after generation. I wonder if they've always known that its strong flavor comes with so very few calories. The sauce is also ideal for Northern Italian Lasagna (page 214).

2 tablespoons olive oil
2 medium-size onions, finely chopped
2 large cloves garlic, finely chopped
1 pound lean (90% to 95%) ground beef
1 pound ground turkey or chicken white meat
2 cans (6 ounces each) tomato paste
2 cans (14 ounces each) unseasoned diced tomatoes
8 ounces white button mushrooms, sliced (about 3 cups)
2 bay leaves
2 tablespoons fresh oregano, or 2 teaspoons dried oregano
2 tablespoons fresh basil, or 2 teaspoons dried basil
1 teaspoon salt, or more to taste
$1/3$ teaspoon freshly ground black pepper, or more to taste
$1/2$ pound baby carrots, sliced
$1/2$ cup cooked whole-wheat pasta for each serving
$1/2$ teaspoon grated Parmesan cheese, preferably imported, for each serving

Nutritional information per $2/3$-cup serving of sauce with $1/2$-cup cooked whole-wheat pasta:

Calories 309
Protein 27.2 grams
Total fat 7.7 grams
Saturated fat 18.1 grams
Total carbohydrates 35.8 grams
Dietary fiber 6.1 grams

1. Place the olive oil in a heavy pot over high heat. Add the onions and garlic and cook until starting to brown, about 5 minutes.

2. Add the beef and turkey or chicken and cook, stirring to break up all lumps, until the meat is browned, about 5 minutes.

3. Stir in the tomato paste, tomatoes, mushrooms, bay leaves, oregano, basil, salt and pepper. Stir in 1 cup of water and bring to a boil. Cover the pot tightly and let simmer for about 2 hours, stirring occasionally. If the sauce sticks to the bottom a little, just scrape it up and stir it in. Check that there's enough liquid for the sauce, adding more water if necessary.

4. Add the carrots and taste for seasoning, adding more salt and/or pepper as needed. Let the sauce simmer, covered, until the carrots are just soft, about 30 minutes. Remove the bay leaves. There should be a total of 10 cups of sauce; check this by measuring the sauce after it has cooled so you won't be eating more calories per serving than you think.

5. Serve the sauce with ½ cup cooked whole-wheat pasta and ½ teaspoon Parmesan cheese per person.

(V)

Northern Italian Lasagna

Makes eight servings about 4 by 2½ by 2 inches

THE LASAGNA OF NORTHERN ITALY and France is lighter than its familiar southern cousin. And substituting a low-calorie béchamel for huge amounts of ricotta is much easier on the waistline.

8 ounces whole-wheat lasagna pasta sheets
2½ cups meat sauce from John's Pasta Supper
   (page 213)
2½ cups "I" Diet Béchamel Sauce
¼ cup grated Parmesan cheese, preferably imported

Nutritional information per serving:

Calories 250

Protein 17.9 grams

Total fat 7.6 grams

Saturated fat 1.8 grams

Total carbohydrates 32.2 grams

Dietary fiber 3.4 grams

1. Have ready a 10 by 8 by 2-inch baking dish. Cook the lasagna pasta as directed on the box. Drain the noodles.

2. While the pasta is cooking, preheat the oven to 425°F.

3. Starting with meat sauce, then noodles, then béchamel sauce, then more noodles, layer the ingredients until all have been used, finishing with a good layer of béchamel. Sprinkle the Parmesan cheese on top.

4. Bake the lasagna until the top is nicely browned, 40 to 50 minutes.

Vegetarian variation: Tomato and broccoli lasagna— Substitute tomato sauce for the meat sauce. Arrange a layer of 2 cups of steamed broccoli on top of one of the layers of tomato sauce.

> **Nutritional information per vegetarian serving:**
> **Calories** 216
> **Protein** 10.7 grams
> **Total fat** 5.2 grams
> **Saturated fat** 1.1 grams
> **Total carbohydrates** 35.1 grams
> **Dietary fiber** 4.6 grams

"I" Diet Béchamel Sauce Ⓥ

Makes 2½ cups

The perfect base for cheese sauce, béchamel sauce is an essential ingredient in this recipe. This version of the old standby is both healthier (less saturated fat) and lower in calories than traditional versions.

2 tablespoons corn or canola oil
¼ cup all-purpose flour
2½ cups nonfat milk
Salt

> **Nutritional information per ¼-cup serving:**
> **Calories** 57
> **Protein** 2.4 grams
> **Total fat** 2.9 grams
> **Saturated fat** 0.3 gram
> **Total carbohydrates** 5.4 grams
> **Dietary fiber** 0.1 gram

Put the oil and flour in a heavy pot over low heat. Cook, stirring until the flour foams, then add the milk all at once and, using a balloon whisk, beat furiously until the milk boils to form a smooth sauce. Let the béchamel sauce simmer for 1 minute, then season with salt to taste. The béchamel sauce can be refrigerated, covered, for up to 2 days. Reheat it over low heat before using.

Stuffed Green Peppers

Makes four servings

STUFFED WITH CHEESE, vegetables and bulgur wheat, green bell peppers make a great-tasting main dish that also feels very substantial. One large pepper cut in half is the perfect size for two individual servings. Leftovers keep well in the refrigerator to make a terrific lunch for another day.

2 large green bell peppers
⅓ cup low-sodium vegetable broth
⅓ cup bulgur wheat
1 tablespoon olive oil
1 small onion, finely chopped
1 clove garlic, finely chopped
1 large carrot, finely chopped
½ rib celery, finely chopped
⅓ cup chopped fresh parsley
1 egg, beaten
¼ teaspoon salt
¼ teaspoon freshly ground black pepper
Cooking oil spray
⅓ cup tomato sauce (optional)
2 ounces low-fat (50% reduced-fat) sharp cheddar cheese, such as Cabot, grated, or ¼ cup grated Parmesan cheese, preferably imported

Nutritional information per ½-pepper serving with tomato sauce:

Calories 169
Protein 7.6 grams
Total fat 7.3 grams
Saturated fat 2.1 grams
Total carbohydrates 19.3 grams
Dietary fiber 5.1 grams

1. Cut the bell peppers in half lengthwise and remove the cores, seeds and ribs. Rinse the peppers under cold running water; set aside to dry.

2. Heat the vegetable broth to boiling. Place the bulgur wheat in a heatproof bowl, pour the broth over it and let it soak for 5 minutes.

3. Preheat the oven to 375°F.

4. Heat the olive oil in a saucepan over medium heat. Add the onion, garlic, carrot, celery and parsley and cook, stirring often, until the vegetables are softened and lightly browned, about 15 minutes. Mix in the soaked bulgur wheat, beaten egg, salt and black pepper.

5. Spray the outsides of the bell pepper halves with cooking oil spray, then place the peppers in a baking dish and spoon the filling inside them, dividing it evenly among the pepper halves. Cover the peppers loosely with aluminum foil and bake until cooked and almost soft, about 1 hour and 15 minutes.

6. Spread the tomato sauce, if using, over the tops of the peppers and sprinkle the grated cheese over the sauce. Broil the peppers until the cheese starts to brown, 3 to 4 minutes. The peppers can be served immediately or kept refrigerated, covered, for a day or two. Reheat a stuffed pepper by microwaving it on high power for about 45 seconds.

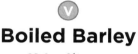

Boiled Barley

Makes 3½ cups

IT MAY NOT SOUND terribly appetizing, but barley is a great substitute for rice when you're dieting. With a rich, nutty flavor, it contains more fiber and is much lower in GI even than brown rice. And it's extra satisfying.

1 cup hulled barley, rinsed and drained

Place the rinsed barley in a saucepan, add water to cover and bring to a boil. Reduce the heat and let the barley simmer until the grains are still a little chewy but plump and cooked through, about 45 minutes. Rinse the cooked barley under cold water to keep the grains from getting sticky. Freeze ½-cup portions for future use. Thaw portions in the microwave on high power for about 1 minute, then let sit until the heat is distributed.

> Nutritional information per
> ¹/₂-cup serving:
>
> **Calories** 95
> **Protein** 2.6 grams
> **Total fat** 0.3 gram
> **Saturated fat** 0 grams
> **Total carbohydrates** 18.0 grams
> **Dietary fiber** 3.7 grams

ⓥ
Mushroom and Barley Risotto

Makes 3½ cups

THIS CLASSIC RISOTTO becomes an "I" Diet favorite just by substituting barley for rice and cutting down on the oil and butter. Working with whole grains is actually much easier: no adding boiling stock bit by bit. Just throw everything in together and put your feet up while the grains cook.

1 package (⅙ ounce) dried porcini mushrooms
1 cup hulled barley, rinsed and drained
4½ teaspoons olive oil
5 ounces white button mushrooms, sliced
½ medium-size red onion, finely chopped
1 small clove garlic
3 tablespoons red wine
2 cups low-sodium chicken or vegetable broth
½ teaspoon salt
¼ teaspoon freshly ground black pepper
3 tablespoons grated Parmesan cheese, preferably imported
2 tablespoons chopped fresh parsley

Nutritional information per ¾-cup serving:
Calories 262
Protein 11.6 grams
Total fat 7.4 grams
Saturated fat 1.9 grams
Total carbohydrates 36.9 grams
Dietary fiber 7.3 grams

1. Place the dried mushrooms in ¼ cup hot water and let soak.

2. Heat ½ teaspoon of olive oil in a saucepan over high heat. Add the mushrooms and cook them for a few minutes until browned. Transfer the mushrooms to a bowl and set aside.

3. Add the remaining 4 teaspoons of olive oil to the pan. Add the onion and garlic and cook over medium heat until lightly browned, about 10 minutes.

4. Stir in the barley and cook briefly for 1 minute, then return the mushrooms to the pan and add the red wine, broth, salt and pepper. Cover the pan and let simmer until the barley is chewy but cooked and most of the liquid is absorbed, about 40 minutes.

5. Stir in the Parmesan cheese and the parsley and taste for seasoning, adding more salt as needed. Serve immediately. Leftovers reheat well.

Keep-Your-Kids-Company "Macaroni and Cheese"

Makes two servings

ON THE NIGHTS WHEN YOUR KIDS ask for macaroni and cheese, consider this recipe for yourself while they get "the real thing." Replacing the pasta with cannellini beans actually works pretty well; the beans have the consistency of pasta but lots more fiber.

> 1 can (15 ounces) no-salt cannellini beans
> 1 package "deluxe" macaroni and cheese with a package of cheese sauce, such as Annie's

Rinse and drain the cannellini beans well. Place the beans in a microwave-safe container and microwave on high power until heated through, about 1 minute and 20 seconds. Mix half of the dry cheese sauce with the beans (use the rest of the cheese sauce with half of the pasta to make 2 servings for the kids).

Nutritional information per serving:	
Calories 256	
Protein 13.6 grams	
Total fat 7.5 grams	
Saturated fat 3.6 grams	
Total carbohydrates 33.7 grams	
Dietary fiber 10.6 grams	

Mixed Vegetable Curry

Makes 7 cups

THE CURRY YOU GET IN RESTAURANTS is death to dieting because of the enormous amount of oil in every dish, but curry is perfect for any dieter who cooks at home. Serve this vegetarian curry with Moong Dal Stew (page 222) and Boiled Barley (page 217) in place of rice, accompanied by Lemon and Date Chutney (page 223) or mango chutney and plain low-fat yogurt.

Save any curry that's left over; it freezes well and can be used as a side with chicken and lamb dishes.

1 medium-size onion, coarsely chopped

4 large cloves garlic, peeled

1 piece (2 inches) fresh ginger, peeled and coarsely chopped

¼ cup canola or corn oil

1½ teaspoons ground turmeric

2 teaspoons ground cumin

3 teaspoons ground coriander

½ teaspoon freshly ground coarse black pepper

1½ teaspoons garam masala

4 cardamom pods

1 bay leaf

1 can (14 ounces) unseasoned, salt-free diced tomatoes

1 tablespoon lemon juice

1 teaspoon salt

9 cups mixed vegetables: carrot slices, cauliflower florets, peas, sliced mushrooms, zucchini slices and red bell pepper slices

¼ cup chopped fresh cilantro (optional)

Nutritional information per 1-cup serving:
Calories 154
Protein 4.5 grams
Total fat 8.6 grams
Saturated fat 0.6 gram
Total carbohydrates 17.5 grams
Dietary fiber 5.8 grams

1. Place the onion, garlic and ginger in a food processor and run the machine until a smooth paste forms (you can add a little water if necessary).

2. Put the onion paste in a heavy-bottomed pot over high heat and cook, stirring, until most of the liquid has evaporated, about 10 minutes.

3. Add the oil and cook, stirring, until the onion paste is starting to brown nicely, then add the turmeric, cumin, coriander and black pepper in that order. Cook, stirring, about 2 minutes over low heat.

4. Add the garam masala, cardamom, bay leaf, tomatoes, lemon juice, salt and 1 cup of water. Let simmer, covered, until the sauce has reduced, about 20 minutes, checking occasionally to see that there's enough liquid.

5. Add the vegetables to the pot: First simmer the carrots, covered, for 5 minutes. Then add the cauliflower, peas, mushrooms and zucchini and let simmer for 5 minutes. Finally add the bell pepper slices and let simmer until everything is cooked, about 10 minutes longer. Remove the cardamom and bay leaf. Serve the curry with the cilantro, if using.

Chickpea Masala

Makes about 3½ cups

IN INDIAN CUISINE, *masala* means a blend of spices, and this recipe for chickpeas masala style lives up to its name. The rich blend of flavors pairs well with Boiled Barley (page 217), Lemon and Date Chutney (page 223) and a side of Cucumber-Mint Raita (page 174).

1 cup dried chickpeas (garbanzo beans)
½ teaspoon baking soda
1 tablespoon canola or corn oil
1 medium-size onion, finely chopped
1 clove garlic, chopped
1½ teaspoons cumin seeds
1 teaspoon ground coriander
⅓ teaspoon freshly ground black pepper
1½ teaspoons garam masala
1 bay leaf
1 cup canned unseasoned, salt-free diced tomatoes
1 tablespoon lemon juice
½ teaspoon salt

> **Nutritional information per ½-cup serving:**
> **Calories** 104
> **Protein** 3.3 grams
> **Total fat** 5.3 grams
> **Saturated fat** 0.4 gram
> **Total carbohydrates** 12.4 grams
> **Dietary fiber** 3.3 grams

1. Soak the chickpeas and the baking soda overnight in plenty of water.

2. The next day, bring the chickpeas to a boil in the soaking liquid and let simmer until they start to soften but are still somewhat firm, about 1 hour. Drain the chickpeas, setting aside 1 cup of the chickpea cooking liquid.

3. Heat the oil in a saucepan over medium heat. Add the onion and garlic and cook, stirring occasionally, until lightly browned, about 15 minutes.

4. Add the cumin seeds and cook for 2 minutes, then add the coriander and pepper and cook for 1 minute. Add the garam masala, bay leaf, tomatoes, lemon juice, salt, chickpeas and reserved chickpea cooking liquid. Let simmer, covered, until the chickpeas are soft and in a nice sauce, about 20 minutes. Remove the lid for the last few minutes if the sauce is too thin; if it's too thick, add a little water. Remove the bay leaf before serving.

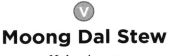

Moong Dal Stew

Makes 4 cups

A MUNG BEAN "STEW," *moong dal* is a very mild but delicious northern Indian dish. Made from split mung beans, also called *moong dal,* it's a snap to prepare and pairs perfectly with Lemon and Date Chutney and Mixed Vegetable Curry (page 219). During weight loss, simple Boiled Barley (page 217) makes a satisfying side dish; non-dieting family members can enjoy rice or chapati (picked up at the store where you get your *moong dal* and spices). When cooking for one or two, make half a recipe or freeze leftovers (add some water when you reheat them).

1 cup (7 ⅕ ounces) moong dal
2 cloves garlic, peeled
¼-inch slice fresh ginger, peeled
2 teaspoons ground turmeric
1 tablespoon lemon juice
½ teaspoon salt
1 pinch asafetida
1 tablespoon corn or canola oil
1 teaspoon cumin seeds
2 tablespoons chopped fresh cilantro (optional)
Lemon and Date Chutney (optional)

> **Nutritional information per ½-cup serving:**
>
> **Calories** 112
> **Protein** 5.6 grams
> **Total fat** 3.8 grams
> **Saturated fat** 0.5 gram
> **Total carbohydrates** 14.7 grams
> **Dietary fiber** 5.6 grams

1. Place the *moong dal* and 4 cups of water in a saucepan and bring to a boil, skimming off any scum that rises to the surface.

2. Add the garlic, ginger and turmeric, cover the pan, lower the heat and let simmer until the dal is soft and creamy, the consistency of thick pea soup, about 40 minutes.

3. Add the lemon juice, salt and asafetida to the dal and stir.

4. Heat the oil in a small pan over low heat, add the cumin seeds and cook until the seeds start to darken, about 15 seconds. Stir the cumin seeds into the dal and serve immediately, garnished with the cilantro, if using, and with chutney on the side, if desired.

Lemon and Date Chutney Ⓥ

Makes 1¼ cups

In India, meals never come with the sweet mango chutney that we know so well. Instead they're accompanied by a sour lime or mango pickle. This recipe is a cross between a chutney and a pickle. If you like a strong lemon flavor, it's a great addition to any Indian meal.

3 ripe organic lemons (see Note)
5 fresh or dried dates, finely chopped
2 tablespoons cider vinegar or wine vinegar
2 tablespoons brown sugar

> **Nutritional information per 1½-teaspoon serving:**
> **Calories** 8
> **Protein** 0 grams
> **Total fat** 0 grams
> **Saturated fat** 0 grams
> **Total carbohydrates** 2.0 grams
> **Dietary fiber** 0.3 gram

1. Rinse the lemons under cold running water. Cut off the ends, score the rinds in quarters and peel them away from the flesh as you would with an orange. Set aside the lemon flesh. Chop the rinds into small pieces the size of half a peanut. Place the lemon rinds and 6 cups of water in a saucepan and bring to a boil. Reduce the heat and let simmer until easily pierced with a fork, about 10 minutes. Drain the lemon rinds. Repeat this step one more time.

2. Drain the lemon rinds again, discarding the cooking liquid. Return the drained rinds to the saucepan. Finely chop the lemon flesh and add it to the saucepan along with 1½ cups of water. Cover the saucepan and let simmer until the lemons are fully soft, about 50 minutes.

3. Add the dates, vinegar and brown sugar to the pan and let simmer until the chutney is a thick sauce, 20 to 30 minutes. Add more water if the chutney becomes *too* thick or leave the lid off if it seems watery.

4. Ladle the chutney into a glass jar with a tight-fitting lid and refrigerate it.

NOTE Check that the lemons are ripe by pinching them in the store. You should feel some give—not a thick, solid skin.

(V)

West African Bean Cakes with Spicy Dip and Green Salad

Makes four servings of six chickpea cakes, plus dip and salad;
there will be chickpea cakes left over

THIS ADAPTATION OF TRADITIONAL West African bean cakes is one of my favorite chickpea recipes—a great way to convince even kids that beans taste good. Bean cakes are a popular treat in West Africa, where they're usually fried since ovens are rare. When you bake chickpea cakes, though, they become a marvelous-tasting, perfect diet food, particularly when served with a salad on the side. This recipe makes a lot, but the cakes freeze well and become beautifully crisp when reheated in a hot oven for three to four minutes.

For the chickpea cakes:

1 cup dried chickpeas (garbanzo beans),
    soaked for 12 hours or overnight
1 small or ½ large onion, chopped
1 teaspoon salt
⅓ teaspoon freshly ground black pepper
1 large egg
Cooking oil spray

For the dip:

1 cup nonfat plain yogurt
1 to 2 teaspoons cayenne pepper sauce, such as Texas Champagne
Juice of ¼ medium-size lemon, or more to taste
Salt and freshly ground black pepper

For one serving of salad:

2 to 3 cups lettuce or other greens
Sliced scallion, cucumber, green bell pepper and the like, as desired
1 teaspoon olive oil
½ teaspoon cider vinegar
Salt and freshly ground black pepper

> **Nutritional information per serving of 6 chickpea cakes, salad and ¼ cup of dip:**
>
> **Calories** 254
>
> **Protein** 14.7 grams
>
> **Total fat** 8.2 grams
>
> **Saturated fat** 1.3 grams
>
> **Total carbohydrates** 33.8 grams
>
> **Dietary fiber** 9.8 grams

1. Preheat the oven to 425°F. Spray a baking sheet with cooking oil spray.

2. Make the chickpea cakes: Drain the soaked chickpeas and blend them in a food processor with the onion, salt, black pepper and egg until the mixture has the consistency of thick mashed potatoes; add a little water if necessary to make a smooth paste.

3. Spoon dollops of about 1 tablespoon of the chickpea mixture onto the prepared baking sheet and form them into small disks approximately 1½ inches across and ¼ inch thick, making sure they're not touching (you will have about 32 cakes). Spray the tops of the cakes lightly with the cooking oil. Bake the chickpea cakes until lightly browned, 13 to 18 minutes.

4. Meanwhile, make the dip: Place the yogurt, pepper sauce and lemon juice in a bowl and stir to mix. Season with salt and black pepper to taste, adding more lemon juice as necessary.

5. Make the salad: Place the lettuce, scallion, cucumber and/or green pepper in a bowl and toss to mix. Add the olive oil and cider vinegar and toss to coat.

6. Serve the chickpea cakes hot with the dip and the salad on the side.

Cooked Vegetables

START THINKING OF COOKED VEGETABLES as totally separate from salads. It's a good idea to have both in a single meal—the variety makes for a more satisfying eating experience and the increased amount of vitamin-rich food is just plain good for you.

Potato Skins ⓥ

Florentine Braised Kale

Healthy Collard Greens ⓥ

A Perfect Ratatouille ⓥ

Classic Red Cabbage with Apples ⓥ

Helen's Red Flannel Cabbage ⓥ

Summer Squash with Butter and Sage ⓥ

Zesty Baked Beans ⓥ

Tuscan Beans with Rosemary and Olive Oil ⓥ

Black-Eyed Peas ⓥ

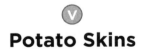

Potato Skins

Makes one serving

I HAVE NEVER FOUND a diet mashed potato recipe that I thought was worth eating. Most such recipes call for potato substitutes and come out not tasting like potatoes, and the texture is never creamy enough. But there is a way you can have real potatoes when you diet—by eating the skins! Fiber is more concentrated in the skins, so if you're honest about scooping out virtually all of the insides (turn them into mashed potatoes for family members), you can have your potatoes and your diet, too.

2 small baked potatoes (see Note)
Dash of salt
1 teaspoon low-fat sour cream

1. Scoop out virtually all of the flesh from the potatoes and set it aside for another use. Both potato skins should fit easily into a ¼-cup measure.

2. Sprinkle the potato skins with the salt and spoon the sour cream on top. Serve immediately.

> **Nutritional information per serving:**
> **Calories** 94
> **Protein** 2.2 grams
> **Total fat** 0.6 gram
> **Saturated fat** 0.4 gram
> **Total carbohydrates** 9.8 grams
> **Dietary fiber** 3.6 grams

NOTE The potatoes will have the best texture if you bake them in the oven, but failing that, use a microwave or a combination of microwaving and baking.

Florentine Braised Kale

Makes 3 cups

GREENS WITH STRONG FLAVORS go well with strong-flavored meat dishes. Try this healthy kale dish with Arista Chicken (page 197).

1 tablespoon olive oil
1 small clove garlic, peeled and crushed
2 thin slices (about 1 ounce) imported prosciutto, chopped
1 pound fresh kale or spinach, rinsed (but not dried) and chopped
Salt and freshly ground black pepper

> **Nutritional information per 1-cup serving:**
> **Calories** 113
> **Protein** 7.7 grams
> **Total fat** 6.5 grams
> **Saturated fat** 1.1 grams
> **Total carbohydrates** 8.6 grams
> **Dietary fiber** 3.3 grams

1. Heat the olive oil in a large saucepan over medium heat. Add the garlic and cook briefly.

2. Add the prosciutto and then the kale and cook, uncovered, until the kale has wilted, 3 to 5 minutes. If necessary, add a little water to keep the kale from sticking to the pan. Season the kale with salt and pepper to taste and serve immediately.

$$\text{(V)}$$

Healthy Collard Greens

Makes 4 cups

SOUTHERN FOOD is too often loaded with fat and sugar; however, many traditional dishes, such as collard greens, can be prepared as tasty diet food. Simply substitute a good strong prosciutto and chicken stock for the fatty pork.

2 teaspoons olive oil
½ medium-size onion, chopped
1 clove garlic, peeled and crushed
1½ thin slices (about ¾ ounce) imported prosciutto (optional)
1 tablespoon red wine vinegar
¾ cup canned low-sodium chicken or vegetable broth
1 pound collard greens, with large stems snapped off, rinsed carefully (but not drained) and chopped
Salt and freshly ground black pepper

Nutritional information per 1-cup serving with prosciutto:
Calories 77
Protein 5.0 grams
Total fat 3.6 grams
Saturated fat 0.5 gram
Total carbohydrates 8.4 grams
Dietary fiber 4.4 grams

1. Heat the olive oil in a saucepan over medium heat. Add the onion and garlic and cook, stirring constantly, until lightly browned, 5 to 10 minutes.

2. Add the prosciutto, if using, and cook briefly, then add the wine vinegar, broth and collard greens. Let simmer, covered, until the greens are tender and there is still some liquid in the bottom of the pan for serving, 20 to 30 minutes, stirring occasionally. Season with salt and pepper to taste, then serve.

$$\text{(V)}$$

A Perfect Ratatouille

Makes 6 cups

RICH-TASTING RATATOUILLE makes low-calorie zucchini feel like substantial food. Try a steaming bowl for lunch, topped with a tablespoon or two of grated Parmesan cheese.

1 tablespoon olive oil or canola oil
1 medium-size onion, coarsely chopped
1 clove garlic, peeled and crushed
1½ teaspoons chopped fresh basil leaves,
    or ½ teaspoon dried basil
1½ teaspoons chopped fresh oregano,
    or ½ teaspoon dried oregano
1 bay leaf
1 cup diced canned tomatoes
2 tablespoons tomato paste
Salt and freshly ground black pepper
4 medium-size zucchini, cut into cubes

> **Nutritional information per 1-cup serving:**
>
> **Calories** 71
> **Protein** 3.3 grams
> **Total fat** 2.7 grams
> **Saturated fat** 0.3 gram
> **Total carbohydrates** 11.1 grams
> **Dietary fiber** 3.7 grams

1. Heat the oil in a saucepan over medium heat. Add the onion and garlic and cook, stirring occasionally, until lightly browned, 5 to 10 minutes.

2. Add the basil, oregano, bay leaf, tomatoes and tomato paste, cover the pan, reduce the heat to low and let simmer until the flavors mix, about 15 minutes.

3. Season the tomato mixture with salt and pepper to taste, add the zucchini and stir to mix. Let simmer, covered, until the zucchini is just cooked, about 10 minutes. As it cooks, check to see if the ratatouille looks dry, adding a little water if necessary. Discard the bay leaf before serving. The ratatouille can be refrigerated, covered, for a few days but does not freeze well.

Ⓥ

Classic Red Cabbage with Apples

Makes 6 cups

YOU MAY THINK YOU DON'T LIKE CABBAGE, but add some oil, sugar, vinegar—and a few other ingredients for extra flavor—and see if you don't change your mind. Low in calories and high in fiber, this tasty dish is filling and makes the beginnings of a great lunch with a slice or two of lean deli meat on the side.

1 tablespoon canola or corn oil
1 medium-size onion, finely chopped
1 clove garlic, chopped
¼ cup cider vinegar
2 tablespoons sugar
2 tablespoons sugar substitute
1 medium-size red cabbage (about 1½ pounds),
    cut in quarters and shredded
1 firm apple, such as Gala or Braeburn,
    peeled and chopped
Salt and freshly ground black pepper

Nutritional information per 1-cup serving:

Calories 60
Protein 1.3 grams
Total fat 1.8 grams
Saturated fat 0.3 gram
Total carbohydrates 11.3 grams
Dietary fiber 2.1 grams

1. Heat the oil over medium heat in a saucepan large enough to hold all the ingredients. Add the onion and garlic and cook, stirring occasionally, until starting to brown, about 5 minutes.

2. Add the vinegar, sugar, sugar substitute and ½ cup of water and stir to mix, then add the cabbage. Let simmer, covered, until the cabbage begins to soften, about 15 minutes.

3. Add the apple and season with salt and pepper to taste. Let simmer, covered, until the cabbage and apple are soft and cooked, 30 to 40 minutes. As the cabbage cooks, check to see if it looks dry, adding a little water if necessary.

(V)

Helen's Red Flannel Cabbage

Makes 7 cups

WHENEVER I SET UP A NEW STUDY at Tufts, I hope that my colleague Helen Rasmussen, R.D., Ph.D., will find the time to help with the menu design— she has no equal when it comes to creating simple but delicious recipes that fit any nutritional composition. This one is classic Helen, turning sustaining "I" Diet ingredients into a filling, tasty side dish that goes well with a wide range of main dishes, including Broiled Tofu (page 208) and Perfect Grill with Creamy Mustard Sauce (page 199).

2 cups thinly sliced onions
1 tablespoon tub margarine
1 tablespoon olive oil
3 tablespoons tomato paste
1/8 teaspoon cayenne pepper
1/2 medium head green cabbage (1 pound), finely shredded
1/2 medium head red cabbage (1 pound), finely shredded
1/4 teaspoon salt

> **Nutritional information per 1-cup serving:**
> **Calories** 83
> **Protein** 2.5 grams
> **Total fat** 4.5 grams
> **Saturated fat** 0.7 gram
> **Total carbohydrates** 15.4 grams
> **Dietary fiber** 3.7 grams

1. Place the onions in a large dry skillet or Dutch oven over medium-low heat. Cook, stirring every 5 minutes, until the onions look slightly dried out, 15 to 20 minutes—don't let them burn.

2. Add the margarine to the skillet. When it has melted, add the olive oil and increase the heat to high. Cook the onions until all of them are browned, about 7 minutes.

3. Mix the tomato paste and cayenne pepper together in a small bowl. Gradually stir in 2/3 cup of water. Add the tomato paste mixture to the onions, then add the green and red cabbage and stir to coat well. Let the cabbage simmer, covered, until tender but not squishy and unrecognizable, about 30 minutes, stirring occasionally. If the cabbage mixture starts to look too dry, add 1/4 cup of water. Season with salt to taste.

(V)

Summer Squash with Butter and Sage

Makes 6 cups

FLAVORFUL, BUTTERY SAGE brings the squash to life in this delectable side dish. Since herbs are loaded with protein and fiber, the sage is good for you, too.

> **Nutritional information per 1-cup serving:**
> **Calories** 64
> **Protein** 1.7 grams
> **Total fat** 3.6 grams
> **Saturated fat** 0.7 gram
> **Total carbohydrates** 8.0 grams
> **Dietary fiber** 2.7 grams

1 tablespoon tub margarine, or 1 tablespoon olive oil
1 small clove garlic, peeled and crushed
3 large yellow summer squash (about 2 pounds), sliced
6 medium-size fresh sage leaves, finely chopped
Salt and freshly ground black pepper

Heat the margarine in a saucepan over low heat. Add the garlic and cook until just beginning to soften, about 1 minute. Add the summer squash, stir to coat, and cook about 2 minutes. Cover the pan and let the squash steam over low heat until just beginning to soften, about 20 minutes. Then remove the lid and let any liquid that has accumulated evaporate. Add the sage, season with salt and pepper to taste and serve immediately.

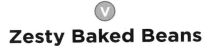

Zesty Baked Beans

Makes 5 cups

LOTS OF BEANS MEANS LOTS OF FIBER, and it's that fiber that makes this protein-packed dish so good—and good for you. Canned beans are used here to make it easier to prepare, and don't be afraid to experiment with other bean varieties. The more color contrast between the beans, the more beautiful the final product.

1 teaspoon canola or similar oil
1 large onion, diced
1 cup beef or vegetable broth
1/4 cup tomato paste
1/4 cup molasses
1 tablespoon Worcestershire sauce
1 1/2 tablespoons dry mustard
1/2 teaspoon salt
1/4 teaspoon freshly ground black pepper
3 cans (15 ounces each) different beans,
    such as Great Northern, pinto and cannellini, rinsed and drained
1 tablespoon orange juice

Nutritional information per 1/2-cup serving:	
Calories 160	
Protein 7.6 grams	
Total fat 1.2 grams	
Saturated fat 0.2 gram	
Total carbohydrates 30.8 grams	
Dietary fiber 9.2 grams	

1. Preheat the oven to 350°F.

2. Heat the oil in an ovenproof or cast-iron pot with a lid over medium heat. Add the onion and cook, stirring occasionally, until lightly browned, about 10 minutes. Add the broth, tomato paste, molasses, Worcestershire sauce, dry mustard, salt, pepper and a scant 1 cup of water and stir to mix until smooth. Stir in the beans.

3. Cover the pot and bake the beans until there's a nice rich sauce and the top is just starting to crust over, 1 to 1¼ hours.

4. Just before serving, stir in the orange juice (it adds a nice piquancy). You can freeze ½-cup servings of the beans, but be sure to thaw them before microwaving them on high power for 1 minute and let them sit for 5 minutes before gently heating them to the desired temperature.

Ⓥ

Tuscan Beans
with Rosemary and Olive Oil

Makes 1½ cups

THIS ADAPTATION OF AN OLD ITALIAN RECIPE makes a wonderful side dish for Arista Chicken (page 197) and is a first-class diet food as well.

1 tablespoon mild extra-virgin olive oil
1 small garlic clove, chopped
1 thin slice (about ½ ounce) imported prosciutto
   (optional), finely chopped
1 can (15 ounces) cannellini beans,
   lightly rinsed and drained
2 large or 4 small fresh sage leaves
Salt and freshly ground black pepper

> Nutritional information per ½-cup serving with prosciutto:
>
> **Calories** 109
> **Protein** 4.9 grams
> **Total fat** 3.5 grams
> **Saturated fat** 0.5 gram
> **Total carbohydrates** 14.8 grams
> **Dietary fiber** 5.5 grams

Place the olive oil in a skillet over medium heat. Add the garlic and cook until softened but not browned, about 1 minute. Add the prosciutto, if using, and stir to mix. Add the cannellini beans and sage and season with salt and pepper to taste. Increase the heat to medium and cook until the beans are heated through, about 3 minutes. Let the beans stand for 10 minutes to allow the flavor to develop before serving.

(V)

Black-Eyed Peas

Makes 2 cups

HERE'S ANOTHER HEALTHY, traditional Southern favorite. More often combined with rice, black-eyed peas are great on their own. Here, cooked with a little prosciutto rather than pork fat, they become a diet staple.

2 teaspoons canola or corn oil
1/2 medium-size onion, finely chopped
1 clove garlic, peeled and crushed
1 1/2 thin slices (about 3/4 ounce) prosciutto (optional)
1 can (15 ounces) black-eyed peas, rinsed well and drained
1/4 cup low-sodium chicken or vegetable broth
Barbecue sauce of your choice for serving

Nutritional information per 1/2-cup serving with prosciutto:

Calories 120
Protein 7.5 grams
Total fat 3.2 grams
Saturated fat 0.5 gram
Total carbohydrates 15.7 grams
Dietary fiber 3.8 grams

Heat the oil in a skillet over medium heat. Add the onion and garlic and cook, stirring occasionally, until the onion is lightly browned, 5 to 10 minutes. Add the prosciutto, if using, and cook briefly. Add the black-eyed peas and broth, cover the skillet and let simmer until the black-eyed peas are soft and have absorbed most of the liquid, about 20 minutes. Serve hot with barbecue sauce.

Desserts

THINK OF A DIET . . . and you'll most likely think about giving up dessert. Well, time to think again. Desserts are crucial to the "I" Diet, and not just as add-ons to keep you happy (though they'll do that, too). On this plan, desserts are a tasty diet medicine—you'll find fiber-packed chocolates, ice creams and fruits that will satisfy your craving for sweets *and* help you lose weight.

"I" Diet Cereal Desserts ⓥ
Chocolate Cereal Dessert
Ice Cream Sundae
Ginger-Pecan Crunch
Chocolate-Raspberry Parfait

Chocolate Pudding I ⓥ

Chocolate Pudding II ⓥ

Chocolate Bread Pudding ⓥ

Orange Flan ⓥ

Indian Barley Pudding ⓥ

Baked Apples with Figs ⓥ

Almost Apple Cobbler ⓥ

Frozen Fruits ⓥ

Chocolate-Tipped Strawberries and Cream ⓥ

Vanilla Spice Cookies ⓥ

Snack Attack Packs ⓥ
Salty Snack Attack Pack
Sweet Snack Attack Pack
Trail Mix Snack Attack Pack

Rhubarb Yogurt ⓥ

Ⓥ

"I" Diet Cereal Desserts

YOU'LL FIND THAT THESE QUICK-AND-EASY DESSERTS will help you feel satisfied and hunger-free, particularly if you're choosing menus with meat during Stage I of the "I" Diet program. Each of these desserts would also make a perfect substitute for a morning or afternoon Snack Attack Pack.

Chocolate Cereal Dessert

Makes one serving

Because the cereal is coated with chocolate, you'll feel as if you're eating more chocolate than you really are.

⅓ cup high-fiber cereal
   (Fiber One or All-Bran Extra Fiber)
1 square (about 10 grams) good bittersweet chocolate, such as Lindt Excellence Intense Dark or Hershey's All Natural Extra Dark (or good milk chocolate if you prefer it and can keep it in your home without eating it at other times)
⅓ cup nonfat or 1% milk
2 drops mint extract (optional)

> Nutritional information per serving of each cereal dessert:
>
> **Calories** 106
>
> **Protein** 4.7 grams
>
> **Total fat** 3.0 grams
>
> **Saturated fat** 1.2 grams
>
> **Total carbohydrates** 24.4 grams
>
> **Dietary fiber** 9.9 grams

Put the cereal in a small microwave-safe bowl with the chocolate on top. Microwave on high power until the chocolate is melted but not bubbling, 20 to 40 seconds. Mix the cereal and chocolate together well with a fork until all of the cereal is nicely coated. Wait a minute or two for it to cool, then add the milk and mint extract, if desired.

Ice Cream Sundae

Makes one serving

Ice cream on a diet? Why not? In our studies at Tufts, we find that giving up ice cream is one hardship some people just can't handle. I think you'll be amazed at our solution. Combine high-fiber cereal with ice cream, as in this no-work recipe, and everybody's happy.

Be careful, though. Since you can't buy ice cream in quarter-cup containers, you need to be able to either keep it in your kitchen without eating more of it or find a pal who's willing to look after the container for you. If you're nervous about bingeing, pass on this dessert until you're a few weeks into your diet, when control should be easier.

> ¼ cup sugar-free ice cream in the flavor of your choice
> ⅓ cup high-fiber cereal (Fiber One or All-Bran Extra Fiber)

Place the ice cream and cereal in a bowl. Using a fork, gently mash them together until the cereal is covered but not broken up. Enjoy immediately!

Variation: If you're using vanilla ice cream, try mixing in a very finely chopped ½-inch square of crystallized ginger.

Ginger-Pecan Crunch
Makes one serving

So good that it feels like a special treat, this crunchy delight is actually an appetite suppressant. The gingerol in ginger is a first cousin of capsaicin, the ingredient in hot peppers that can cut calorie intake by an average of 8% per meal.

> 1 cube (¾ inch) crystallized ginger, finely chopped
> ⅓ cup high-fiber cereal (Fiber One or All-Bran Extra Fiber)
> 3 ounces (½ container) sugar-free fruit yogurt of your choice,
>   such as Dannon Light & Fit, or nonfat plain Greek yogurt
> 2 pecan halves, coarsely chopped

Mix the cereal with the ginger and yogurt, then sprinkle the chopped pecans on top.

Chocolate-Raspberry Parfait
Makes one serving

Chocolate and raspberries go together beautifully and pair easily with high-fiber cereal. Although fresh raspberries are wonderful, I often use frozen because they're so convenient to have on hand.

⅓ cup high-fiber cereal (Fiber One or All-Bran Extra Fiber)
1 square (about 10 grams) bittersweet or dark chocolate
¼ cup fresh or thawed frozen raspberries
3 ounces (½ container) nonfat yogurt (see Note)

Put the cereal in a small microwave-safe bowl with the chocolate on top. Microwave on high power until the chocolate is melted but not bubbling, 20 to 40 seconds. Mix the cereal and chocolate together well with a fork until all of the cereal is nicely coated. Let cool a minute, then add the raspberries and yogurt and stir to mix.

NOTE You can use either nonfat plain yogurt—regular or Greek style— or a nonfat vanilla yogurt flavored with an artificial sweetener, such as Dannon Light & Fit.

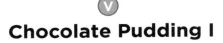

Chocolate Pudding I

Makes one serving

THIS RICH TREAT will help you feel full and satisfied at the same time. Since fiber is increased slowly in Stage I, protein is the filling ingredient here. Double or triple the recipe if you want to make more than one serving.

2 teaspoons Dutch-process cocoa,
    such as Droste
¼ cup nonfat ricotta cheese
Sugar substitute equivalent to
    2 teaspoons sugar
¼ teaspoon vanilla extract
1 tablespoon light whipped cream, for garnish

Nutritional information per serving:
Calories 91
Protein 7.1 grams
Total fat 2.7 grams
Saturated fat 1.9 grams
Total carbohydrates 9.5 grams
Dietary fiber 3.0 grams

1. Place the cocoa and 1 tablespoon of water in a microwave-safe bowl and microwave on high power for about 10 seconds. Add the ricotta, sugar substitute and vanilla and stir until the pudding has a uniformly smooth consistency.

2. Transfer the pudding to an individual serving bowl and garnish it with a squirt of whipped cream. Served immediately, the pudding will be thick in consistency; refrigerate it if you want a firmer texture.

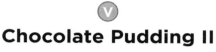

Chocolate Pudding II

Makes one serving

LOADED WITH THE PROTEIN AND FIBER that you need in Stage II, this luscious creamy pudding is a breeze to make and leaves you feeling happy and satisfied.

1½ teaspoons Dutch-process cocoa, such as Droste
⅓ cup nonfat or 1% milk
¼ cup oat bran
Sugar substitute equivalent to 1 tablespoon sugar
¼ teaspoon vanilla extract
1 tablespoon light whipped cream, for garnish

> **Nutritional information per serving:**
>
> **Calories** 130
> **Protein** 8.9 grams
> **Total fat** 10.3 grams
> **Saturated fat** 2.4 grams
> **Total carbohydrates** 23.6 grams
> **Dietary fiber** 5.9 grams

1. Place the cocoa and about 2 teaspoons of the milk in a microwave-safe bowl and stir until they form a nice smooth paste (you can do this in an individual size ramekin that the pudding will be served in). Add the remaining milk and microwave on high power until almost boiling, about 30 seconds.

2. Add the oat bran, sugar substitute and vanilla and mix everything together. Let the pudding stand for a minute or so until it thickens, or microwave it on high power for about 10 seconds so that it sets right away. Serve the pudding with a squirt of whipped cream for garnish.

Chocolate Bread Pudding

Makes six servings

IMAGINE A CROSS BETWEEN chocolate custard and bread pudding but with bran taking the place of the bread. Trust me—delicious! You can freeze any leftover pudding for the next time it's on your menu.

You will need six small ceramic ramekins that hold one-half cup or less.

1¼ cups coarse bran (from regular red wheat, not white wheat)

1¼ cups nonfat or 1% milk

1 ounce good-quality bittersweet chocolate, such as imported Belgian chocolate

½ cup Egg Beaters, or 2 egg whites

2 to 3 teaspoons Dutch-process cocoa, such as Droste

Sugar substitute equivalent to 5 tablespoons sugar

2 tablespoons sugar

1½ teaspoons vanilla extract, or ½ teaspoon orange extract

6 tablespoons light whipped cream (optional), for serving

> **Nutritional information per serving with whipped cream:**
>
> **Calories** 116
> **Protein** 6.4 grams
> **Total fat** 3.3 grams
> **Saturated fat** 1.4 grams
> **Total carbohydrates** 20.9 grams
> **Dietary fiber** 5.8 grams

1. Preheat the oven to 300°F.

2. Bring ½ cup of water to a boil. Mix in the bran, cover and let stand for 5 minutes.

3. Heat the milk in a saucepan over medium heat. Turn off the heat, add the bittersweet chocolate and let it melt. Mix well with a whisk or fork.

4. Place the Egg Beaters or egg whites, cocoa, sugar substitute, sugar and vanilla or orange extract in a bowl and stir to mix. Add the milk with the melted chocolate and the soaked bran to the egg mixture and mix well.

5. Divide the pudding among 6 ramekins, spooning about ⅓ cup into each, and keep stirring to distribute the bran evenly. Place the ramekins in a roasting pan and add ¾ inch of cold water to the pan.

6. Bake the puddings until just set in the middle, 40 minutes to 1 hour (the time they take to set is very variable). Let cool slightly before topping with whipped cream, if desired. Frozen puddings can be thawed by microwaving them on high power for 30 seconds, letting them stand for 2 minutes and then microwaving them again for 30 seconds.

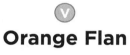

Orange Flan

Makes five servings

FLAN IS THE SPANISH NAME for what the French call *crème caramel—* a rich custard pudding with a caramel topping that's a long way from any normal diet food. Here is our "I" Diet version, indulgent in taste and high in fiber, great on its own or with a few tablespoons of fresh fruit salad. Freeze any extras.

You will need five small ceramic ramekins that hold one-half cup.

3 tablespoons sugar
$^1/_2$ cup Egg Beaters, or 2 egg whites
Sugar substitute equivalent to 4 tablespoons sugar
$^1/_2$ teaspoon vanilla extract
Grated zest of 1 orange
1 ounce ($^1/_4$ cup) corn bran (see Note)
$1^1/_2$ teaspoons cornstarch
$1^1/_4$ cups nonfat or 1% milk

> **Nutritional information per serving:**
> **Calories** 93
> **Protein** 5.4 grams
> **Total fat** 0.7 gram
> **Saturated fat** 0.4 gram
> **Total carbohydrates** 18.3 grams
> **Dietary fiber** 5.1 grams

1. Preheat the oven to 300°F.

2. Place 2 tablespoons of the sugar and $^1/_4$ cup of water in a small saucepan and heat, stirring, over medium heat until the sugar dissolves, then let come to a boil and boil until the water evaporates and the sugar turns light brown.

3. Pour another $^1/_4$ cup of water into the saucepan of caramel and stir to dissolve, then let boil until you have about 3 tablespoons of caramel liquid. Pour an equal amount of the caramel into each ramekin.

4. Place the Egg Beaters or egg whites, sugar substitute, vanilla, orange zest, corn bran and the remaining 1 tablespoon of sugar in a bowl and stir to mix.

5. Place the cornstarch in a small bowl, add a little of the milk and stir until a paste forms.

6. Place the remaining milk in a saucepan and heat it almost to a boil over medium heat. Stir the cornstarch paste again and add it to the pan, stirring until it comes to a boil and thickens slightly. Pour the milk mixture over the Egg Beaters or egg white mixture and stir well. Divide the flan among the 5 ramekins, spooning a generous ⅓ cup into each.

7. Place the ramekins in a roasting pan and add ¾ inch of cold water to the pan. Bake the flans until just set, 40 minutes to 1 hour (the time they take to set is very variable).

8. Remove the flans from the roasting pan and cover them as they cool. To serve, run a knife around the inside of each ramekin and invert it quickly so the caramel is on the top. Frozen flans can be thawed by microwaving them on high power for 30 seconds and then letting them stand at room temperature for about 30 minutes.

NOTE One source for corn bran is www.honeyvillegrain.com.

Indian Barley Pudding

Makes five ⅓-cup servings

A CONVENTIONAL INDIAN PUDDING starts with cornmeal, but use barley instead, cut down on the cream, keep the molasses and wonderful spices— and you end up with a sublime dessert (and a peak hedonic experience). Indian Barley Pudding makes a fine low-calorie diet finish to any Stage II dinner.

½ cup hulled barley
1½ cups nonfat or 1% milk,
    plus milk for serving
2 tablespoons molasses
Sugar substitute equivalent to 2 tablespoons sugar
    (optional)
½ teaspoon ground ginger
½ teaspoon ground cinnamon
¼ teaspoon ground nutmeg

Nutritional information per ⅓-cup serving with 2 tablespoons milk:	
Calories 150	
Protein 6.7 grams	
Total fat 1.0 gram	
Saturated fat 0.4 gram	
Total carbohydrates 28.8 grams	
Dietary fiber 3.1 grams	

1. Put the barley and 1¼ cups water in a pot with a tight-fitting lid and bring to a boil. Turn off the heat and let stand until the water is completely absorbed, about 20 minutes.

2. Add the milk, cover the pot and let simmer over low heat until the barley is cooked and the liquid is mostly absorbed, about 40 minutes.

3. Add the molasses, sugar substitute, if using, ginger, cinnamon and nutmeg and stir. There should be a nice thick sauce, and the grains of barley should be plump (if the sauce is a little thin, cover the pot again and let the pudding sit for about 15 minutes to thicken).

4. Serve the pudding warm or cold with a little milk.

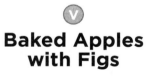

Baked Apples with Figs

Makes six servings

EVEN THOUGH FIGS ARE THOUGHT to be the first cultivated food, predating cereals like barley and wheat, they came to the Americas only about 200 years ago. I'm glad they did! This yummy source of fiber—with nearly one gram per small fig—is also a great source of minerals such as iron and zinc. Here, black mission figs are matched up with apples and spices to make a delicious dessert that you'll never tire of. (P.S. Try this one on company.)

5 to 6 dried black mission figs

Finely grated zest of 1 large orange,
   or ½ teaspoon orange extract

Sugar substitute equivalent to 3 tablespoins sugar
   (optional)

1 tablespoon dark brown sugar

2 teaspoons ground cinnamon

¼ teaspoon grated nutmeg

6 small to medium-size cooking apples,
   such as Cortland or Rome

> **Nutritional information per serving:**
>
> **Calories** 135
>
> **Protein** 0.5 gram
>
> **Total fat** 0.5 gram
>
> **Saturated fat** 0.1 gram
>
> **Total carbohydrates** 23.8 grams
>
> **Dietary fiber** 4.3 grams

1. Preheat the oven to 350°F.

2. Cut up the figs into small pieces and mix them with the orange zest or orange extract, sugar substitute, if using, brown sugar, cinnamon and nutmeg.

3. Core the apples (this is really easy to do with a corer, but if you don't have one, just cut a hole through the center of each apple to remove the core). Score the skin around the middle of each apple to give it a "belt," which will keep the apple from disintegrating when it bakes.

4. Put the apples in a baking dish just large enough to fit them snugly, spoon the fig filling into the holes that you've made in each one and then pour ⅓ cup water into the baking dish. If there is more fig mixture than will fit in the apples, just put the extra filling in the water.

5. Cover the baking dish tightly with aluminum foil and bake the apples until softened, 45 to 55 minutes (when done, the apples can be easily pierced with a skewer). Don't worry if the apples mush up some despite having been scored; they will still taste great. When the apples have finished baking, the sauce may be too liquid; if so, boil it until some of the liquid has evaporated, then pour it over the apples. The apples keep well in the refrigerator for several days.

Variation: For dinner parties, I sometimes add a dash of brandy to the filling for the apples.

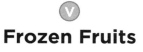

Almost Apple Cobbler

Makes one serving

IF IT SOUNDS TOO GOOD TO BE TRUE, it probably is—except in this case. This instant dessert is so close to the real thing that you'll be amazed at how good it tastes. While it can be made with store-bought applesauce, do use the homemade variety (page 140) if you have some handy.

½ cup unsweetened applesauce
¼ cup raw oat bran
A little sugar substitute (optional)
2 tablespoons sweetened light whipped cream

Place the applesauce and oat bran in a bowl and stir to mix. Add sugar substitute to taste if needed. Serve the "cobbler" with the whipped cream on top.

> **Nutritional information per serving:**
> **Calories** 140
> **Protein** 3.5 grams
> **Total fat** 2.5 grams
> **Saturated fat** 1.3 grams
> **Total carbohydrates** 27 grams
> **Dietary fiber** 5.0 grams

Frozen Fruits

Makes four ¼-cup servings

FROZEN FRUITS ARE FINE DIET FOOD because they take a long time to eat and help you spin out a meal while you wait to feel full.

1 cup assorted fruits, such as grapes, thinly sliced watermelon, thin bite-size pieces of pineapple and/or sliced strawberries

Arrange the fruits in a single layer on a baking sheet and freeze them. Transfer the frozen fruits to a plastic freezer bag for storage.

> **Average nutritional information per ¼-cup serving:**
> **Calories** 18
> **Protein** 0.2 gram
> **Total fat** 0 grams
> **Saturated fat** 0 grams
> **Total carbohydrates** 6.5 grams
> **Dietary fiber** 0.7 gram

(V)
Chocolate-Tipped Strawberries and Cream
Makes two servings

BY MAKING THIS DESSERT at home with bittersweet chocolate, you can turn a diet no-no into a fabulous low-cal treat.

2 cups ripe strawberries, hulls removed,
    rinsed and dried well
1½ squares (about 15 grams) best bittersweet
    chocolate
¼ cup light whipped cream (optional),
    for serving

Nutritional information
per serving with whipped
cream:

Calories 90	
Protein 1.2 grams	
Total fat 2.8 grams	
Saturated fat 1.2 grams	
Total carbohydrates 17.5 grams	
Dietary fiber 3.7 grams	

Line a baking sheet with wax paper. Melt the chocolate in a microwave on high power for about 20 seconds; be sure not to overheat the chocolate or it will burn. Quickly dip the tips of the strawberries in the chocolate, placing each on the baking sheet as it's done. If the chocolate gets hard before you've finished dipping all the fruit, you can remelt it in the microwave. Let the strawberries stand for a few minutes so the chocolate hardens. Serve them with the light whipped cream, if desired.

(V)
Vanilla Spice Cookies
Makes thirty-six cookies

COOKIES ARE USUALLY OFF THE MENU for dieters because they're so high in calories and easy to overeat. This recipe makes cookie eating a no-guilt activity. The cookies are good and easy to prepare, while the extra fiber and healthy oils keep you satisfied longer than a regular cookie would.

1 cup good granola (vanilla or cinnamon-flavored),
    not low-fat

²/₃ cup flaxseed meal

1 cup chickpea (garbanzo bean) flour

¹/₂ cup (2 ounces) corn bran (see Note)

Sugar substitute equivalent to 1 cup sugar

¹/₂ cup lightly packed dark brown sugar

¹/₂ teaspoon baking soda

¹/₄ teaspoon ground cinnamon

¹/₂ teaspoon ground mace (optional if you're using
    cinnamon-flavored granola)

2 teaspoons vanilla extract

4 ounces tub margarine, melted

2 large eggs, beaten

A little sugar, for sprinkling on the cookies

> **Nutritional information per cookie:**
>
> **Calories** 70
>
> **Protein** 1.9 grams
>
> **Total fat** 3.7 grams
>
> **Saturated fat** 0.8 gram
>
> **Total carbohydrates** 8.2 grams
>
> **Dietary fiber** 2.6 grams

1. Preheat the oven to 325°F.

2. Grind the granola in a food processor until small pieces form; it should not be chunky but it should also not have the consistency of flour.

3. Place the granola in a bowl and add the flaxseed meal, chickpea flour, corn bran, sugar substitute, brown sugar, baking soda, cinnamon and mace, if using.

4. Stir the vanilla into the margarine, pour the mixture over the dry ingredients and mix well with a fork. Add the eggs and stir to form a soft batter, kneading it a bit while it firms up.

5. Divide the dough into 36 balls about the size of whole walnuts, place them on a baking sheet and flatten them with a fork until they're about 3 inches in diameter. Bake the cookies until just set, about 6 minutes for soft cookies, or until they are starting to brown lightly around the edges, about 10 minutes for crisp cookies. Sprinkle each cookie with about ¹/₄ teaspoon sugar immediately after they come out of the oven. These cookies store well in plastic bags.

NOTE One source for corn bran is www.honeyvillegrain.com.

ⓥ Snack Attack Packs

Makes one serving

HOW DO YOU COUNTER a hunger attack? You can walk into the nearest deli and buy an 800-calorie brownie . . . or you can plan ahead and carry a Snack Attack Pack with you at all times. These convenient snacks show up in the Stage II menus when you need to keep fiber intake high but may not want to have high-fiber cereal at both breakfast and dinner.

Salty Snack Attack Pack

¼ cup high-fiber cereal
   (Fiber One or All-Bran Extra Fiber)
2 tablespoons roasted salted peanuts
Seasoning powder, such as nacho,
   Cajun or barbecue flavor (optional;
   see Note)

Put the cereal and peanuts in a plastic bag. Add seasoning powder, if using, mix everything together and you have a snack to go.

NOTE One source for seasoning powders is www.spicesetc.com.

Sweet Snack Attack Pack

¼ cup high-fiber cereal
   (Fiber One or All-Bran Extra Fiber)
1 square (about 10 grams) bittersweet
   chocolate
4 pecan halves, chopped

Put the cereal in a small microwave-safe bowl with the chocolate square on top. Microwave on high power until the chocolate is melted but not bubbling—this usually takes 20 to 40 seconds. Then mix the cereal and chocolate together well with a fork until all of the cereal is nicely coated. Let cool completely, mix in the chopped pecans and put this sweet snack in a bag to take with you the next time you go out.

Trail Mix Snack Attack Pack

¼ cup high-fiber cereal
   (Fiber One or All-Bran Extra Fiber)
1 tablespoon raisins
2 teaspoons sunflower seeds
2 pecan halves, chopped

Just put the cereal, raisins, sunflower seeds and chopped pecans in a plastic bag and they're ready to go.

Nutritional information per Snack Attack Pack:	
Calories 125	
Protein 2.7 grams	
Total fat 8.2 grams	
Saturated fat 2.1 grams	
Total carbohydrates 18.1 grams	
Dietary fiber 8.1 grams	

Rhubarb Yogurt

Makes four servings

IT SEEMS THAT RHUBARB WAS USED in ancient China for medicinal purposes. I can't speak to that, but I can tell you that the fruit's high acid content slows down digestion, making it a good diet food. Here's a simple but delicious way to prepare it, suitable for either breakfast or dessert. I especially like Greek yogurt with the rhubarb because its high protein content makes it luxuriously creamy, as well as extra-satisfying.

1 pound rhubarb stalks
Sugar substitute equivalent to ¼ cup sugar,
   or more to taste (optional)
4 teaspoons sugar
2 cups 0% (nonfat) or 2% plain Greek yogurt

Nutritional information per serving:

Calories 90	
Protein 7.3 grams	
Total fat 1.7 grams	
Saturated fat 1.1 grams	
Total carbohydrates 18.3 grams	
Dietary fiber 2.0 grams	

Cut the rhubarb stalks into 1-inch lengths. Place them in a pot with a tight-fitting lid, add ⅓ cup water and bring to a simmer over low heat. Cook the rhubarb, covered, until it's soft but not broken up, about 10 minutes, then remove it from the heat and stir in the sugar substitute, if using, and sugar. Let the rhubarb sauce cool to room temperature, then refrigerate it until it's thoroughly chilled. To serve, place ½ cup yogurt in 4 bowls and add ½ cup cold rhubarb sauce to each.

Drinks

WE ALL KNOW THAT WATER is the perfect drink (no calories), but often we crave something a little more interesting. Since many non-dieters get as much as 22% or even more of their calories from what they drink and liquid calories aren't as satisfying as solid ones, a lot of calories can be saved by switching to good-tasting, healthy options like the ones that follow.

Refreshing Limonata Ⓥ

Fennel Infusion Ⓥ

Kenyan Chai Ⓥ

Masala Tea Ⓥ

"I" Diet Hot or Cold Chocolate Ⓥ

See also Bonus Recipes, page 270

Ⓥ

Refreshing Limonata

Makes one serving

A CLASSIC ITALIAN THIRST-QUENCHER, *limonata* can be made with still or sparkling water; it's great either way. One advantage of this drink is its acidity, which slows digestion and leads to more prolonged fullness.

1 very small ripe lemon, cut in half
Ice
Still or sparkling water
Sugar substitute equivalent to 1 teaspoon sugar
(optional)

Squeeze the lemon into a tall glass and add ice and water. Add a little sugar substitute if you need it, but you may also like the drink without.

> **Nutritional information per serving:**
>
> **Calories** 6
> **Protein** 0.1 gram
> **Total fat** 0 grams
> **Saturated fat** 0 grams
> **Total carbohydrates** 1 gram
> **Dietary fiber** 0.1 gram

Fennel Infusion

Makes one serving

IT'S IMPORTANT TO HAVE A DRINK with every meal and every snack. If you get a little tired of, say, herbal tea, try this fragrant alternative.

> 2 teaspoons fennel seeds
> Sugar substitute (optional)

Bring 1 cup of water almost to a boil. Place the fennel seeds in a mug and pour the hot water over them. Let steep for 10 to 15 minutes. If you like, reheat the infusion a bit before drinking it and add some sugar substitute if you want it to be sweet. It can also be served with ice.

Nutritional information per serving:

Calories 0	
Protein 0 grams	
Total fat 0 grams	
Saturated fat 0 grams	
Total carbohydrates 0 grams	
Dietary fiber 0 grams	

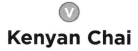

Kenyan Chai

Makes 4 cups

REAL CHAI IS NOTHING LIKE the thin, hot tea with hot spices that sometimes goes by that name. This recipe is an authentic version of true Kenyan chai—aromatic, thick and intensely sweet. You can make up a biggish batch and keep some in the refrigerator. It's great for people who need a sweet fix at the end of a meal. Serve the chai in small cups—four ounces is plenty.

> 15 green cardamom pods (see Note)
> 3 tea bags of good regular or decaf black tea,
>   such as Twinings Darjeeling
> 2 cups nonfat or 1% milk
> ¼ cup sugar substitute (optional),
>   or more to taste

Nutritional information per ½-cup serving:

Calories 27	
Protein 2.0 grams	
Total fat 0.7 gram	
Saturated fat 0.4 gram	
Total carbohydrates 3.4 grams	
Dietary fiber 0 grams	

Bring 2 cups of water nearly to a boil in a small pot. Turn off the heat, add the cardamom pods, cover the pot and let steep for about ½ hour. Add the tea bags and let steep for 5 minutes. Remove the tea bags, add the milk and sugar substitute, if using, and bring to a boil. If you refrigerate the chai, heat each serving in the microwave on high power for about 1 minute before drinking.

NOTE Cardamom pods are inexpensive if you buy them in an Indian supermarket.

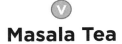

Masala Tea

Makes enough masala powder
for many cups of tea

IF YOU ENJOY TEA, this is a drink to fall in love with. Masala powder, a well-known Tanzanian spice mix, takes a little while to make, but you'll feel as if you're in an African bazaar as you stand over the roasting spices (and your home will smell wonderful for hours!). The powder stores well in an airtight jar away from light, and then delicious spicy tea is yours anytime you want it. Masala tea makes a great snack with a piece of fruit. Many spices contain natural chemicals that seem to help modulate blood glucose, which means they may be good for weight control, too.

For the masala powder:
- 4 large cinnamon sticks
- 4 whole nutmegs
- ¼ cup green cardamom pods
- 2 tablespoons plus 1 teaspoon whole black peppercorns
- 2 tablespoons ground ginger
- 2 tablespoons whole cloves

Nutritional information per ½-cup serving:

Calories 27

Protein 2.0 grams

Total fat 0.7 gram

Saturated fat 0.4 gram

Total carbohydrates 3.4 grams

Dietary fiber 0 grams

For the tea:

3 tea bags of good regular or decaf black tea, such as Twinings Darjeeling
Nonfat or 1% milk
Sugar substitute (optional)

1. Make the masala powder: Break the cinnamon sticks into pieces and crush the nutmegs. Toast the cinnamon sticks, nutmegs, cardamom pods, peppercorns, ginger and cloves in a heavy pan over medium heat, stirring frequently, until they roast but don't brown, 10 to 15 minutes. Grind the spices in a spice mill or coffee grinder and store in a closed dark jar.

2. Make the tea: Bring 2 cups of water to a boil, turn off the heat, then add the tea bags and 1 generous teaspoon of masala powder and let steep for 5 to 10 minutes. Strain the infused tea.

3. For each serving, scald ¼ cup of milk and mix with ¼ cup of the infused tea. Sweeten the tea to taste with sugar substitute, if desired. You can save leftover infused tea in the refrigerator for a couple of days.

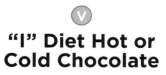

"I" Diet Hot or Cold Chocolate

Makes one serving

MOST TYPES OF HOT CHOCOLATE are the last thing you need when you're trying to lose weight—they're packed full of bad carbohydrates and not much else. This recipe is scientifically formulated with two ingredients that make it ideal for weight loss. The first is Dutch-process cocoa powder; unlike other cocoa powders, it's loaded with fiber. The second ingredient is the enriched nonfat (or, if you prefer, 1%) milk, which tastes richer than regular skim. I've used this recipe as a snack in the "I" Diet menus, but an eight-ounce serving with a piece of "carb-style" toast and a side of fruit also makes a great breakfast.

1½ teaspoons Dutch-process cocoa,
    such as Droste
Sugar substitute equivalent to 2 teaspoons sugar,
    or more to taste
1 cup enriched nonfat milk

Nutritional information
per 1-cup serving:

Calories 122

Protein 11.3 grams

Total fat 1.5 grams

Saturated fat 1 gram

Total carbohydrates 15.0 grams

Dietary fiber 2.2 grams

Blend the cocoa, sugar substitute and about 1 tablespoon of milk together in a microwave-safe cup until really smooth—Dutch-process cocoa powder needs a little vigorous mixing with a small amount of milk.

For hot chocolate: Add the rest of the milk, then microwave on high power until hot, about 1 minute and 30 seconds. Stir the hot chocolate well and taste for sweetness, adding more sugar substitute as needed. If you're making hot chocolate for fussy kids as well as yourself, you can strain the hot chocolate before serving in case there are a few remaining lumps in the bottom.

For cold chocolate: Stir the cocoa mixture, then add the remaining cold milk. If you want it really cold, you can make the chocolate in advance and refrigerate it or add an ice cube.

Variations: Orange chocolate—Add ¼ teaspoon of orange extract before serving.

Mint chocolate—Add ⅛ teaspoon of peppermint extract before serving.

Vanilla chocolate—Add ½ teaspoon of vanilla extract before serving.

Christmas Eve chocolate—Add 2 teaspoons of brandy or rum before serving; great for an afternoon snack while wrapping presents!

A Celebration Dinner for Eight

JUST BECAUSE YOU'RE DIETING doesn't mean you shouldn't be entertaining guests with food that looks spectacular and tastes great. With this menu—simple enough for even a novice chef to pull off—your guests will never suspect that they're eating diet-friendly food. They'll have a wonderful time, enjoy a fabulous meal and thank you the next day when they get on the scale without any of that next-day dread.

Menu

Potage St. Germaine

Roast Tenderloin of Beef
with Porcini Mushroom Gravy

Lemon-Braised Artichoke Hearts

Green Beans with Caramelized Onions

Warmed bread with butter, for people
who are not dieting

Kirsch-Marinated Peaches

Fine chocolates

Potage St. Germaine

Makes 8 cups

THIS SOPHISTICATED THICK SOUP is packed full of satisfying vegetables. And it's so easy to make.

2 large leeks, white parts only
1 tablespoon tub margarine
1 tablespoon canola oil
5 cups good-quality store-bought chicken stock
2 packages (10 ounces each) frozen peas
3 cups chopped Bibb lettuce
Salt and freshly ground black pepper
1/4 cup half-and-half
1 cup store-bought low-fat croutons
1/4 cup finely shredded fresh mint leaves

Nutritional information per 1-cup serving:

Calories 121
Protein 5.7 grams
Total fat 4.8 grams
Saturated fat 1.1 grams
Total carbohydrates 14.5 grams
Dietary fiber 4.7 grams

1. Split the leeks in half lengthwise and rinse them under cold running water. Chop the leeks, place them with the margarine and oil in a large pot and cook, stirring occasionally, over very low heat until the leeks are wilted but not browned, about 10 minutes.

2. Add the chicken stock, peas and lettuce and let simmer until thickened, about 5 minutes, then season with salt and pepper to taste. Refrigerate the soup, covered, until you're ready to serve.

3. Reheat the soup, if necessary, on the stove over medium-low heat. Ladle a cup of soup into each of 8 bowls and drizzle a little half-and-half over each serving. Scatter about 1/4 cup of croutons in the middle of each bowl and sprinkle a little mint on top.

Roast Tenderloin of Beef with Porcini Mushroom Gravy

Makes enough to serve eight generously,
with leftovers for a salad the next day

SO TASTY, YOU'D NEVER KNOW YOU WERE ON A DIET!

1 beef tenderloin (4 to 5 pounds), trimmed of fat
around the outside
Salt, freshly ground black pepper, garlic powder and
paprika
Olive oil or canola oil spray
1 medium-size carrot, peeled and chopped
1 medium-size onion, peeled and cut in quarters
1 rib celery, roughly chopped
1½ cups good-quality store-bought beef stock
½ ounce dried porcini mushrooms
½ cup mellow red wine
3 tablespoons port wine
2 tablespoons canola oil
3 tablespoons all-purpose flour
Watercress (optional), for garnish

> **Nutritional information per 4½-ounce serving of beef:**
> **Calories** 264
> **Protein** 28.1 grams
> **Total fat** 12.4 grams
> **Saturated fat** 3.7 grams
> **Total carbohydrates** 4.7 grams
> **Dietary fiber** 0.5 gram

1. Preheat the oven to 350°F.

2. Rinse the tenderloin under cold running water and pat it dry with paper towels. Place the tenderloin in a roasting pan and sprinkle a little salt, pepper, garlic powder and paprika on top, then lightly spray it with oil. Add the carrot, onion and celery to the roasting pan.

3. Bake the tenderloin until done to your liking. When it's cooked to medium-rare, an instant-read thermometer inserted in the center of the tenderloin will read 135°F after about 50 minutes.

4. While the meat is cooking, heat the beef stock until almost boiling and soak the mushrooms in it for about 20 minutes. Remove the mushrooms and chop them finely. Drain the stock into a separate bowl, being careful to leave behind any sand from the mushrooms, and set it aside.

5. Remove the meat from the roasting pan and let it rest while you make the gravy. Skim all of the fat out of the roasting pan and discard. Add the red wine and port and heat on the stove top until boiling, stirring up any meat drippings from the bottom of the pan. Discard the vegetables.

6. Place the oil and flour in a pot and heat over low heat, stirring to blend, until sandy in appearance but not browning, 2 to 3 minutes. Using a balloon whisk, add the reserved stock, the chopped mushrooms and the wine mixture and let come to a boil. Taste for seasoning, adding salt and pepper as needed. If the gravy is too thin, let it boil until reduced.

7. To serve, cut thick slices of the tenderloin, arrange them on a platter and pour some of the gravy on top. Garnish with watercress around the edges, if using, and pass around the remaining gravy.

(V)

Lemon-Braised Artichoke Hearts

Makes about 6 cups

PREPARING ARTICHOKE HEARTS REQUIRES SOME WORK, because you have to remove all the outer leaves, but your guests will love you for it. (Those from a salad bar taste completely different and can't be used here.)

About 4 lemons
10 large artichokes
1 tablespoon tub margarine
1 tablespoon canola oil
Salt

Nutritional information per $3/4$-cup serving:
Calories 97
Protein 4.7 grams
Total fat 3.4 grams
Saturated fat 0.4 gram
Total carbohydrates 15.8 grams
Dietary fiber 7.2 grams

1. Squeeze the juice of ½ lemon into a bowl of cold water. Cut the stem off 1 artichoke, pull off all the leaves and, using a spoon, remove the fibrous center, leaving the good central heart. Place the heart in the bowl of lemon water. Repeat with the remaining artichokes.

2. About 1 hour before dinner is to be served, cut each choke into 8 wedges. Place the margarine and oil in a heavy pot over low heat. Add the artichoke wedges and cook, turning occasionally, until soft but not browned, about 45 minutes.

3. Add the juice of 2 lemons to the pot, season with salt to taste, cover the pot tightly and cook until the hearts are tender, about 30 minutes. You shouldn't need to add water if the pot lid fits really well, but check every 5 minutes or so, adding water if necessary.

4. Taste for seasoning, adding more lemon juice as needed; the artichoke hearts should have a strong but not overpowering lemon taste.

(V)

Green Beans with Caramelized Onions

Makes 8 cups

CARAMELIZED ONIONS make so many dishes special. This recipe caramelizes about twice as much onion as you need for the green beans, so you can be indulgent and use the leftovers to liven up salads, grilled meats, hamburgers and vegetables over the next few days.

3 large onions
1 tablespoon (½ ounce) real butter
1½ tablespoons canola oil
¾ teaspoon salt
1 teaspoon sugar (optional)
2½ pounds green beans, trimmed
    (about 10 cups before trimming)

> **Nutritional information per 1-cup serving:**
>
> **Calories** 48
> **Protein** 1.8 grams
> **Total fat** 1.6 grams
> **Saturated fat** 0.3 gram
> **Total carbohydrates** 8.2 grams
> **Dietary fiber** 3.3 grams

1. Peel and quarter the onions, then thinly slice the quarters. Melt the butter in the oil in a saucepan over very low heat. Add the onions and salt and cook, stirring often, without browning at all until the onions are completely wilted and cooked, about 1 hour.

2. Increase the heat to medium and let the onions brown, stirring frequently, until they're uniformly golden brown. You can add the sugar and 2 tablespoons of water if the pan bottom browns, rather than the onions. Cover the caramelized onions and set them aside until ready to serve or let them cool and then refrigerate them, covered, for up to 2 days.

3. Steam the green beans in a little water until almost tender, about 5 minutes.

4. Remove the green beans to a serving bowl, mix them with about ¼ cup of the caramelized onions and then garnish them with another ¼ cup of onions.

(V)

Kirsch-Marinated Peaches

Makes 8 cups

THIS DESSERT is a real after-dinner pick-me-up. Try it for breakfast, too, without the kirsch and topped with a little 2% Greek yogurt.

12 small peaches in season (2½ to 3 pounds)
¼ cup kirsch
2 tablespoons sugar
Sugar substitute (optional)

Nutritional information per 1-cup serving:
Calories 95
Protein 1 gram
Total fat 0.1 gram
Saturated fat 0 grams
Total carbohydrates 21.8 grams
Dietary fiber 2.9 grams

1. To cut a peach in half without mashing the flesh, first cut a ring around the outside down to the pit. Then firmly twist the halves in opposite directions. Remove and discard the pit, thinly slice the peach and place the slices in a bowl. Repeat with the remaining peaches. (It's not necessary to peel the peaches.)

2. Pour the kirsch over the peaches, add the sugar and mix well. Cover the bowl and let the peaches marinate for 1 to 2 hours. Just before serving, taste for sweetness, adding sugar substitute to taste if desired.

Bonus Recipes

(V)

Mint-Cilantro Dipping Sauce

Makes 1 cup

OH, GOODNESS, this pungent sauce from central Asia is a fabulous diet treat that will set your taste buds dancing. It's delicious as a dip for raw veggies or Spicy Sesame Cracker Chips (page 182), or you can use it as a salad dressing. The high vinegar content is great for weight loss, since acidic foods slow digestion and the return of hunger before the next meal.

1 ounce fresh mint leaves with thin stems
   (about 1 cup)
1 ounce fresh cilantro leaves with thin stems
   (about 1 cup)
2 large cloves garlic
1 fresh serrano (small green) pepper, stemmed,
   cut in half, seeds removed
³/₈ cup cider vinegar
1 teaspoon sugar
¹/₂ teaspoon salt

Nutritional information per 2-tablespoon serving:
Calories 8
Protein 0.3 gram
Total fat 0 grams
Saturated fat 0 grams
Total carbohydrates 1.4 grams
Dietary fiber 0.4 gram

1. Wash the mint and cilantro leaves under running water; drain well.

2. Place the garlic, serrano pepper, vinegar, sugar and salt in a blender and blend to a liquid. Add the mint and cilantro leaves and blend again until the mixture is smooth. Add up to ¹/₈ cup of water if necessary to make a nice creamy sauce. The sauce keeps well in the refrigerator for 3 to 4 days but does not freeze well.

Rosemary-Thyme Dressing

Makes two servings

THIS SIMPLE, MAKE-AND-SERVE DRESSING takes no time and is a wonderful aromatic addition to almost any salad.

2 teaspoons extra-virgin olive oil
1 teaspoon white wine vinegar
½ teaspoon fresh rosemary leaves, finely chopped
½ teaspoon fresh thyme, finely chopped
Salt and freshly ground black pepper, to taste

Drizzle the oil over salad greens of your choice and mix in well. Add the vinegar and mix again. Add the rosemary leaves, thyme, salt and pepper, and give the salad a final good toss. Serve immediately.

Nutritional information per serving of dressing:

Calories 40	
Protein 0 grams	
Total fat 4.5 grams	
Saturated fat 0.6 gram	
Total carbohydrates 0 grams	
Dietary fiber 0 grams	

Italian Meatballs

Makes 15 meatballs

WHO DOESN'T LOVE rich, satisfying Italian meatballs? And now you can enjoy them while you lose weight, because this recipe is scientifically formulated with "I" Diet principles. The recipe doubles easily, and the meatballs freeze well. And here's another bonus: Kids love them!

For the meatballs:
½ cup coarse wheat bran
½ cup seltzer
4 mushrooms
1 small red onion
1 large clove garlic
1 teaspoon olive oil
½ pound extra-lean (95%) ground beef (see Note)
½ large egg, beaten

2 tablespoons finely chopped parsley

⅛ teaspoon paprika

⅛ teaspoon dried basil

⅔ teaspoon salt

¼ teaspoon freshly ground black pepper

Cooking oil spray

For each 3-meatball serving:

1 ounce 100% whole-wheat pasta, uncooked

⅓ cup tomato sauce (Bertolini is my favorite commercial brand)

2 teaspoons grated Parmesan cheese, preferably imported

> **Nutritional information per 3-meatball serving with fixings:**
>
> **Calories** 240
>
> **Protein** 18.3 grams
>
> **Total fat** 6.0 grams
>
> **Saturated fat** 1.7 grams
>
> **Total carbohydrates** 32.0 grams
>
> **Dietary fiber** 7.2 grams

1. Preheat the oven to 425°F.

2. Mix the wheat bran and seltzer. Leave the mixture to soak.

3. Place the mushrooms, onion and garlic in a food processor and blend until very fine.

4. Heat a nonstick skillet until very hot. Add the olive oil and the mushroom mixture, and sauté for 2 to 3 minutes, or until browned. Turn off the heat and add the bran mixture to the mushroom mixture, scraping any brown bits off the bottom.

5. In a large bowl, mix the ground beef, egg and seasonings with the mushroom-bran mixture. Let sit for 5 minutes to firm up.

6. Form the meatballs, each about 1½ inches in diameter.

7. Line a baking tray with foil and spray lightly with cooking oil. Place the meatballs on the tray and bake for 15 to 20 minutes, or until the meatballs are lightly browned but not overdone.

8. Meanwhile, prepare the pasta according to package directions. When done, top with the meatballs, tomato sauce and cheese.

NOTE If necessary, ask your butcher to grind lean bottom round (after first removing any visible fat).

The Ultimate "I" Burger

Makes four burgers

WHEN HENRY LOUIS GATES JR. came to me wanting advice on losing weight, (see his story on pages xx–xxi), one of his nonnegotiables was a real hamburger. (His love of big, juicy, satisfying hamburgers is so well known around the Harvard campus that a famous burger place down the street has one named for him!) I created this recipe especially for Professor Gates, to give him a gourmet hamburger experience at a fraction of the usual calories. The patties freeze well when individually wrapped, so make up a large batch and have some on hand for a great standby lunch or dinner.

For the burgers:

1 medium onion, very finely chopped

½ large apple, preferably Cortland, peeled and grated

12 ounces extra-lean (95%) ground beef

4 teaspoons egg white

¼ teaspoon salt

⅛ teaspoon freshly ground black pepper

Cooking oil

For serving, per burger:

1 high-fiber hamburger roll, such as a Country Kitchen Light Wheat Roll

1 lettuce leaf

1 large slice fresh tomato

2 teaspoons ketchup

Pickles, as desired

Nutritional information per burger with roll, ketchup, lettuce and tomato slice:

Calories 238

Protein 23.2 grams

Total fat 5.9 grams

Saturated fat 1.9 grams

Total carbohydrates 26.8 grams

Dietary fiber 5.8 grams

1. In a heavy nonstick skillet, cook the onion without oil over high heat, stirring often, for about 3 minutes, or until it starts to brown.

2. Turn off the heat, add the grated apple to the skillet and scrape up all the brown mixture.

3. Mix the beef, egg white, salt and pepper with the onion-apple mixture. Shape into 4 patties, each 4 inches in diameter.

4. Place some cooking oil on a paper towel and wipe the inside of a nonstick skillet. Fry the patties for 2 to 3 minutes, or until cooked through and browned on both sides.

5. Assemble the burgers with lettuce, tomato, ketchup and pickles, if desired.

Ⓥ

Mexican Black Beans with Chips, Salsa and Sour Cream

Makes 4³⁄₄ cups
(just over nine ¹⁄₂-cup servings)

BEANS ARE PACKED with both fiber and protein, making them perfect "I" Diet fare. This foolproof, authentic Mexican recipe is great for either lunch or dinner and allows chips to be a legitimate part of your diet. I often make this dish on weekends so I can have a super-satisfying meal available for a busy weekday. Individual portions freeze well and can be microwaved for a minute or two to reheat.

For black bean mixture:
1 very large onion, finely chopped
3 garlic cloves, finely chopped
2 teaspoons olive oil
2 cups (13 ounces) dried black beans,
    soaked overnight in water to cover
    or soaked in hot water for 30 minutes
6 cups bean-soaking liquid
1¹⁄₂ teaspoons kosher salt
¹⁄₄ cup chopped cilantro

Nutritional information per ¹⁄₂-cup serving of beans with accompaniments:

Calories 287
Protein 13.1 grams
Total fat 6.2 grams
Saturated fat 2.0 grams
Total carbohydrates 47.2 grams
Dietary fiber 12.9 grams

For each serving of ¹/₂ cup cooked beans:

1 teaspoon grated Parmesan cheese (optional)

2 to 3 ounces baked tortilla chips such as Baked Tostitos
    (about 10 chips, or 80 calories worth depending on the brand)

¹/₄ cup salsa

1 tablespoon low-fat sour cream

1 cup or more iceberg lettuce "dippers"

1. In a nonstick skillet, sauté the onion and garlic in the olive oil over high heat for 5 minutes, or until browned. Add the beans, bean-soaking liquid and salt. Cover and simmer for about 2½ hours. Add the cilantro and simmer for another ½ hour, or until very soft. If the bean mixture is too watery, remove the lid for the last few minutes.

2. For each serving, spoon ½ cup of the beans into a small bowl and sprinkle with Parmesan cheese to melt on top, if desired. Serve with chips, salsa, sour cream and lettuce "dippers." The lettuce adds volume to the meal, which will make the moderate number of chips go a long way.

Belgian-Style Beef Stew

Makes 6 cups
(eight ³/₄-cup servings)

THE BELGIANS REALLY KNOW how to eat well, and this "I" version of their classic beef stew is great comfort food and a wonderful dinner-party dish, particularly when served on a cold winter night. You'll find the stew truly easy to prepare. Make lots—it freezes well for easy weeknight dinners. And add potatoes for non-dieting family members.

¹/₂ cup yellow split peas, soaked in 3 cups hot water
    for 1 hour or overnight

2 teaspoons olive oil

1¹/₂ pounds extra-lean cubed beef (see Note)

10 ounces (1 box) baby bella or white mushrooms, rinsed well

2 medium onions (12 ounces), chopped into ¹/₄-inch pieces

3 cloves garlic, peeled and chopped

1 cup Guinness or other rich stout
1 medium fresh tomato, skinned and finely chopped
1¾ cups beef stock
¾ teaspoon dried thyme
1 teaspoon kosher salt
½ teaspoon freshly ground black pepper
2 large carrots (10 ounces), peeled and cut into
    1-inch chunks
2 medium red potatoes with skins (11 ounces),
    cut into 1-inch chunks (optional for non-dieters)

> **Nutritional information per ³⁄₄-cup serving (without potatoes):**
>
> **Calories** 221
>
> **Protein** 25.2 grams
>
> **Total fat** 5.0 grams
>
> **Saturated fat** 1.3 grams
>
> **Total carbohydrates** 18.1 grams
>
> **Dietary fiber** 5.6 grams

1. Preheat the oven to 300°F.

2. Place the split peas in a saucepan with enough water to cover and bring to a boil, then lower the heat and let simmer for 10 to 15 minutes while you prepare the beef.

3. Heat ½ teaspoon of the olive oil in a Dutch oven or nonstick pan over high heat until very hot. Add the cubes of beef and brown on all sides; remove from pan. Add another ½ teaspoon of the oil to the pan and add the mushrooms; brown on all sides and remove. Reduce the heat to medium, add the remaining 1 teaspoon of oil and sauté the onions and garlic for about 10 minutes, or until lightly browned.

4. Return the beef and mushrooms to the pan. Add the stout and bring to a boil. Lower the heat and simmer for 2 minutes to reduce the alcohol.

5. Add the split peas, tomato, beef stock, thyme, salt and pepper to the pan. Cover and bake for 2½ hours. (If you've been using a nonstick pan, transfer the ingredients to a covered casserole dish before baking.)

6. Add the carrots and the potatoes, if using, and bake for about 60 minutes longer, or until the vegetables are cooked and the sauce is nicely thick.

NOTE There should be no visible fat or internal marbling. Bottom round, which your butcher can cut into fat-free chunks, is ideal.

Afghan Stuffed Peppers

Makes two servings

ENJOYING THE FOOD OF AFGHANISTAN is about as close as most of us will get to visiting. Upon being introduced to some delicious national dishes by thriller author extraordinaire Joe Finder and the Helmand Restaurant in Boston, I was not surprised to discover that the food is a fusion of European, Indian and Mongolian influences. What did surprise me was the "I" Diet appropriateness of many of the dishes I sampled, including this simple traditional recipe.

3 large green bell peppers
2 medium onions, finely chopped
1 jalapeño pepper, stemmed and finely chopped
1½ tablespoons corn oil
1 teaspoon cumin seeds
1 piece (1½ inches long and 1 inch in diameter)
    fresh ginger, peeled and chopped very fine
⅔ cup yellow split peas, soaked in hot water for
    1 hour and drained well
1¼ cups water
1 tablespoon coriander seeds, ground to a fine powder
2 tablespoons chopped fresh cilantro
1/16 teaspoon cayenne pepper
1 teaspoon kosher salt
½ teaspoon freshly ground black pepper
2 tablespoons plain yogurt mixed with pinch of salt (optional), for serving

Nutritional information per 1½ pepper halves (not including yogurt):

Calories 231	
Protein 10.2 grams	
Total fat 8.2 grams	
Saturated fat 0.7 gram	
Total carbohydrates 42.0 grams	
Dietary fiber 12.4 grams	

1. Cut the bell peppers in half lengthwise and remove the cores, seeds and ribs. Rinse the peppers under cold running water; set aside to dry.

2. Preheat the oven to 350°F.

3. In a large skillet, sauté the onions and jalapeño pepper in the corn oil over medium heat for about 10 minutes, or until lightly browned. Add the cumin seeds and ginger, and sauté for 2 minutes more.

4. Add the split peas plus the remaining herbs and seasonings to the pan and let simmer, covered, for about 1 hour, or until the peas are soft and all the water is absorbed. If necessary, leave the lid off at the end to make sure no water remains.

5. Place the peppers in an ovenproof dish, pile on the split-pea mixture and bake, covered, for 45 to 55 minutes, or until the peppers are just cooked but still slightly firm.

6. Transfer the baked peppers to the broiler and broil briefly to lightly brown the tops. Serve immediately. Top with yogurt, if desired.

(V)

Easy Bean-and-Cheese Burritos

Makes two servings
(1½ burritos each)

THIS IS A GREAT RECIPE for when you want something good in no time at all. Use high-fiber wraps, such as Cedar's Whole Wheat or Joseph's Flax, Oat Bran and Whole Wheat tortillas, to ensure the "I" Diet composition that will leave you full and satisfied. Substitute white wraps and cheddar cheese for non-dieting family members.

1 cup canned black beans, rinsed well and drained
3 tablespoons grated Parmesan cheese
3 high-fiber wraps (see Note)
4 tablespoons salsa
3 tablespoons nonfat sour cream
²/₃ cup or more shredded iceberg lettuce
Hot sauce, as desired

Nutritional information per
per 1½-burrito serving:

Calories 301	
Protein 24.1 grams	
Total fat 8.1 grams	
Saturated fat 3.8 grams	
Total carbohydrates 42.6 grams	
Dietary fiber 17.1 grams	

1. Place the beans and cheese in a microwave-proof container and microwave for 30 seconds to 1 minute. Cover the wraps with a damp towel and warm them on a microwave-proof plate. Pile all the fillings into the three wraps, close the wraps tightly and roll them up in aluminum foil for mess-free enjoyment. Each serving is 1½ burritos, so cut one in half. The half-burrito is a little awkward to eat but makes you super-full, so it's worth the mess!

NOTE Check out the Nutrition Facts on the package. The wraps should have 80 calories each, and grams of protein plus grams of fiber should add up to at least 8 grams.

Strawberry-Blueberry Smoothie

Makes 2¾ cups

MY WONDERFUL DAUGHTER, DIANA, introduced me to delectable Greek yogurt smoothies. This frozen slush of hers works best with frozen berries, so you can make it all year round.

1 cup 0% (nonfat) plain Greek yogurt
1¼ cups frozen strawberries
1¼ cup frozen blueberries
Sugar substitute equivalent to 1 tablespoon sugar, or more to taste
¼ cup nonfat or 1% milk

Place all the ingredients in a blender and blend to a smooth slush. You may need to stop the blender once or twice to move the fruit around so that it's well mixed. Serve immediately.

Nutritional information per scant 1-cup serving:
Calories 104
Protein 7.9 grams
Total fat 0.7 gram
Saturated fat 0.1 gram
Total carbohydrates 20.7 grams
Dietary fiber 3.1 grams

APPENDICES

Body Mass Index (BMI) Table

Using the table below, you can see right away whether your weight falls within the normal range for your height or indicates an overweight or obese condition. Just find your height in the left column and move across the table until you come to the column that includes your approximate weight. If that number falls in the white area, your weight is considered normal. Light gray represents a problem with overweight, and the darker gray shows up the more serious problem of obesity.

	Healthy Weight						Overweight										
BMI	**19**	**20**	**21**	**22**	**23**	**24**	**25**	**26**	**27**	**28**	**29**	**30**	**31**	**32**	**33**	**34**	**35**
Height	**Body Weight (pounds)**																
4'10"	91	96	100	105	110	115	119	124	129	134	138	143	148	153	158	162	167
4'11"	94	99	104	109	114	119	124	128	133	138	143	148	153	158	163	168	173
5'0"	97	102	107	112	118	123	128	133	138	143	148	153	158	163	168	174	179
5'1"	100	106	111	116	122	127	132	137	143	148	153	158	164	169	174	180	185
5'2"	104	109	115	120	126	131	136	142	147	153	158	164	169	175	180	186	191
5'3"	107	113	118	124	130	135	141	146	152	158	163	169	175	180	186	191	197
5'4"	110	116	122	128	134	140	145	151	157	163	169	174	180	186	192	197	204
5'5"	114	120	126	132	138	144	150	156	162	168	174	180	186	192	198	204	210
5'6"	118	124	130	136	142	148	155	161	167	173	179	186	192	198	204	210	216
5'7"	121	127	134	140	146	153	159	166	172	178	185	191	198	204	211	217	223
5'8"	125	131	138	144	151	158	164	171	177	184	190	197	203	210	216	223	230
5'9"	128	135	142	149	155	162	169	176	182	189	196	203	209	216	223	230	236
5'10"	132	139	146	153	160	167	174	181	188	195	202	209	216	222	229	236	243
5'11"	136	143	150	157	165	172	179	186	193	200	208	215	222	229	236	243	250
6'0"	140	147	154	162	169	177	184	191	199	206	213	221	228	235	242	250	258
6'1"	144	151	159	166	174	182	189	197	204	212	219	227	235	242	250	257	265
6'2"	148	155	163	171	179	186	194	202	210	218	225	233	241	249	256	264	272
6'3"	152	160	168	176	184	192	200	208	216	224	232	240	248	256	264	272	279
6'4"	156	164	172	180	189	197	205	213	221	230	238	246	254	263	271	279	287

Obese

36	37	38	39	40	41	42	43	44	45	46	47	48	49	50	51	52	53
172	177	181	186	191	196	201	205	210	215	220	224	229	234	239	244	248	253
178	183	188	193	198	203	208	212	217	222	227	232	237	242	247	252	257	262
184	189	194	199	204	209	215	220	225	230	235	240	245	250	255	261	266	271
190	195	201	206	211	217	222	227	232	238	243	248	254	259	264	269	275	280
196	202	207	213	218	224	229	235	240	246	251	256	262	267	273	278	284	289
203	208	214	220	225	231	237	242	248	254	259	265	270	278	282	287	293	299
209	215	221	227	232	238	244	250	256	262	267	273	279	285	291	296	302	308
216	222	228	234	240	246	252	258	264	270	276	282	288	294	300	306	312	318
223	229	235	241	247	253	260	266	272	278	284	291	297	303	309	315	322	328
230	236	242	249	255	261	266	274	280	287	293	299	306	312	319	325	331	338
236	243	249	256	262	269	276	282	289	295	302	308	315	322	328	335	341	348
243	250	257	263	270	277	284	291	297	304	311	318	324	331	338	345	351	358
250	257	264	271	278	285	292	299	306	313	320	327	334	341	348	355	362	369
257	265	272	279	286	293	301	308	315	322	329	338	343	351	358	365	373	379
265	272	279	287	294	302	309	316	324	331	338	346	353	361	368	375	383	390
272	280	288	295	302	310	318	325	333	340	348	355	363	371	378	386	393	401
280	287	295	303	311	319	326	334	342	350	358	365	373	381	389	396	404	412
287	295	303	311	319	327	335	343	351	359	367	375	383	391	399	407	415	423
295	304	312	320	328	336	344	353	361	369	377	385	394	402	410	418	426	435

Typical Daily Calorie Requirements Before and After Weight Loss

Find your height and the figure for your weight that corresponds to your activity level (see key at bottom of page), then factor in your age according to decade. For example, if you're in your forties, you can use the figures as they appear in the tables. If you're younger or older, follow the instructions that accompany each table.

Women: Calorie Requirements Before Weight Loss at Age 40

Height	Activity Level	90 Pounds	105 Pounds	120 Pounds	135 Pounds	150 Pounds	165 Pounds
5'0"	A	1,539	1,616	1,694	1,771	1,849	1,927
	B	1,764	1,854	1,944	2,034	2,124	2,214
	C	1,919	2,018	2,116	2,215	2,313	2,412
5'1"	A	1,554	1,632	1,710	1,787	1,865	1,942
	B	1,782	1,872	1,962	2,052	2,142	2,232
	C	1,939	2,038	2,136	2,235	2,333	2,432
5'2"	A	1,570	1,648	1,725	1,803	1,880	1,958
	B	1,801	1,891	1,981	2,071	2,161	2,251
	C	1,959	2,058	2,156	2,255	2,353	2,452
5'3"	A	1,586	1,663	1,741	1,819	1,896	1,974
	B	1,819	1,909	1,999	2,089	2,179	2,269
	C	1,979	2,078	2,176	2,275	2,373	2,472
5'4"	A	1,602	1,679	1,757	1,834	1,912	1,989
	B	1,837	1,927	2,017	2,107	2,197	2,287
	C	1,999	2,097	2,196	2,295	2,393	2,492
5'5"	A	1,617	1,695	1,772	1,850	1,928	2,005
	B	1,855	1,945	2,035	2,125	2,215	2,305
	C	2,019	2,117	2,216	2,314	2,413	2,511
5'6"	A	1,633	1,711	1,788	1,866	1,943	2,021
	B	1,874	1,964	2,054	2,144	2,233	2,323
	C	2,039	2,137	2,236	2,334	2,433	2,531
5'7"	A	1,649	1,726	1,804	1,882	1,959	2,037
	B	1,892	1,982	2,072	2,162	2,252	2,342
	C	2,059	2,157	2,256	2,354	2,453	2,551
5'8"	A	1,665	1,742	1,820	1,897	1,975	2,052
	B	1,910	2,000	2,090	2,180	2,270	2,360
	C	2,079	2,177	2,276	2,374	2,473	2,571
5'9"	A	1,680	1,758	1,835	1,913	1,991	2,068
	B	1,928	2,018	2,108	2,198	2,288	2,378
	C	2,099	2,197	2,296	2,394	2,493	2,591
5'10"	A	1,696	1,774	1,851	1,929	2,006	2,084
	B	1,947	2,037	2,126	2,216	2,306	2,396
	C	2,119	2,217	2,316	2,414	2,513	2,611
5'11"	A	1,712	1,789	1,867	1,944	2,022	2,100
	B	1,965	2,055	2,145	2,235	2,325	2,415
	C	2,139	2,237	2,336	2,434	2,533	2,631

A = Sedentary. B = Light activity (30 minutes of moderate activity, such as walking, on most days of

(Add 80 calories for each decade below 40; subtract 80 calories for each decade above 40.)

180 Pounds	195 Pounds	210 Pounds	225 Pounds	240 Pounds	255 Pounds	270 Pounds	285 Pounds
2,004	2,082	2,159	2,237	2,314	2,392	2,470	2,547
2,304	2,394	2,484	2,574	2,664	2,754	2,844	2,934
2,510	2,609	2,707	2,806	2,904	3,003	3,101	3,200
2,020	2,097	2,175	2,253	2,330	2,408	2,485	2,563
2,322	2,412	2,502	2,592	2,682	2,772	2,862	2,952
2,530	2,629	2,727	2,826	2,924	3,023	3,121	3,220
2,036	2,113	2,191	2,268	2,346	2,423	2,501	2,579
2,340	2,430	2,520	2,610	2,700	2,790	2,880	2,970
2,550	2,649	2,747	2,846	2,944	3,043	3,141	3,240
2,051	2,129	2,206	2,284	2,362	2,439	2,517	2,594
2,359	2,449	2,539	2,629	2,719	2,809	2,899	2,989
2,570	2,669	2,767	2,866	2,964	3,063	3,161	3,260
2,067	2,145	2,222	2,300	2,377	2,455	2,532	2,610
2,377	2,467	2,557	2,647	2,737	2,827	2,917	3,007
2,590	2,689	2,787	2,886	2,984	3,083	3,181	3,280
2,083	2,160	2,238	2,315	2,393	2,471	2,548	2,626
2,395	2,485	2,575	2,665	2,755	2,845	2,935	3,025
2,610	2,709	2,807	2,906	3,004	3,103	3,201	3,300
2,098	2,176	2,254	2,331	2,409	2,486	2,564	2,641
2,413	2,503	2,593	2,683	2,773	2,863	2,953	3,043
2,630	2,728	2,827	2,925	3,024	3,123	3,221	3,320
2,114	2,192	2,269	2,347	2,424	2,502	2,580	2,657
2,432	2,522	2,612	2,702	2,792	2,882	2,972	3,062
2,650	2,748	2,847	2,945	3,044	3,142	3,241	3,339
2,130	2,207	2,285	2,363	2,440	2,518	2,595	2,673
2,450	2,540	2,630	2,720	2,810	2,900	2,990	3,080
2,670	2,768	2,867	2,965	3,064	3,162	3,261	3,359
2,146	2,223	2,301	2,378	2,456	2,533	2,611	2,689
2,468	2,558	2,648	2,738	2,828	2,918	3,008	3,098
2,690	2,788	2,887	2,985	3,084	3,182	3,281	3,379
2,161	2,239	2,317	2,394	2,472	2,549	2,627	2,704
2,486	2,576	2,666	2,756	2,846	2,936	3,026	3,116
2,710	2,808	2,907	3,005	3,104	3,202	3,301	3,399
2,177	2,255	2,332	2,410	2,487	2,565	2,642	2,720
2,505	2,595	2,685	2,775	2,865	2,955	3,044	3,134
2,730	2,828	2,927	3,025	3,124	3,222	3,321	3,419

the week). **C** = At least 30 minutes of strenuous activity on most days.

Typical Daily Calorie Requirements Before and After Weight Loss (continued)

Men: Calorie Requirements Before Weight Loss at Age 40

Height	Activity Level	120 Pounds	135 Pounds	150 Pounds	165 Pounds	180 Pounds	195 Pounds
5'5"	A	2,115	2,208	2,301	2,394	2,487	2,581
	B	2,286	2,391	2,495	2,600	2,704	2,808
	C	2,530	2,650	2,770	2,891	3,011	3,131
5'6"	A	2,125	2,218	2,312	2,405	2,498	2,591
	B	2,298	2,403	2,507	2,611	2,716	2,820
	C	2,544	2,664	2,784	2,904	3,025	3,145
5'7"	A	2,136	2,229	2,322	2,415	2,509	2,602
	B	2,310	2,415	2,519	2,623	2,728	2,832
	C	2,557	2,677	2,798	2,918	3,038	3,158
5'8"	A	2,146	2,239	2,333	2,426	2,519	2,612
	B	2,322	2,426	2,531	2,635	2,740	2,844
	C	2,571	2,691	2,811	2,932	3,052	3,172
5'9"	A	2,157	2,250	2,343	2,436	2,530	2,623
	B	2,334	2,438	2,543	2,647	2,751	2,856
	C	2,584	2,705	2,825	2,945	3,065	3,186
5'10"	A	2,167	2,261	2,354	2,447	2,540	2,633
	B	2,346	2,450	2,554	2,659	2,763	2,868
	C	2,598	2,718	2,839	2,959	3,079	3,199
5'11"	A	2,178	2,271	2,364	2,458	2,551	2,644
	B	2,357	2,462	2,566	2,671	2,775	2,879
	C	2,612	2,732	2,852	2,972	3,093	3,213
6'0"	A	2,188	2,282	2,375	2,468	2,561	2,655
	B	2,369	2,474	2,578	2,682	2,787	2,891
	C	2,625	2,746	2,866	2,986	3,106	3,227
6'1"	A	2,199	2,292	2,385	2,479	2,572	2,665
	B	2,381	2,486	2,590	2,694	2,799	2,903
	C	2,639	2,759	2,880	3,000	3,120	3,240
6'2"	A	2,210	2,303	2,396	2,489	2,582	2,676
	B	2,393	2,497	2,602	2,706	2,811	2,915
	C	2,653	2,773	2,893	3,013	3,134	3,254
6'3"	A	2,220	2,313	2,407	2,500	2,593	2,686
	B	2,405	2,509	2,614	2,718	2,822	2,927
	C	2,666	2,787	2,907	3,027	3,147	3,268
6'4"	A	2,231	2,324	2,417	2,510	2,604	2,697
	B	2,417	2,521	2,625	2,730	2,834	2,939
	C	2,680	2,800	2,920	3,041	3,161	3,281

A = Sedentary. **B** = Light activity (30 minutes of moderate activity, such as walking, on most days of

(Add 100 calories for each decade below 40; subtract 100 calories for each decade above 40.)

210 Pounds	225 Pounds	240 Pounds	255 Pounds	270 Pounds	285 Pounds	300 Pounds	315 Pounds
2,674	2,767	2,860	2,953	3,047	3,140	3,233	3,326
2,913	3,017	3,122	3,226	3,330	3,435	3,539	3,644
3,251	3,372	3,492	3,612	3,732	3,853	3,973	4,093
2,684	2,778	2,871	2,964	3,057	3,150	3,244	3,337
2,925	3,029	3,133	3,238	3,342	3,447	3,551	3,655
3,265	3,385	3,506	3,626	3,746	3,866	3,987	4,107
2,695	2,788	2,881	2,975	3,068	3,161	3,254	3,347
2,937	3,041	3,145	3,250	3,354	3,459	3,563	3,667
3,279	3,399	3,519	3,639	3,760	3,880	4,000	4,120
2,706	2,799	2,892	2,985	3,078	3,172	3,265	3,358
2,948	3,053	3,157	3,262	3,366	3,470	3,575	3,679
3,292	3,413	3,533	3,653	3,773	3,894	4,014	4,134
2,716	2,809	2,903	2,996	3,089	3,182	3,275	3,369
2,960	3,065	3,169	3,273	3,378	3,482	3,587	3,691
3,306	3,426	3,546	3,667	3,787	3,907	4,027	4,148
2,727	2,820	2,913	3,006	3,100	3,193	3,286	3,379
2,972	3,076	3,181	3,285	3,390	3,494	3,598	3,703
3,320	3,440	3,560	3,680	3,801	3,921	4,041	4,161
2,737	2,830	2,924	3,017	3,110	3,203	3,297	3,390
2,984	3,088	3,193	3,297	3,401	3,506	3,610	3,715
3,333	3,453	3,574	3,694	3,814	3,934	4,055	4,175
2,748	2,841	2,934	3,027	3,121	3,214	3,307	3,400
2,996	3,100	3,204	3,309	3,413	3,518	3,622	3,726
3,347	3,467	3,587	3,708	3,828	3,948	4,068	4,189
2,758	2,852	2,945	3,038	3,131	3,224	3,318	3,411
3,008	3,112	3,216	3,321	3,425	3,530	3,634	3,738
3,360	3,481	3,601	3,721	3,841	3,962	4,082	4,202
2,769	2,862	2,955	3,049	3,142	3,235	3,328	3,421
3,019	3,124	3,228	3,333	3,437	3,541	3,646	3,750
3,374	3,494	3,615	3,735	3,855	3,975	4,096	4,216
2,779	2,873	2,966	3,059	3,152	3,246	3,339	3,432
3,031	3,136	3,240	3,344	3,449	3,553	3,658	3,762
3,388	3,508	3,628	3,748	3,869	3,989	4,109	4,229
2,790	2,883	2,976	3,070	3,163	3,256	3,349	3,443
3,043	3,147	3,252	3,356	3,461	3,565	3,669	3,774
3,401	3,522	3,642	3,762	3,882	4,003	4,123	4,243

the week). **C** = At least 30 minutes of strenuous activity on most days.

Typical Daily Calorie Requirements Before and After Weight Loss (continued)

According to our research at Tufts, energy requirements after weight loss are slightly lower than those for the same body weights before weight loss. For example, the daily requirement for a 5'3", 120-pound woman with a sedentary lifestyle is 1,741 calories before weight loss and 1,567 calories after weight loss.

Women: Calorie Requirements After Weight Loss at Age 40

Height	Activity Level	90 Pounds	105 Pounds	120 Pounds	135 Pounds	150 Pounds	165 Pounds
5'0"	A	1,385	1,455	1,524	1,594	1,664	1,734
	B	1,588	1,669	1,750	1,831	1,912	1,993
	C	1,727	1,816	1,905	1,993	2,082	2,170
5'1"	A	1,399	1,469	1,539	1,608	1,678	1,748
	B	1,604	1,685	1,766	1,847	1,928	2,009
	C	1,745	1,834	1,922	2,011	2,100	2,188
5'2"	A	1,413	1,483	1,553	1,623	1,692	1,762
	B	1,621	1,702	1,783	1,863	1,944	2,025
	C	1,763	1,852	1,940	2,029	2,118	2,206
5'3"	A	1,427	1,497	1,567	1,637	1,707	1,776
	B	1,637	1,718	1,799	1,880	1,961	2,042
	C	1,781	1,870	1,958	2,047	2,136	2,224
5'4"	A	1,441	1,511	1,581	1,651	1,721	1,791
	B	1,653	1,734	1,815	1,896	1,977	2,058
	C	1,799	1,888	1,976	2,065	2,154	2,242
5'5"	A	1,456	1,525	1,595	1,665	1,735	1,805
	B	1,670	1,751	1,832	1,913	1,994	2,075
	C	1,817	1,906	1,994	2,083	2,172	2,260
5'6"	A	1,470	1,540	1,609	1,679	1,749	1,819
	B	1,686	1,767	1,848	1,929	2,010	2,091
	C	1,835	1,924	2,012	2,101	2,190	2,278
5'7"	A	1,484	1,554	1,624	1,693	1,763	1,833
	B	1,703	1,784	1,865	1,946	2,027	2,108
	C	1,853	1,942	2,030	2,119	2,208	2,296
5'8"	A	1,498	1,568	1,638	1,708	1,777	1,847
	B	1,719	1,800	1,881	1,962	2,043	2,124
	C	1,871	1,960	2,048	2,137	2,226	2,314
5'9"	A	1,512	1,582	1,652	1,722	1,791	1,861
	B	1,735	1,816	1,897	1,978	2,059	2,140
	C	1,889	1,978	2,066	2,155	2,244	2,332
5'10"	A	1,526	1,596	1,666	1,736	1,806	1,875
	B	1,752	1,833	1,914	1,995	2,076	2,157
	C	1,907	1,996	2,084	2,173	2,262	2,350
5'11"	A	1,541	1,610	1,680	1,750	1,820	1,890
	B	1,768	1,849	1,930	2,011	2,092	2,173
	C	1,925	2,014	2,102	2,191	2,280	2,368

A = Sedentary. **B** = Light activity (30 minutes of moderate activity, such as walking, on most days of

(Add 80 calories for each decade below 40; subtract 80 calories for each decade above 40.)

180 Pounds	195 Pounds	210 Pounds	225 Pounds	240 Pounds	255 Pounds	270 Pounds	285 Pounds
1,804	1,874	1,943	2,013	2,083	2,153	2,223	2,292
2,074	2,155	2,236	2,317	2,398	2,478	2,559	2,640
2,259	2,348	2,436	2,525	2,614	2,702	2,791	2,880
1,818	1,888	1,957	2,027	2,097	2,167	2,237	2,307
2,090	2,171	2,252	2,333	2,414	2,495	2,576	2,657
2,277	2,366	2,454	2,543	2,632	2,720	2,809	2,898
1,832	1,902	1,972	2,041	2,111	2,181	2,251	2,321
2,106	2,187	2,268	2,349	2,430	2,511	2,592	2,673
2,295	2,384	2,472	2,561	2,650	2,738	2,827	2,916
1,846	1,916	1,986	2,056	2,125	2,195	2,265	2,335
2,123	2,204	2,285	2,366	2,447	2,528	2,609	2,690
2,313	2,402	2,490	2,579	2,668	2,756	2,845	2,934
1,860	1,930	2,000	2,070	2,140	2,209	2,279	2,349
2,139	2,220	2,301	2,382	2,463	2,544	2,625	2,706
2,331	2,420	2,508	2,597	2,686	2,774	2,863	2,952
1,874	1,944	2,014	2,084	2,154	2,224	2,293	2,363
2,156	2,237	2,318	2,399	2,480	2,561	2,642	2,723
2,349	2,438	2,526	2,615	2,704	2,792	2,881	2,970
1,889	1,958	2,028	2,098	2,168	2,238	2,307	2,377
2,172	2,253	2,334	2,415	2,496	2,577	2,658	2,739
2,367	2,456	2,544	2,633	2,722	2,810	2,899	2,988
1,903	1,973	2,042	2,112	2,182	2,252	2,322	2,391
2,189	2,269	2,350	2,431	2,512	2,593	2,674	2,755
2,385	2,474	2,562	2,651	2,740	2,828	2,917	3,006
1,917	1,987	2,057	2,126	2,196	2,266	2,336	2,406
2,205	2,286	2,367	2,448	2,529	2,610	2,691	2,772
2,403	2,492	2,580	2,669	2,758	2,846	2,935	3,024
1,931	2,001	2,071	2,141	2,210	2,280	2,350	2,420
2,221	2,302	2,383	2,464	2,545	2,626	2,707	2,788
2,421	2,510	2,598	2,687	2,776	2,864	2,953	3,041
1,945	2,015	2,085	2,155	2,224	2,294	2,364	2,434
2,238	2,319	2,400	2,481	2,562	2,643	2,724	2,805
2,439	2,528	2,616	2,705	2,793	2,882	2,971	3,059
1,959	2,029	2,099	2,169	2,239	2,308	2,378	2,448
2,254	2,335	2,416	2,497	2,578	2,659	2,740	2,821
2,457	2,545	2,634	2,723	2,811	2,900	2,989	3,077

the week). **C** = At least 30 minutes of strenuous activity on most days.

Typical Daily Calorie Requirements Before and After Weight Loss (continued)

According to our research at Tufts, energy requirements after weight loss are slightly lower than those for the same body weights before weight loss. For example, the daily requirement for a 5´10″, 150-pound man with a sedentary lifestyle is 2,354 calories before weight loss and 2,118 calories after weight loss.

Men: Calorie Requirements After Weight Loss at Age 40

Height	Activity Level	120 Pounds	135 Pounds	150 Pounds	165 Pounds	180 Pounds	195 Pounds
5'5"	A	1,903	1,987	2,071	2,155	2,239	2,323
	B	2,058	2,152	2,246	2,340	2,434	2,528
	C	2,277	2,385	2,493	2,602	2,710	2,818
5'6"	A	1,913	1,996	2,080	2,164	2,248	2,332
	B	2,068	2,162	2,256	2,350	2,444	2,538
	C	2,289	2,397	2,506	2,614	2,722	2,830
5'7"	A	1,922	2,006	2,090	2,174	2,258	2,342
	B	2,079	2,173	2,267	2,361	2,455	2,549
	C	2,302	2,410	2,518	2,626	2,734	2,843
5'8"	A	1,932	2,016	2,099	2,183	2,267	2,351
	B	2,090	2,184	2,278	2,372	2,466	2,560
	C	2,314	2,422	2,530	2,638	2,747	2,855
5'9"	A	1,941	2,025	2,109	2,193	2,277	2,361
	B	2,100	2,194	2,288	2,382	2,476	2,570
	C	2,326	2,434	2,542	2,651	2,759	2,867
5'10"	A	1,951	2,035	2,118	2,202	2,286	2,370
	B	2,111	2,205	2,299	2,393	2,487	2,581
	C	2,338	2,447	2,555	2,663	2,771	2,879
5'11"	A	1,960	2,044	2,128	2,212	2,296	2,380
	B	2,122	2,216	2,310	2,404	2,498	2,592
	C	2,351	2,459	2,567	2,675	2,783	2,892
6'0"	A	1,970	2,054	2,137	2,221	2,305	2,389
	B	2,132	2,226	2,320	2,414	2,508	2,602
	C	2,363	2,471	2,579	2,688	2,796	2,904
6'1"	A	1,979	2,063	2,147	2,231	2,315	2,399
	B	2,143	2,237	2,331	2,425	2,519	2,613
	C	2,375	2,483	2,592	2,700	2,808	2,916
6'2"	A	1,989	2,073	2,156	2,240	2,324	2,408
	B	2,154	2,248	2,342	2,436	2,529	2,623
	C	2,387	2,496	2,604	2,712	2,820	2,928
6'3"	A	1,998	2,082	2,166	2,250	2,334	2,418
	B	2,164	2,258	2,352	2,446	2,540	2,634
	C	2,400	2,508	2,616	2,724	2,833	2,941
6'4"	A	2,008	2,092	2,175	2,259	2,343	2,427
	B	2,175	2,269	2,363	2,457	2,551	2,645
	C	2,412	2,520	2,628	2,737	2,845	2,953

A = Sedentary. B = Light activity (30 minutes of moderate activity, such as walking, on most days of

(Add 100 calories for each decade below 40; subtract 100 calories for each decade above 40.)

210 Pounds	225 Pounds	240 Pounds	255 Pounds	270 Pounds	285 Pounds	300 Pounds	315 Pounds
2,406	2,490	2,574	2,658	2,742	2,826	2,910	2,994
2,622	2,716	2,809	2,903	2,997	3,091	3,185	3,279
2,926	3,035	3,143	3,251	3,359	3,467	3,576	3,684
2,416	2,500	2,584	2,668	2,752	2,835	2,919	3,003
2,632	2,726	2,820	2,914	3,008	3,102	3,196	3,290
2,939	3,047	3,155	3,263	3,371	3,480	3,588	3,696
2,425	2,509	2,593	2,677	2,761	2,845	2,929	3,013
2,643	2,737	2,831	2,925	3,019	3,113	3,207	3,301
2,951	3,059	3,167	3,276	3,384	3,492	3,600	3,708
2,435	2,519	2,603	2,687	2,771	2,854	2,938	3,022
2,654	2,747	2,841	2,935	3,029	3,123	3,217	3,311
2,963	3,071	3,180	3,288	3,396	3,504	3,612	3,721
2,444	2,528	2,612	2,696	2,780	2,864	2,948	3,032
2,664	2,758	2,852	2,946	3,040	3,134	3,228	3,322
2,975	3,084	3,192	3,300	3,408	3,516	3,625	3,733
2,454	2,538	2,622	2,706	2,790	2,873	2,957	3,041
2,675	2,769	2,863	2,957	3,051	3,145	3,239	3,333
2,988	3,096	3,204	3,312	3,421	3,529	3,637	3,745
2,463	2,547	2,631	2,715	2,799	2,883	2,967	3,051
2,685	2,779	2,873	2,967	3,061	3,155	3,249	3,343
3,000	3,108	3,216	3,325	3,433	3,541	3,649	3,757
2,473	2,557	2,641	2,725	2,809	2,892	2,976	3,060
2,696	2,790	2,884	2,978	3,072	3,166	3,260	3,354
3,012	3,120	3,229	3,337	3,445	3,553	3,662	3,770
2,483	2,566	2,650	2,734	2,818	2,902	2,986	3,070
2,707	2,801	2,895	2,989	3,083	3,177	3,271	3,364
3,024	3,133	3,241	3,349	3,457	3,566	3,674	3,782
2,492	2,576	2,660	2,744	2,828	2,911	2,995	3,079
2,717	2,811	2,905	2,999	3,093	3,187	3,281	3,375
3,037	3,145	3,253	3,361	3,470	3,578	3,686	3,794
2,502	2,585	2,669	2,753	2,837	2,921	3,005	3,089
2,728	2,822	2,916	3,010	3,104	3,198	3,292	3,386
3,049	3,157	3,265	3,374	3,482	3,590	3,698	3,807
2,511	2,595	2,679	2,763	2,847	2,931	3,014	3,098
2,739	2,833	2,927	3,021	3,115	3,209	3,302	3,396
3,061	3,169	3,278	3,386	3,494	3,602	3,711	3,819

the week). **C** = At least 30 minutes of strenuous activity on most days.

Nutrient Content of Common Foods

It's useful to have a general idea of the nutrient content and calorie count of foods you're likely to eat. Here are some values to get you started.

DAIRY	PORTION SIZE	CALORIES
Cheese, blue	1 ounce	100
Cheese, cream, low-fat	1 tablespoon	35
Cheese, feta	1 tablespoon	25
Cheese, Parmesan, grated	1 tablespoon	22
Cream, half-and-half	1 tablespoon	20
Cream, sour, reduced-fat	1 tablespoon	20
Egg, hard-boiled	1 large	78
Margarine, 80% fat	1 teaspoon	33
Milk, nonfat	1 cup	83
Milk, nonfat, enriched to taste like 2%	1 cup	101
Milk, 1%	1 cup	102
Milk, 1%, enriched to taste like full-fat milk	1 cup	118
Yogurt, plain, nonfat	½ cup	54
Yogurt, plain, nonfat Greek, strained	½ cup	60
Yogurt, plain, 2% fat	½ cup	67
Yogurt, plain, 2% fat Greek, strained	½ cup	75
FRUIT*	PORTION SIZE	CALORIES
Apple, with skin	1 medium	95
Applesauce, canned, unsweetened	½ cup	52
Apricot	1 medium	17
Avocado	1 medium	322
Banana	1 medium	105
Blackberries	½ cup	31
Blueberries	½ cup	42
Carambola (star fruit), cubed	½ cup	28

* Figures apply to raw fruit unless otherwise noted.

FIBER (grams)	PROTEIN (grams)	CARBOHYDRATES (grams)	FAT (grams)	SATURATED FAT (grams)
0.0	6.1	0.7	8.2	5.3
0.0	1.6	1.1	2.6	1.7
0.0	1.3	0.4	2.0	1.4
0.0	1.9	0.2	1.4	0.9
0.0	0.4	0.7	1.7	1.1
0.0	0.4	0.6	1.8	1.1
0.0	6.3	0.6	5.3	1.6
0.0	0.0	0.0	3.8	0.7
0.0	8.3	12.2	0.2	0.1
0.0	9.7	13.7	0.6	0.4
0.0	8.2	12.2	2.4	1.5
0.0	9.7	13.6	2.9	1.8
0.0	6.0	8.0	0.2	0.1
0.0	10.0	4.5	0.0	0.0
0.0	5.4	8.0	1.7	1.0
0.0	9.5	4.5	2.3	1.5
FIBER (grams)	PROTEIN (grams)	CARBOHYDRATES (grams)	FAT (grams)	SATURATED FAT (grams)
4.4	0.5	25.1	0.3	0.0
1.5	0.2	13.8	0.1	0.0
0.7	0.5	3.9	0.1	0.0
13.5	4.0	17.1	29.5	4.3
3.1	1.3	27.0	0.4	0.1
3.8	1.0	6.9	0.4	0.0
1.8	0.6	10.7	0.2	0.0
2.5	1.0	6.2	0.3	0.0

Nutrient Content of Common Foods (continued)

FRUIT*	PORTION SIZE	CALORIES
Cherries, sweet	1/2 cup	43
Figs, dried	1/4 cup	93
Grapefruit, pink, red or white	1/2 medium	53
Grapes, red or green, seedless	1/2 cup	52
Mango	1 medium	135
Melon balls	1/2 cup	29
Nectarine	1 medium	62
Orange	1 medium	62
Papaya, cubed	1/2 cup	27
Peach	1 medium	58
Pear	1 medium	103
Pear, Asian	1 large	116
Pineapple, cubed fresh	1/2 cup	41
Plum	1 medium	30
Raisins, seedless	1 tablespoon	28
Raspberries	1/2 cup	32
Strawberries	1/2 cup	23
Watermelon balls	1/2 cup	23

VEGETABLES**	PORTION SIZE	CALORIES
Artichoke (globe or French) hearts, cooked	1/2 cup	45
Asparagus, boiled	8 spears	26
Beans, green, boiled	1 cup	38
Beets, boiled, sliced	1/2 cup	37
Broccoli, boiled	1 medium stalk	63
Brussels sprouts, boiled	6 sprouts	45
Cabbage, sliced, boiled	1 cup	34

* Figures apply to raw fruit unless otherwise noted.
** Figures apply to raw vegetables unless otherwise noted; no salt used in cooking.

FIBER (grams)	PROTEIN (grams)	CARBOHYDRATES (grams)	FAT (grams)	SATURATED FAT (grams)
1.4	0.7	11.1	0.1	0.0
3.7	1.2	23.8	0.4	0.1
1.8	1.1	13.4	0.2	0.0
0.7	0.5	13.7	0.1	0.0
3.7	1.1	35.2	0.6	0.1
0.6	0.7	6.9	0.2	0.0
2.4	1.5	15.0	0.5	0.0
3.1	1.2	15.4	0.2	0.0
1.3	0.4	6.9	0.1	0.0
2.2	1.4	14.3	0.4	0.0
5.5	0.7	27.5	0.2	0.0
9.9	1.4	29.3	0.6	0.0
1.2	0.5	10.8	0.1	0.0
0.9	0.5	7.5	0.2	0.0
0.3	0.3	7.5	0.0	0.0
4.0	0.7	7.3	0.4	0.0
1.4	0.5	5.5	0.2	0.0
0.3	0.5	5.8	0.1	0.0
FIBER (grams)	**PROTEIN (grams)**	**CARBOHYDRATES (grams)**	**FAT (grams)**	**SATURATED FAT (grams)**
7.2	2.4	10.0	0.3	0.0
2.4	2.9	4.9	0.3	0.1
4.0	2.0	8.7	0.2	0.1
1.7	1.4	8.5	0.2	0.0
5.9	4.3	12.9	0.7	0.1
3.3	3.2	9.0	0.6	0.1
2.9	1.9	8.3	0.1	0.0

Nutrient Content of Common Foods (continued)

VEGETABLES**	PORTION SIZE	CALORIES
Carrots, baby	1 cup	55
Cauliflower, boiled	1 cup	29
Celery, chopped	3 medium stalks	19
Corn, sweet, white, boiled	1 medium ear	111
Cucumber, peeled	1 cup slices	14
Hearts of palm, canned	1 cup	41
Kale, chopped, boiled	1 cup	36
Leek white parts, boiled	1 leek	38
Lettuce, cos or romaine, shredded	1 cup	8
Lettuce, green leaf, shredded	1 cup	5
Lettuce, iceberg, shredded	1 cup	10
Marinara pasta sauce	½ cup	111
Mung beans, mature seeds, sprouted, boiled	½ cup	16
Mushrooms, white, sliced	1 cup	15
Oil, vegetable	1 tablespoon	119
Okra, boiled	1 cup	35
Olives, ripe, canned	3 small	11
Onion, chopped	¼ cup	16
Peas, boiled	1 cup	83
Peppers, sweet, chopped	1 cup	30
Pickles, dill or kosher dill	1 medium	8
Potato with skin, baked	1 large	278
Potato without skin, boiled	1 large	258
Rutabaga, cubed, boiled	1 cup	66
Spinach	1 cup	7
Spinach, boiled	1 cup	65
Squash, summer, sliced, boiled	1 cup	36

** Figures apply to raw vegetables unless otherwise noted; no salt used in cooking.

FIBER (grams)	PROTEIN (grams)	CARBOHYDRATES (grams)	FAT (grams)	SATURATED FAT (grams)
4.6	1.0	12.9	0.2	0.0
2.9	2.3	5.1	0.6	0.1
1.9	0.8	3.6	0.2	0.0
2.9	3.4	25.9	1.3	0.2
0.8	0.7	2.6	0.2	0.0
3.5	3.7	6.8	0.9	0.2
2.6	2.5	7.3	0.5	0.1
1.2	1.0	9.5	0.3	0.0
1.0	0.6	1.6	0.1	0.0
0.5	0.5	1.0	0.1	0.0
0.9	0.7	2.1	0.1	0.0
3.3	2.3	17.6	3.4	0.9
0.9	1.6	3.1	0.1	0.0
0.7	2.2	2.3	0.2	0.0
0.0	0.0	0.0	13.5	1.9
4.0	3.0	7.2	0.3	0.1
0.3	0.1	0.6	1.0	0.1
0.7	0.4	3.7	0.0	0.0
5.0	5.6	14.4	0.6	0.1
2.5	1.3	6.9	0.3	0.1
0.7	0.4	2.0	0.1	0.0
6.6	7.5	63.2	0.4	0.1
6.0	5.1	60.0	0.3	0.1
3.1	2.2	14.9	0.4	0.0
0.7	0.9	1.0	0.1	0.0
7.0	7.6	9.1	1.7	0.3
2.5	1.6	7.8	0.6	0.1

Nutrient Content of Common Foods (continued)

VEGETABLES**	PORTION SIZE	CALORIES
Squash, winter, frozen, baked, cubed	1 cup	80
Tomato	1 medium	22
Turnip greens, frozen, boiled	1 cup	48

CARBOHYDRATES AND GRAINS	PORTION SIZE	CALORIES
Bagel, plain	1 large	283
Beans, baked, canned, plain or vegetarian	½ cup	119
Beans, black, boiled	½ cup	114
Beans, kidney, red, boiled	½ cup	112
Beans, navy, boiled	½ cup	127
Beans, pinto, boiled	½ cup	122
Bread, whole-wheat, commercially prepared	1 slice	69
Cereal, oat, regular, quick and instant, cooked	½ cup	74
Cereal, Fiber One (General Mills)	⅓ cup	40
Cereal, All-Bran Extra Fiber (Kellogg's)	⅓ cup	34
Chickpeas (garbanzo beans), boiled	½ cup	134
Couscous, cooked	½ cup	88
Crackers, whole-wheat	4 medium	71
Granola bar, soft, uncoated, plain	1 bar	124
Hummus, commercial	¼ cup	104
Lentils, boiled	½ cup	113
Lima beans, baby, boiled	½ cup	94
Oat bran, raw	¼ cup	59
Peas, split, boiled	½ cup	116
Popcorn, air-popped	1 cup	31
Refried beans, canned	½ cup	118
Rice cake, brown rice, plain	1 cake	35

* Figures apply to raw vegetables unless otherwise noted; no salt used in cooking.

FIBER (grams)	PROTEIN (grams)	CARBOHYDRATES (grams)	FAT (grams)	SATURATED FAT (grams)
5.7	1.8	17.9	1.3	0.3
1.5	1.1	4.8	0.3	0.0
5.6	5.5	8.3	0.7	0.2
FIBER (grams)	PROTEIN (grams)	CARBOHYDRATES (grams)	FAT (grams)	SATURATED FAT (grams)
2.4	11.0	55.6	1.8	0.4
5.2	6.0	26.9	0.5	0.1
7.5	7.6	20.4	0.5	0.1
5.7	7.7	20.2	0.4	0.1
9.6	7.5	23.7	0.6	0.1
7.7	7.7	22.4	0.6	0.1
1.9	3.6	11.6	0.9	0.2
2.0	3.0	2.3	1.2	0.2
9.5	1.3	16.8	0.7	0.1
8.7	2.0	13.3	0.7	0.0
6.2	7.3	22.5	2.1	0.2
1.1	3.0	18.2	0.1	0.0
1.7	1.4	11.0	2.8	0.5
1.3	2.1	18.8	4.8	2.0
3.8	5.0	8.9	6.0	0.9
7.8	8.9	19.3	0.4	0.1
5.4	6.0	17.5	0.3	0.0
3.6	4.1	15.6	1.7	0.3
8.1	8.2	20.7	0.4	0.0
1.2	1.0	6.2	0.4	0.0
6.7	6.9	19.6	1.6	0.6
0.4	0.7	7.3	0.3	0.1

Nutrient Content of Common Foods (continued)

CARBOHYDRATES AND GRAINS	PORTION SIZE	CALORIES
Rice, brown, long-grain, cooked	½ cup	109
Rice, white, long-grain, cooked	½ cup	103
Tofu, light firm (nigari)	4 ounces	57
Wild rice, cooked	½ cup	83

NUTS	PORTION SIZE	CALORIES
Almonds, whole	2 tablespoons	103
Cashews, whole	2 tablespoons	94
Peanuts	2 tablespoons	108
Pecans, halved	2 tablespoons	86
Pine nuts, dried, whole	2 tablespoons	114
Sunflower seed kernels	2 tablespoons	102
Walnuts, English, halved	2 tablespoons	82

MEAT, POULTRY AND SEAFOOD	PORTION SIZE	CALORIES
Beef, tenderloin, broiled	4 ounces	244
Chicken, breast only, skinless	4 ounces	185
Chicken, dark meat only, skinless, roasted	4 ounces	215
Haddock, broiled	4 ounces	125
Ham, lean, sliced, boiled	2 ounces	60
Lamb, leg, roasted	4 ounces	241
Lobster, steamed	4 ounces	110
Pork, leanest tenderloin, broiled	4 ounces	130
Salmon, broiled	4 ounces	156
Shrimp, boiled	4 ounces	111
Swordfish, broiled	4 ounces	174
Tuna, light, water-packed	4 ounces	130
Turkey, breast, skinless, roasted	4 ounces	151
Veggie burger, frozen patty	1 medium	124

FIBER (grams)	PROTEIN (grams)	CARBOHYDRATES (grams)	FAT (grams)	SATURATED FAT (grams)
1.8	2.5	22.4	0.9	0.2
0.3	2.1	22.3	0.2	0.0
0.0	10.0	1.4	2.1	0.0
1.5	3.3	17.5	0.3	0.0

FIBER (grams)	PROTEIN (grams)	CARBOHYDRATES (grams)	FAT (grams)	SATURATED FAT (grams)
2.2	3.8	3.9	8.8	0.7
0.5	2.7	4.9	7.7	1.4
1.7	5.1	2.8	9.5	1.6
1.2	1.1	1.7	8.9	0.9
0.6	2.3	2.2	11.6	0.8
1.5	3.6	3.5	9.0	0.9
0.8	1.9	1.7	8.2	0.8

FIBER (grams)	PROTEIN (grams)	CARBOHYDRATES (grams)	FAT (grams)	SATURATED FAT (grams)
0.0	30.9	0.0	12.5	4.8
0.0	34.7	0.0	4.0	1.1
0.0	29.1	4.3	10.1	2.7
0.0	27.1	5.1	1.0	0.2
0.0	10.6	0.4	1.5	0.4
0.0	28.6	0.0	13.2	6.0
0.0	23.0	4.1	0.7	0.1
0.0	24.2	0.9	3.5	1.2
0.0	26.3	0.0	4.8	1.1
0.0	23.4	0.0	1.2	0.3
0.0	28.4	0.0	5.8	1.6
0.0	28.6	0.0	0.9	0.3
0.0	33.7	0.0	0.8	0.3
3.4	11.0	10.0	4.4	1.0

Portion Sizes of 100-Calorie Free Choices

Plenty of "non-diet" foods can be enjoyed as Stage II free-choice treats. Brands differ, so always check the product label to work out exactly how much you can eat for your 100 calories. Here are some suggestions.

FOOD	APPROXIMATE PORTION FOR 100 CALORIES
Bagel, white	$1/2$ 3" bagel or $1/3$ medium 4" bagel
Beer	1 cup
Bread, white	1 large slice
Cake, plain	1 ounce or $1/2$ small slice
Chicken nuggets	2 nuggets
Chips, baked	10 Lay's Crisps
Chips, regular	9 tortilla chips, 9 Pringles or 11 SunChips
Chocolate, dark or milk	4 Hershey's Kisses, 2 Hershey's Miniatures
Cocktail	$1/4$ cup
Cookie	$1/2$ medium cookie
Doughnut, glazed	$1/2$ small doughnut
French fries	$1/5$ large or $1/4$ medium fries
Frozen yogurt, low-fat	$1/3$ cup
Frozen drink	$2/3$ cup Coolatta or $1/2$ cup smoothie
Ice cream, premium	3 tablespoons
Ice cream, sugar-free	$1/2$ cup
Latte with low-fat milk	12 ounces
Macaroni and cheese	$1/4$ cup
Mashed potato (no butter)	$2/3$ cup
Muffins	$1/2$ large muffin or 2 mini-muffins
Nuts, roasted	2 tablespoons
Pie	$1/3$ slice (slice = $1/8$ of 9" pie)
Pizza, typical cheese	$1/3$ slice from 14" pizza, $1/6$ personal pan
Pretzels, hard	3 rods, 15 tiny twists or 48 small sticks
Pretzel, soft	$1/2$ small or $1/5$ large pretzel
Steak fries	6 fries
Trail mix	3 tablespoons
Wine	5 ounces

Savvy Shopper Supermarket Directory

Here's a list of some important supermarket items that will help your diet. It's a good idea to memorize your supermarket's layout or even draw a small diagram like the one below. This way, you can make out a shopping list that will take you up and down the aisles in an orderly fashion without having to search the shelves and leave yourself open to temptation along the way.

A TYPICAL SUPERMARKET LAYOUT

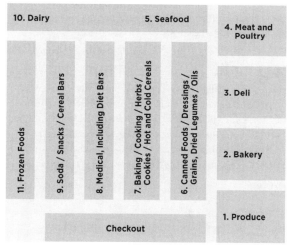

1. PRODUCE

Dried fruit. When used in small amounts, raisins, black mission figs, prunes (dried plums) and crystallized ginger are good for livening up high-fiber cereals.

Fresh fruit and veggies. All fruits are interchangeable in our menus except bananas (not good for a diet), so go for variety and enjoy! Look for small apples and oranges (large ones are often so big they add unwanted calories). All veggies are interchangeable, too, except potatoes and yams unless specified in the menus.

Fresh prepared fruit and veggies. Cut-up fruits such as melon, watermelon, pineapple and mango and cut-up cauliflower and broccoli are good choices. Washed salad greens are now widely available to make your life easier (for a higher price). The store-prepared packages and raw washed produce are fine, but avoid containers of fruit packed in juice and fresh fruit packed in containers with rich sauces; they have many more calories.

Herbs. Fresh herbs are wonderful but also pretty expensive. I have to admit that I sometimes chop up leftover fresh herbs and freeze them for another day. These are not as good as fresh, but they're better than dried and *lots* better than none at all!

Nuts in shells. These are good for limiting nut consumption because it takes more work to eat them.

Salad bar meals. Great diet aids, these offer effort-free variety. Be careful to stick to raw veggies, the specified amounts of high-protein foods in the menu, just a teaspoon of high-calorie items like bacon bits and sunflower seeds, and low-fat dressings (or half as much regular dressing as amounts specified in the menu).

Tofu. There are several kinds of tofu, and they differ in firmness and calories. Look for the words "firm light" on the package to get the kind that's lower in calories and higher in protein.

2 AND 3. BAKERY AND DELI

Low-carbohydrate bread. Supermarket breads vary enormously in composition. What you need is low-carbohydrate, fiber-enriched bread, which is sometimes called "carb style," "low net carbs" or simply "high fiber." Look for packages with orange logos and lots of fiber. The bread should have between 60 and 80 calories per slice or piece. Loaves and rolls are usually in the regular bread section, while pita bread and tortillas are most often found on the shelf in front of the deli counter. Here are some brands that have a good composition:

> Arnold 100 Calorie Sandwich Bread
> Cedar's Whole Wheat Wraps
> Country Kitchen Light Wheat Rolls
> Joseph's Flax, Oat Bran & Whole Wheat Pita Bread
> Joseph's Flax, Oat Bran & Whole Wheat Tortillas
> Pepperidge Farm Carb Style Bread
> Pepperidge Farm 7 Grain Deli Flats
> Pepperidge Farm Whole Grain Double Fiber Bread

I also count real pumpernickel (in the flat packages of thin slices that are made up of squashed grains, not the bread product with the same name) as a low-carb product, even though it really isn't. Because it's digested so slowly, it has the same metabolic effects as low-carb bread.

100% whole-wheat bread. This is for people using the vegetarian menus (where there is so much fiber and bulk that low carbs are less important) and for people using the with-meat menus who don't find themselves always hungry. Try to choose products made with coarse flour (look for lots of coarse particles and whole grains inside the loaf) so you get the benefits of lower insulin and blood glucose. Check calories per slice to find a brand with 80 calories per slice at most; some brands run much higher. During Stage III (weight maintenance), 100% whole-wheat bread is fine if you don't get hungry too quickly or too often.

Lean cold cuts. Sliced turkey and lean ham are great for easy salads and sandwiches. Ask for "very thin sliced" so you get more slices for your portion. Slice thickness and size vary so much that it's better to go by ounces rather than number of slices to keep to your portion sizes.

Cooked salads and vegetables. Items such as garbanzo bean salad, black bean salad, tabbouleh, grilled vegetables and wheat berry salad are all good meat-free diet staples.

Light Alfredo sauce. With a popular taste and only 45 calories per 2 tablespoons, this is a great sauce for livening up entrées and hot sandwiches. Sometimes it's found in the cheese section rather than the deli section.

Cooked entrées. Plain grilled skinless chicken breast and fish are staples of with-meat weight loss meals. Hummus is good diet food when served in controlled amounts with plenty of veggies on the side. Avoid anything that looks fried or has breading on it.

4. MEAT AND POULTRY

Lean choices. Look for meat with no visible fat on the outside of the cut and no marbling inside. Ground beef should be 90% to 95% lean. Chicken breasts should be skinless. For franks, opt for chicken or turkey rather than beef—you'll save a lot of calories.

6. CANNED FOODS, DRESSINGS, GRAINS AND DRIED LEGUMES

Legumes (plain). Go for variety to increase your enjoyment of this important food group. Try these beans: pinto, garbanzo (chickpeas), White Northern, cannellini, black, kidney and refried. Cooked beans in cans are easy to prepare. Dried beans that you soak and cook take more time but taste really good and cost less.

Baked beans. Look for a product with no more than 140 calories per half-cup serving, such as:

Bush's Onion Baked Beans
Campbell's Pork & Beans

Soups. There's a confusing array of cans and cup-o'-soups on supermarket shelves. Some are useful for weight loss, but others are loaded with calories. Spend a little time browsing Nutrition Facts labels to choose the following:

• *Broth-based soups:* Low calorie content is the name of the game here. Look for vegetable and broth soups with 80 calories or less per cup, such as:

Campbell's Healthy Request Vegetable Barley
Progresso French Onion
Progresso Light Italian-Style Vegetable

• *Hearty soups:* As a main dish with a protein source like lean meat or a legume, the soup should contain 160 or less calories per cup, such as:

Progresso Hearty Black Bean
Progresso Vegetable Classics Lentil
Progresso Traditional Beef Barley

Salad dressings. Another dizzying array here, and again the bottom line is calories:

• *Low-calorie dressings:* These are labeled "reduced fat," "light," "lite" and "sugar-free." Choose those with fewer than 80 calories per 2 tablespoons.

• *Non-fat dressings:* These have even fewer calories than low-cal dressings (typically 35 calories at most per 2 tablespoons or less), so they're good for an extra salad snack and in some recipes. Look for dressings such as:

> Ken's Lite Italian Dressing
> Newman's Own Light Italian Dressing
> Newman's Own Light Caesar Dressing

Tomato sauce. There are big variations here. Look for products that have fewer than 70 calories per half-cup serving, such as:

> Barilla Tomato & Basil
> Classico Tomato & Basil

Tuna. Water-packed tuna is a fine standby to keep in the cupboard. *Note:* The individual plastic packages of other fish or shrimp found in the same store location also make good protein helpings for salads.

7. BAKING AND HOT AND COLD CEREALS

Artificial sweeteners. There are several brands with different chemical ingredients (aspartame, sucralose, saccharine). If you find sweeteners helpful, try them all out in a coffee shop to decide which you prefer.

Coarse bran (wheat). An important recipe ingredient, this is particularly good for mixing with oatmeal in hot cereal. (See our recipe on page 135.)

Cocoa. Dutch-process cocoa (such as Droste brand) has more fiber than regular cocoa and is the starting point for "I" Diet Hot or Cold Chocolate (page 253).

High-fiber cereals. These are important diet aids and are a "free" food if you get hungry, so go for variety and make sure you never run out. Look for brands containing at least 13 grams of fiber per half-cup serving, such as:

> General Mills Fiber One (Original)
> Kellogg's All-Bran Extra Fiber

• *"Complete" high-fiber cereals:* These cereals are high in fiber but also higher in calories than the fiber-only cereals and therefore are eaten like a regular cereal in amounts of about a cup. Look for cereals such as:

> General Mills Fiber One Honey Clusters
> Kashi GOLEAN

Maple (or pancake) syrup. This is used in two Stage II breakfasts: "I" Diet Instant Hot Cereal (page 135) and Orange-Crumbed French Toast (page 138). If you like the taste of sugar-free pancake syrup, go ahead and get some. New Englanders and others who have grown up with the real stuff may prefer Grade B maple syrup in smaller amounts.

Oat bran. Use this for making our Almost Apple Cobbler dessert (page 245).

Oatmeal. Irish (steel-cut) oatmeal is definitely better for weight control than the instant oatmeal, because the larger particle sizes take longer to digest and cause less insulin secretion. However, Irish oatmeal takes an age to cook and another age to clean the pan afterwards. The "I" Diet Instant Hot Cereal recipe (page 135) microwaves quick-cooking oatmeal with coarse bran and milk to make a very passable, satisfying hot cereal.

Barley. A useful substitute for rice when you're dieting, this comes with different degrees of "pearling." Try to buy it in clear plastic bags so you can see the grains, and be sure to choose the hulled kind with bran that looks light brown rather than cream-colored.

Whole-wheat pasta. Look for "100% whole wheat" on the package and avoid those with words like "multigrain" or "enriched," which suggest that a product might be 100% whole-grain when it's actually not.

8. DIET PRODUCTS

Liquid meal replacements. I'm not a big fan of these products, but if you find them useful for emergencies, be sure to choose one with plenty of protein, such as:

Atkins Advantage Chocolate Royale Shake

Meal and snack bars. Though not good as real meals, these can be okay for occasional use in emergencies. The "small" bars in our menus contain 80 to 100 calories or less, and if the bar you want has too many calories, you can always cut off a chunk and save it for another meal.

• *High-fiber, high-protein bars:* Look for bars such as:

Atkins Advantage Chocolate Peanut Butter Bar
Atkins Advantage Morning Apple Crisp
Snickers Marathon caramel nut protein bar
Snickers Marathon low-carb peanut butter
South Beach chocolate peanut butter bar
South Beach caramel peanut crisp

• *High-protein bars:* When you're limiting fiber at the start of your diet, look for:

Odwalla Super Protein Bar
South Beach Living Chocolate High Protein Cereal Bar

9. SNACKS AND CEREAL BARS

Nuts. All shelled raw, roasted, dry-roasted, salted and salt-free nuts are fine, but avoid the ones with honey, yogurt or candy coatings (which add calories).

Peanut butter. Think natural here. Without any real proof, I suspect that crunchy is better than smooth for suppressing hunger (surely it takes longer to digest).

Cereal snack bars. These are generally not as good (i.e., lower in protein and fiber) for weight loss as the bars in the diet section.

10. DAIRY

Milk. Nonfat and 1% milk modified to taste like 2% or whole milk, such as Hood's Simply Smart, are recommended for their creamier taste and more favorable composition for weight loss.

Low-fat yogurt. Sugar-free, low-fat yogurt (any brand) is recommended during weight loss.

• *Greek nonfat or low-fat plain yogurt.* The best for its creamy taste, it's also much higher in protein and lower in carbs, so it's good for satiety.

• *Plain nonfat or 1% yogurt:* All brands from major companies are good.

• *Sugar-free sweetened nonfat yogurt:* This makes a reasonable substitute for with-sugar regular fruit yogurts.

Whipped light cream. This doesn't sound like diet food, but it has only about 15 calories per two tablespoons, so it's an indulgence with a small footprint. Some people I know claim that a quarter-cup of whipped cream is the best vehicle for high-fiber cereals like Fiber One. If this is what it takes for you to enjoy your fiber, go right ahead.

Cheese. Used carefully, cheese is useful for snacks and can make entrées delicious.

• *Low-fat cottage cheese:* This is a good low-calorie snack, and there are handy individual 4-ounce containers in various flavors.

• *Low-fat cream cheese:* There's no reason to go with full-fat when even low-fat has plenty of calories.

• *Grated Parmesan:* This cheese is great for dieting because its stronger taste means you can use less. Imported brands are wonderfully tasty, but generally go for the fluffy finely grated kind, not the shreds or blocks, which can add too many calories.

• *Part-skim mozzarella cheese sticks:* Low in calories, these are wonderfully portable—they can be taken anywhere and eaten without mess.

11. FROZEN FOODS

Frozen foods may not be as tasty as fresh, but for busy people they can be useful and help to keep good food at home without the risk of its going bad.

Frozen fruit. Plain frozen raspberries, blackberries and strawberries taste good and are usually much cheaper than fresh for most of the year. 100% frozen fruit bars are an okay substitute for dessert.

Frozen entrées. Items like plain grilled skinless chicken breast and salmon are useful for easy dinners. There are also more elaborate products, like Oven Poppers Cod Stuffed with Broccoli and Cheese, that have 150 calories or less but come with enough protein (15 grams or more) to make them good entrées.

Frozen meal replacements. Frozen "complete" meals with plenty of protein and few calories can be substituted for menu meals whenever "emergency" meals are needed. Keep calorie guidelines in mind and choose a replacement meal with about 50 calories less than your total meal allowance so you can round it out with some vegetables or fruit (the meals usually feel rather small). Here are some reasonable products:

CALORIE GUIDELINES FOR REPLACEMENT MEALS AND SNACKS			
	1,200-Calorie Menu	1,600-Calorie Menu	1,800-Calorie Menu
Breakfast	250	400	400
Snacks	150	150	150
Lunch and dinner	300	350	450
Dessert	100	100	100

Lean Cuisine Salmon in Basil; Chicken Parmesan; Roast Turkey with Vegetables; Steak Tips Portabello; Glazed Chicken
South Beach Caprese-Style Chicken with Broccoli; Chicken Monterey Wrap

Frozen waffles. The only products I'm aware of that are halfway okay diet food are Kashi GOLEAN Original Waffles and Blueberry Waffles. If you find they make you hungry, give them a pass for now.

Frozen vegetarian burgers and sausages. Brands such as Boca provide easy meat-free substitutes for common favorites.

Frozen veggies. The key here is to buy plain veggies, not those in sauce.

Weight-Healthy Meal Suggestions for Stage III of the "I" Diet Program

In addition to any Stage I or Stage II meal, any of the meals below can be enjoyed when you reach Stage III, according to your daily calorie needs. You can also calculate calories, fiber and nutrients in your favorite dishes by using one of the web programs such as www.calorieking.com.

BREAKFASTS	300 CALORIES
Any regular cereal mixed with high-fiber cereal and 1% milk (or nonfat or 2% plain or sugar-free yogurt); fruit; coarse whole-grain toast and healthy spreads such as peanut butter, fruit butter or low-fat cream cheese for higher calorie levels.	3/4 cup any cereal mixed with 1/3 cup high-fiber cereal and 1 cup milk 1 piece fruit
Coarse 100% whole-grain bread with preserves or low-fat cream cheese and fresh fruit salad.	1 large or 2 small slices bread with 1 tablespoon low-fat cream cheese or 1 teaspoon tub margarine and 2 teaspoons preserves 1/2 cup fresh fruit salad
Whole-wheat bagel with low-fat cream cheese; apple or fresh fruit salad.	1/2 bagel with 2 teaspoons low-fat cream cheese 1 apple or 1 cup fruit salad
Hot oat bran cereal with pecans or raisins, fresh fruit, brown sugar, 1% milk or half as much half-and-half and cinnamon to taste.	1 cup hot cereal with 1 1/2 tablespoons pecans or raisins, 1/2 cup fresh fruit, 1 tablespoon brown sugar and 2 tablespoons milk or 1 tablespoon half-and-half
Eggs; Canadian bacon; fresh fruit and/or lightly buttered low-carb coarse 100% whole-wheat or "I" Diet Soda Bread (page 160).	2 eggs, any style 1 1/2 slices Canadian bacon 1/2 cup fresh fruit or 1/2 slice toast

380 CALORIES	460 CALORIES	540 CALORIES
1 cup any cereal mixed with 1/3 cup high-fiber cereal and 1 cup milk	1 1/2 cups any cereal mixed with 1/3 cup high-fiber cereal and 1 cup milk	1 1/2 cups any cereal mixed with 1/3 cup high-fiber cereal and 1 cup milk
1 piece fruit	1 piece fruit	1 1/2 pieces fruit
1/2 slice bread with spread	1 slice bread with spread	1 large slice bread with spread
1 1/2 large or 3 small slices bread with 1 tablespoon low-fat cream cheese or 1 teaspoon tub margarine and 2 teaspoons preserves	3 small or 1 1/2 large slices bread with 1 1/2 tablespoons low-fat cream cheese or 1 teaspoon tub margarine and 1 tablespoon preserves	4 small or 2 large slices bread with 2 tablespoons low-fat cream cheese or 1 teaspoon tub margarine and 1 tablespoon preserves
2/3 cup fresh fruit salad	2/3 cup fresh fruit salad	1 cup fresh fruit salad
3/4 bagel with 3 teaspoons low-fat cream cheese	1 bagel with 4 teaspoons low-fat cream cheese	1 bagel with 4 teaspoons low-fat cream cheese
1 apple or 1 cup fruit salad	1 apple or 1 cup fruit salad	1 1/2 cups fruit salad
1 1/2 cups hot cereal with 2 tablespoons pecans or raisins, 2/3 cup fresh fruit, 1 tablespoon brown sugar and 2 tablespoons milk or 1 tablespoon half-and-half	1 1/2 cups hot cereal with 3 tablespoons pecans or raisins, 1 cup fresh fruit, 1 1/2 tablespoons brown sugar and 2 tablespoons milk or 1 tablespoon half-and-half	1 1/2 cups hot cereal with 3 tablespoons pecans or raisins, 1 1/3 cups fresh fruit, 2 tablespoons brown sugar and 1/4 cup milk or 2 tablespoons half-and-half
2 eggs, any style	2 eggs, any style	2 eggs, any style
3 slices Canadian bacon	3 slices Canadian bacon	3 slices Canadian bacon
2/3 cup fresh fruit or 1 slice toast	2/3 cup fresh fruit or 1 slice toast	1 1/2 cups fresh fruit or 1 slice toast

Weight-Healthy Meal Suggestions for Stage III of the "I" Diet Program

LUNCHES	375 CALORIES
Large green salad with lean turkey breast, beans, oil-and-vinegar dressing, toppings; coarse 100% whole-grain, low-carb or "I" Diet Soda Bread (page 160) for higher calorie levels; fruit. Use a variety of light or regular, Chinese-style and Thai dressings. Substitute any of the following for each 2 ounces turkey: 2 ounces plain grilled chicken, 1 hard-boiled egg, $\frac{1}{2}$ cup cottage cheese made with 1% milk, $\frac{1}{3}$ cup water-packed tuna, 2 1" squares grilled tofu, $1\frac{1}{3}$ slices low-fat cheese or $\frac{2}{3}$ slice of regular cheese.	2+ cups salad greens, $\frac{1}{2}$ cup beans, 1 slice (1 ounce) turkey breast and 1 tablespoon regular or 2 tablespoons low-fat dressing 1 piece fruit
Sandwich made with coarse 100% whole-wheat, low-carb or "I" Diet Soda Bread (page 160) with side salad and apple. Substitute any of the following for each 2 ounces lean ham: 2 ounces plain grilled chicken, 1 hard-boiled egg, $\frac{1}{3}$ cup water-packed tuna, 2 1" squares grilled tofu, $1\frac{1}{3}$ slices low-fat cheese or $\frac{2}{3}$ slice of regular cheese.	2 small slices bread, 1 medium slice (1 ounce) lean ham or equivalent, 1 slice reduced-fat cheese and 1 teaspoon low-fat mayo Salad with lots of green and non-starchy veggies and 1 tablespoon low-fat dressing 1 apple
Thick, non-creamy soup such as bean, lentil, minestrone, beef barley or pea with ham; coarse whole-grain, low-carb or "I" Diet Soda Bread (page 160); side salad and fruit; pecans and raisins for higher calorie levels.	$1\frac{1}{2}$ cups soup 1 slice bread Side salad with 1 tablespoon low-fat dressing or 1 piece fruit
Picnic-style lunch: raw or steamed veggies with oil and vinegar; hummus or equivalent; whole-wheat pita bread; fruit, nuts/seeds/raisins for higher calorie levels. Substitute any of the following for $\frac{1}{4}$ cup hummus: $\frac{1}{2}$ cup low-fat cottage cheese made with 1% milk, 2 slices (2 ounces) lean turkey or ham, 1 hard-boiled egg, 2 1" squares tofu, 1 low-fat mozzarella cheese stick.	$1\frac{1}{2}$ cups veggies with drizzle of oil and vinegar $\frac{1}{4}$ cup hummus or equivalent $\frac{1}{4}$ pita bread 1 piece fruit

425 CALORIES	600 CALORIES	650 CALORIES
3+ cups salad greens, 1/3 cup beans, 1 slice (1 ounce) turkey breast and 1 1/2 tablespoons any dressing 1/2 slice bread 1 piece fruit	3+ cups salad greens, 1/2 cup beans, 2 slices (2 ounces) turkey breast and 1 1/2 tablespoons any dressing 1 slice bread 1 piece fruit	3+ cups salad greens, 1/2 cup beans, 2 slices (2 ounces) turkey breast and 2 tablespoons any dressing 1 slice bread lightly buttered or with a little olive oil for dipping 1 piece fruit
2 small slices bread, 2 medium slices (2 ounces) lean ham or equivalent, 1 slice reduced-fat cheese and 1 teaspoon low-fat mayo Salad with lots of green and non-starchy veggies and 1 tablespoon low-fat dressing 1 apple	2 slices bread, 3 slices (3 ounces) lean meat or equivalent, 1 slice reduced-fat cheese and 2 teaspoons low-fat mayo Lots of veggies with low-fat dressing 1 apple	3 slices bread, 4 slices (4 ounces) lean meat, 2 slices reduced-fat cheese and 2 teaspoons low-fat mayo Lots of veggies with 1 tablespoon any dressing 1 apple
1 1/2 cups soup 1 slice bread Side salad with 1 tablespoon low-fat dressing 1 piece fruit	2 cups soup 2 slices bread Side salad with 1 tablespoon low-fat dressing 1 piece fruit 2 tablespoons pecans and raisins	2 cups soup 2 slices bread Side salad with 1 tablespoon any dressing 1 piece fruit 3 tablespoons pecans and raisins
1 1/2 cups veggies with drizzle of oil and vinegar 1/4 cup hummus or equivalent 1/2 pita bread 1 piece fruit 1 tablespoon nuts/seeds/raisins	2 cups veggies with drizzle of oil and vinegar 1/3 cup hummus or equivalent 1/2 pita bread 1 piece fruit 2 tablespoons nuts/seeds/raisins	2 cups veggies with drizzle of oil and vinegar 1/3 cup hummus or equivalent 1 pita bread 1 piece fruit 3 tablespoons nuts/seeds/raisins

Weight-Healthy Meal Suggestions for Stage III of the "I" Diet Program

DINNERS	375 CALORIES
Roast chicken breast with gravy; green veggies lightly dressed with ½ teaspoon margarine or olive oil; baked sweet potato; side of coarse 100% whole-wheat, low-carb or "I" Diet Soda Bread (page 160) for higher calorie level. Substitute the same amount of lean pork or beef with no visible fat or vegetarian sausage for chicken.	4 ounces roast chicken with 2 tablespoons gravy 1½ cups green veggies Small baked sweet potato
Casseroles such as chili con carne or bean or beef stew; brown basmati rice; salad.	¾ cup chili or stew ⅓ cup brown rice 2 cups salad with 1 tablespoon low-fat dressing
100% whole-wheat pasta with tomato or low-fat meat sauce and grated Parmesan cheese; salad.	1 cup cooked pasta with ⅓ cup tomato or meat sauce and 1 tablespoon grated cheese 2 cups salad with 1 tablespoon low-fat dressing
Extra-lean (90–95%) hamburger with lettuce, tomato, ketchup and relish on a 100% whole-wheat bread roll; side salad. Substitute the following for 4 ounces of hamburger: 1 veggie burger and ½ cup bean salad.	4 ounces hamburger on a whole-wheat roll with ketchup and relish 2 cups salad with 1 tablespoon low-fat dressing

SNACKS (one per day or divided into two)	150 CALORIES
Fresh fruit such as a red or green crispy apple, orange, green or red grapes, cut-up mango, pineapple, kiwi, peach, nectarine, pear; nuts.	1 piece or 1 cup fresh fruit 1 tablespoon nuts
Cut-up fresh veggies with small side of hummus or low-fat cottage cheese; latte or "I" Diet Hot or Cold Chocolate (page 253) for higher calorie levels.	1 cup cut-up veggies ¼ cup hummus or ½ cup cottage cheese

304

425 CALORIES	600 CALORIES	650 CALORIES
5 ounces roast chicken with 3 tablespoons gravy	6 ounces roast chicken with 3 tablespoons gravy	6 ounces roast chicken with 4 tablespoons gravy
1½ cups green veggies	2 cups green veggies	2 cups green veggies
Small baked sweet potato with low-fat sour cream	Medium baked sweet potato with low-fat sour cream	Medium baked sweet potato with low-fat sour cream
		1 slice bread
1 cup chili or stew	1½ cups chili or stew	1½ cups chili or stew
⅓ cup brown rice	½ cup brown rice	¾ cup brown rice
2 cups salad with 1 tablespoon low-fat dressing	2 cups salad with 1 tablespoon any dressing	2 cups salad with 1 tablespoon any dressing
1¼ cups cooked pasta with ½ cup tomato or meat sauce and 1 tablespoon grated cheese	1⅔ cups cooked pasta with ¾ cup tomato or meat sauce and 2 tablespoons grated cheese	1¾ cups cooked pasta with ¾ cup tomato or meat sauce and 2 tablespoons grated cheese
2 cups salad with 1 tablespoon low-fat dressing	2 cups salad with 1 tablespoon any dressing	2 cups salad with 1 tablespoon any dressing
5 ounces hamburger on a whole-wheat roll	6 ounces hamburger on a whole-wheat roll	6 ounces hamburger with 1 slice low-fat cheese on a whole-wheat roll
2 cups salad with 1 tablespoon low-fat dressing	3 cups salad with 1½ tablespoons any dressing	3 cups salad with 1½ tablespoons any dressing

190 CALORIES	240 CALORIES	270 CALORIES
1 piece or 1 cup fresh fruit	2 pieces or 2 cups fresh fruit	2 pieces or 2 cups fresh fruit
2 tablespoons nuts	1½ tablespoons nuts	2 tablespoons nuts
1½ cups cut-up veggies	1 cup cut-up veggies	1½ cups cut-up veggies
⅓ cup hummus or ⅔ cup low-fat cottage cheese	¼ cup hummus or ½ cup cottage cheese	⅓ cup hummus or 1 cup low-fat cottage cheese
	8-ounce latte or "I" Diet Hot or Cold Chocolate	8-ounce latte or "I" Diet Hot or Cold Chocolate

(continued)

Weight-Healthy Meal Suggestions for Stage III of the "I" Diet Program

Trail mix or dried unsweetened fruit such as figs, prunes, raisins, dried apple slices. (Three tablespoons trail mix is equivalent to 5 black mission figs, 9 bite-size pitted prunes, 1/4 cup raisins or 8 dried unsweetened apple rings.) Additional fresh fruit for higher calorie levels.	3 tablespoons trail mix or equivalent amount of dried fruit
Low-fat cheese sticks	1 1/2 cheese sticks

4½ tablespoons trail mix or equivalent amount of dried fruit	2 tablespoons trail mix or equivalent amount of dried fruit	4½ tablespoons trail mix or equivalent amount of dried fruit
	1 piece fresh fruit	1 piece fresh fruit
2 cheese sticks	2½ cheese sticks	3 cheese sticks

Emergency Meals

An emergency meal can keep your diet on track with few calories and good composition when you don't have time to cook even the simple meal you planned. The lunches and dinners below are for the "I" Diet 1,200-calorie plan and make a whole meal when served with a piece of fruit such as an apple or orange and water or a low-calorie drink like coffee or tea. Increase amounts by a third if you're on the 1,600-calorie menu and by 50% for the 1,800-calorie menu.

GRILLED CHICKEN SANDWICH

3 ounces grilled skinless chicken breast (keep frozen cooked chicken breasts for this dish) with 2 slices low-carb bread, a teaspoon of low-fat mayo or BBQ sauce, 2 to 3 lettuce leaves, cucumber and onion slices if available.

STANDBY EGGS

2 large eggs or ½ cup Egg Beaters cooked with 1 teaspoon tub margarine and 2 slices of low-carb bread.

TUNA CASSEROLE

½ cup chickpeas (garbanzo beans) or cannellini beans warmed in the microwave with a 6-ounce can of water-packed solid tuna (drained). Optional: 1 tablespoon BBQ sauce on the side.

WHOLE-WHEAT PASTA WITH TOMATO SAUCE

1 cup cooked whole-wheat pasta (save frozen ahead of time for this dish), ½ cup tomato sauce and 1 tablespoon grated Parmesan cheese.

APPLES AND CHEESE

2 low-fat mozzarella cheese sticks, 1 apple and 1 "I" Diet cereal dessert (page 236).

VANILLA-COFFEE SHAKE

1 scoop vanilla or chocolate whey protein blended with 1 scoop sugar-free Crystal Light powder, 8 ounces skim milk and 3 teaspoons instant coffee powder.

CHOCOLATE TOAST

If you're a chocolaholic and miss chocolate croissants, try this very reasonable diet substitute. Toast 2 slices low-carb bread. Melt 2 squares (20 grams) dark chocolate, spread on the toast and make a sandwich. It needs a glass of milk as well as a piece of fruit for best enjoyment.

Restaurant Survival Guide

Let's face it, eating out is a big challenge to your diet. Besides the enormous portion sizes, there's the problem of figuring out which menu items fit into your daily calorie allowance. And even if you find something that looks promising, its nutrient composition usually leaves a lot to be desired, which means you'll be less satisfied and hungry again sooner. Check the guidelines here and the specific menu suggestions below to help you eat out at restaurants and still keep calories down. It also helps to check out the websites of places you visit, but keep in mind that some restaurants may serve bigger portions than indicated by their calorie listings.

CALORIE GUIDELINES FOR EATING OUT WHILE LOSING WEIGHT			
	1,200-Calorie Menu	1,600-Calorie Menu	1,800-Calorie Menu
Breakfast	250	400	400
Mid-morning snack	150	150	150
Lunch	300	350	450
Mid-afternoon snack	100	100	100
Dinner	300	400	500
Dessert and free choice	100	200	200

Lunch and Dinner 300 Calories

RESTAURANT	OPTIONS
Applebee's	Cajun Lime Tilapia.
	Grilled Chili-Lime Chicken Salad.
Au Bon Pain	Chef Salad with fat-free raspberry vinaigrette.
	Half a Roast Beef Caesar sandwich with small broth-and-vegetable soup such as Garden Vegetable.
Burger King	Chili. Bring a piece of fruit to go with it.
	Whopper Jr. Low Carb or Chicken Whopper Low Carb Side Salad with fat-free ranch or light Italian dressing. Bring a piece of *good* fruit.
Denny's	Grilled Chicken Salad with fat-free dressing.
Domino's Pizza	1 slice Crunchy Thin Crust pizza with regular (not extra) cheese and vegetable toppings and Garden Fresh Salad with light Italian dressing.
KFC	Roasted BLT Salad with light or nonfat dressing (no croutons). Bring an apple.
McDonald's	Chicken Caesar Salad with Newman's Own Low Fat Balsamic dressing. Bring an apple.
	4 Chicken Nuggets with one-half container BBQ or sweet-and-sour sauce and Side Salad with Newman's Own Low Fat Balsamic dressing. Bring a small apple.
P.F. Chang's China Bistro	Half-order of Cantonese scallops with half-order of Buddha's Feast, Steamed.
	Half-order of Cantonese Shrimp plus half-order Sichuan-Style Asparagus.

Ruby Tuesday	Petite (7-ounce) Sirloin with side of Premium Baby Green Beans.
	White Bean Chicken Chili with side Caesar Salad (ask to substitute light ranch for Caesar dressing).
Starbucks	Fiesta Salad.
	Vegetable vinaigrette salad.
Subway	Ham or roasted chicken breast salad with fat-free dressing and side of minestrone.
	Chili soup.
	6" chicken breast or ham sandwich on whole wheat (no mayo or cheese but all the vegetables you like).
Taco Bell	Crunchy Taco and order of Pintos 'n Cheese.
Uno Chicago Grill	Grilled Chicken with Mango Salsa, side of steamed seasonal vegetables or broccoli and house salad with fat-free vinaigrette or low-fat blueberry pomegranate vinaigrette and breadstick.
	Chicken Caesar Salad with fat-free vinaigrette or low-fat blueberry pomegranate vinaigrette.
Wendy's	Small (8 ounce) Chili and side salad with fat-free French-style dressing.
	Jr. Hamburger without cheese (discard the bun) and side salad with fat-free French-style dressing. Bring an apple.

Lunch and Dinner 400 Calories

RESTAURANT	OPTIONS
Applebee's	Confetti Chicken.
	Steak and Portobellos with side salad and fat-free dressing.
Au Bon Pain	Chicken Caesar sandwich and spinach Sonoma salad with fat-free raspberry vinaigrette or discard the croutons and add light ranch dressing.
	Half a Roast Beef Caesar sandwich with small helping of any non-cream soup.
Burger King	Whopper Jr. Low-Carb and side garden salad with nonfat ranch or light Italian dressing, half a small fries (discard other half or give to a friend). Bring along a small piece of *good* fruit.
	4 Chicken Tenders with BBQ sauce and side garden salad with dressing. Bring a piece of *good* fruit.
Cheesecake Factory	Half a "weight management salad." Bring an apple.
Denny's	Chef salad with fat-free dressing.
	Grilled chicken dinner with vegetable blend and side of fruit medley.

Domino's Pizza	1 slice Crunchy Thin Crust pizza with regular (not extra) cheese and vegetable toppings and garden fresh salad with light Italian dressing. Bring an apple.
KFC	Roasted Caesar salad with light or nonfat dressing (no croutons). Bring an apple.
	Chicken breast without skin or breading, house salad with light Italian or fat-free ranch and side of baked beans or large corn on the cob.
McDonald's	Bacon Chicken Ranch Salad with Newman's Own Low Fat Balsamic dressing. Bring an apple.
	1 smallest hamburger (discard one side of roll) and side salad with Newman's Own Low Fat Balsamic dressing. Bring a small apple.
	1 small fries with 2 packets ketchup and side salad with Newman's Own Low Fat Balsamic dressing. Bring an apple. *Note:* This isn't healthy or as good for your diet as other choices, but if you have to have fries this is a better way to have them.
P.F. Chang's China Bistro	Cantonese shrimp plus half a serving of Buddha's Feast steamed or Sichuan-style asparagus.
	Half-order of Cantonese scallops plus Buddha's Feast steamed or Sichuan-style asparagus.
Ruby Tuesday	Creole Catch with side of Premium Baby Green Beans.
	Petite sirloin steak (7 ounces) with side of Premium Baby Green Beans and a tomato and mozzarella salad.
Starbucks	Half a turkey and Swiss sandwich. Bring a piece of fruit.
	Fiesta Salad with one Crisp Cinnamon Twist.
Subway	6" ham, chicken breast or roast beef sandwich on whole wheat (no mayo or cheese) with minestrone.
	Cold-cut combo salad with tomato garden vegetable soup.
Taco Bell	Grilled Steak Taquitos with Salsa and half-order of Pintos 'n Cheese.
	Bean Burrito. Bring an apple.
Uno Chicago Grill	Seven-ounce filet mignon with side of steamed seasonal vegetables or broccoli, house salad with fat-free vinaigrette or low-fat blueberry pomegranate vinaigrette and breadstick or glass of wine.
	Chicken lettuce wraps with side of steamed vegetables and breadstick or glass of wine.
Wendy's	Ultimate Chicken Grill Sandwich without cheese (discard half the bun) and side salad with fat-free French-style dressing.
	One quarter-pound hamburger without cheese (discard the bun) and side salad with fat-free French-style dressing. Bring an apple.
	Half an order of small fries with ketchup and side salad with fat-free French-style dressing. Bring an apple. (This is not good nutrition, just a way to have the fries if you want to give in this time.)

Sample Food Diary

A precise record of everything you eat will give you all the details you need to make an honest assessment of your daily food intake. Be sure to include the exact amount of each food, as well as relevant nutrient content and brand names, including helpful label descriptions.

GOOD:

7 A.M.	8 ounces orange juice (Tropicana, no pulp)
	2 slices low-carb toast (Country Light Wheat)
	1 tablespoon low-fat plain cream cheese (Philadelphia)
	8 ounces coffee with 2 tablespoons whole milk

NOT GOOD:

7 A.M.	orange juice
	2 slices toast
	1 tablespoon cream cheese
	1 coffee

DATE: _____

TIME	FOOD DESCRIPTION *(Start a new line for each item.)*

SCIENTIFIC REFERENCES

Additional references are listed on our website, www.instinctdiet.com.

Ackroff, K., Touzani, K., Peets, T.K. & Sclafani, A. (2001). Flavor preferences conditioned by intragastric fructose and glucose: differences in reinforcement potency. *Physiology & Behavior, 72*(5), 691–703.

Alfenas, R.C.G. & Mattes, R.D. (2003). Effect of fat sources on satiety. *Obesity Research, 11*(2), 183–87.

Anderson, G.H., Catherine, N.L.A., Woodend, D.M. & Wolever, T.M.S. (2002). Inverse association between the effect of carbohydrates on blood glucose and subsequent short-term food intake in young men. *American Journal of Clinical Nutrition, 76*(5), 1023–30.

Anderson, G.H. & Moore, S.E. (2004). Dietary proteins in the regulation of food intake and body weight in humans. *Journal of Nutrition, 134*(4), S974–79.

Anderson, G.H., Tecimer, S.N., Shah, D. & Zafar, T.A. (2004). Protein source, quantity, and time of consumption determine the effect of proteins on short-term food intake in young men. *Journal of Nutrition, 134*(11), 3011–15.

Arosio, M., Ronchi, C.L., Beck-Peccoz, P., Gebbia, C., Giavoli, C., Cappiello, V., et al. (2004). Effects of modified sham feeding on ghrelin levels in healthy human subjects. *Journal of Clinical Endocrinology & Metabolism, 89*(10), 5101–04.

Bathalon, G.P., Hays, N.P., Meydani, S.N., Dawson-Hughes, B., Schaefer, E.J., Lipman, R., et al. (2001). Metabolic, psychological, and health correlates of dietary restraint in healthy postmenopausal women. *Journals of Gerontology Series A—Biological Sciences & Medical Sciences, 56*(4), M206–11.

Bathalon, G.P., Tucker, K.L., Hays, N.P., Vinken, A.G., Greenberg, A.S., McCrory,

M.A., et al. (2000). Psychological measures of eating behavior and the accuracy of 3 common dietary assessment methods in healthy postmenopausal women. *American Journal of Clinical Nutrition, 71*(3), 739–45.

Beglinger, C. & Degen, L. (2006). Gastrointestinal satiety signals in humans—physiologic roles for GLP-1 and PYY? *Physiology & Behavior, 89*(4), 460–64.

Bellisle, F., Guy-Grand, B. & Le Magnen, J. (2000). Chewing and swallowing as indices of the stimulation to eat during meals in humans: effects revealed by the edogram method and video recordings. *Neuroscience & Biobehavioral Reviews, 24*(2), 223–28.

Bellisle, F., Lucas, F., Amrani, R. & Le Magnen, J. (1984). Deprivation, palatability and the micro-structure of meals in human subjects. *Appetite, 5*(2), 85–94.

Benoit, S.C., Air, E.L., Wilmer, K., Messerschmidt, P., Hodge, K.M., Jones, M.B., et al. (2003). Two novel paradigms for the simultaneous assessment of conditioned taste aversion and food intake effects of anorexic agents. *Physiology & Behavior, 79*(4/5), 761–66.

Berthoud, H.-R. (2004a). Mind versus metabolism in the control of food intake and energy balance. *Physiology & Behavior, 81*(5), 781–93.

——. (2004b). Neural control of appetite: cross-talk between homeostatic and non-homeostatic systems. *Appetite, 43*(3), 315–17.

Berthoud, H.-R., Sutton, G.M., Townsend, R.L., Patterson, L.M. & Zheng, H. (2006). Brainstem mechanisms integrating gut-derived satiety signals and descending forebrain information in the control of meal size. *Physiology & Behavior, 89*(4), 517–24.

Birch, L.L. & Deysher, M. (1986). Caloric compensation and sensory specific satiety: evidence for self-regulation of food intake by young children. *Appetite, 7*(4), 323–31.

Birch, L.L., McPhee, L., Steinberg, L. & Sullivan, S. (1990). Conditioned flavor preferences in young children. *Physiology & Behavior, 47*(3), 501–05.

Borzoei, S., Neovius, M., Barkeling, B., Teixeira-Pinto, A. & Rossner, S. (2006). A comparison of effects of fish and beef protein on satiety in normal-weight men. *European Journal of Clinical Nutrition, 60*(7), 897–902.

Bray, G.A. (2000). Afferent signals regulating food intake. *Proceedings of the Nutrition Society, 59*(3), 373–84.

Brunstrom, J.M. (2004). Does dietary learning occur outside awareness? *Consciousness & Cognition, 13*(3), 453–70.

Burton, P. & Lightowler, H.J. (2006). Influence of bread volume on glycaemic response and satiety. *British Journal of Nutrition, 96*(5), 877–82.

Butryn, M.L., Phelan, S., Hill, J.O. & Wing, R.R. (2007). Consistent self-monitoring of weight: a key component of successful weight loss maintenance. *Obesity, 15*(12), 3091–96.

Buyckx, M., Dupont, J.L., Durnin, J.V., Ferro-Luzzi, A., Roberts, S.B., Schurch, B., et al. (1996). Report of the working group on general principles of assessing energy requirements. *European Journal of Clinical Nutrition, 50*(Suppl 1), 186–87.

Cabanac, M. (1971). Physiological role of pleasure. *Science, 173*(4002), 1103–07.

Chapelot, D., Marmonier, C., Aubert, R., Allegre, C., Gausseres, N., Fantino, M., et al. (2006). Consequence of omitting or adding a meal in man on body composition, food intake, and metabolism. *Obesity, 14*(2), 215–27.

Clifton, P.M., Keogh, J.B. & Noakes, M. (2008). Long-term effects of a high-protein weight-loss diet. *American Journal of Clinical Nutrition, 87*(1), 23–29.

Das, S.K., Gilhooly, C.H., Golden, J.K., Pittas, A.G., Fuss, P.J., Cheatham, R.A., et al. (2007). Long-term effects of 2 energy-restricted diets differing in glycemic load on dietary adherence, body composition, and metabolism in CALERIE: a 1-y randomized controlled trial. *American Journal of Clinical Nutrition, 85*(4), 1023–30.

Das, S.K., Saltzman, E., McCrory, M.A., Hsu, L.K.G., Shikora, S.A., Dolnikowski, G., et al. (2004). Energy expenditure is very high in extremely obese women. *Journal of Nutrition, 134*(6), 1412–16.

Di Chiara, G., Bassareo, V., Fenu, S., De Luca, M.A., Spina, L., Cadoni, C., et al. (2004). Dopamine and drug addiction: the nucleus accumbens shell connection. *Neuropharmacology, 47*(Suppl 1), 227–41.

Drewnowski, A. (1998). Energy density, palatability, and satiety: implications for weight control. *Nutrition Reviews, 56*(12), 347–53.

Eisenstein, J., Roberts, S.B., Dallal, G. & Saltzman, E. (2002). High-protein weight-loss diets: are they safe and do they work? A review of the experimental and epidemiologic data. *Nutrition Reviews, 60*(7 Pt 1), 189–200.

Elder, S.J. & Roberts, S.B. (2007). The effects of exercise on food intake and body fatness: a summary of published studies. *Nutrition Reviews, 65*(1), 1–19.

Epstein, L.H., Paluch, R., Smith, J.D. & Sayette, M. (1997). Allocation of attentional resources during habituation to food cues. *Psychophysiology, 34*(1), 59–64.

Epstein, L.H., Truesdale, R., Wojcik, A., Paluch, R.A. & Raynor, H.A. (2003). Effects of deprivation on hedonics and reinforcing value of food. *Physiology & Behavior, 78*(2), 221–27.

Erlanson-Albertsson, C. (2005). How palatable food disrupts appetite regulation. *Basic & Clinical Pharmacology & Toxicology, 97*(2), 61–73.

Fedoroff, I., Polivy, J. & Peter Herman, C. (2003). The specificity of restrained versus unrestrained eaters' responses to food cues: general desire to eat, or craving for the cued food? *Appetite, 41*(1), 7–13.

Fischer, K., Colombani, P.C. & Wenk, C. (2004). Metabolic and cognitive coefficients in the development of hunger sensations after pure macronutrient ingestion in the morning. *Appetite, 42*(1), 49–61.

Foreyt, J.P. & Kennedy, W.A. (1971). Treatment of overweight by aversion therapy. *Behaviour Research & Therapy, 9*(1), 29–34.

Foster, G.D., Wyatt, H. R., Hill, J.O., McGuckin, B.G., Brill, C., Mohammed, B.S., et al. (2003). A randomized trial of a low-carbohydrate diet for obesity. *New England Journal of Medicine, 348*(21), 2082–90.

Gangwisch, J.E., Malaspina, D., Boden-Albala, B. & Heymsfield, S.B. (2005). Inadequate sleep as a risk factor for obesity: analyses of the NHANES I. *Sleep, 28*(10), 1289–96.

Geliebter, A. (1988). Gastric distension and gastric capacity in relation to food intake in humans. *Physiology & Behavior, 44*(4–5), 665–68.

Gibson, E.L. & Desmond, E. (1999). Chocolate craving and hunger state: implications for the acquisition and expression of appetite and food choice. *Appetite, 32*(2), 219–40.

Gibson, E.L., Wainwright, C.J. & Booth, D.A. (1995). Disguised protein in lunch after low-protein breakfast conditions food-flavor preferences dependent on recent lack of protein intake. *Physiology & Behavior, 58*(2), 363–71.

Gibson, E.L. & Wardle, J. (2003). Energy density predicts preferences for fruit and vegetables in 4-year-old children. *Appetite, 41*(1), 97–98.

Gilhooly, C.H., Das, S.K., Golden, J.K., McCrory, M.A., Dallal, G.E., Saltzman, E., et al. (2007). Food cravings and energy regulation: the characteristics of craved foods and their relationship with eating behaviors and weight change during 6 months of dietary energy restriction. *International Journal of Obesity, 31*(12), 1849–58.

Goldstein, G.L., Daun, H. & Tepper, B.J. (2005). Adiposity in middle-aged women is associated with genetic taste blindness to 6-n-propylthiouracil. *Obesity Research, 13*(6), 1017–23.

Gottfried, J.A., O'Doherty, J. & Dolan, R.J. (2003). Encoding predictive reward value in human amygdala and orbitofrontal cortex. *Science, 301*(5636), 1104–07.

Grieve, F.G. & Vander Weg, M.W. (2003). Desire to eat high- and low-fat foods following a low-fat dietary intervention. *Journal of Nutrition Education & Behavior, 35*(2), 98–102.

Hall, W.L., Millward, D.J., Long, S.J. & Morgan, L.M. (2007). Casein and whey exert different effects on plasma amino acid profiles, gastrointestinal hormone secretion and appetite. *British Journal of Nutrition, 89*(02), 239–48.

Halton, T.L. & Hu, F.B. (2004). The effects of high-protein diets on thermogenesis, satiety and weight loss: a critical review. *Journal of the American College of Nutrition, 23*(5), 373–85.

Hays, N.P., Bathalon, G.P., McCrory, M.A., Roubenoff, R., Lipman, R. & Roberts, S.B. (2002). Eating behavior correlates of adult weight gain and obesity in healthy women aged 55–65 y. *American Journal of Clinical Nutrition, 75*(3), 476–83.

Hays, N.P., Bathalon, G.P., Roubenoff, R., McCrory, M.A. & Roberts, S.B. (2006). Eating behavior and weight change in healthy postmenopausal women: results of a 4-year longitudinal study. *Journals of Gerontology Series A–Biological Sciences & Medical Sciences, 61*(6), 608–15.

Hays, N.P. & Roberts, S.B. (2008). Aspects of eating behaviors: disinhibition and restraint are related to weight gain and BMI in women. *Obesity, 16,* 52–58.

Hetherington, M.M. (1996). Sensory-specific satiety and its importance in meal termination. *Neuroscience & Biobehavioral Reviews, 20*(1), 113–17.

Heyman, M.B., Young, V.R., Fuss, P., Tsay, R., Joseph, L. & Roberts, S.B. (1992). Underfeeding and body weight regulation in normal-weight young men. *American Journal of Physiology, 263*(2 Pt 2), R250–57.

Hill, S.W. & McCutcheon, N.B. (1984). Contributions of obesity, gender, hunger, food preference, and body size to bite size, bite speed, and rate of eating. *Appetite, 5*(2), 73–83.

Hlebowicz, J., Darwiche, G., Bjorgell, O. & Almer, L.-O. (2007). Effect of cinnamon on postprandial blood glucose, gastric emptying, and satiety in healthy subjects. *American Journal of Clinical Nutrition, 85*(6), 1552–56.

Holland, P.C. & Petrovich, G.D. (2005). A neural systems analysis of the potentiation of feeding by conditioned stimuli. *Physiology & Behavior, 86*(5), 747–61.

Holt, S.H., Miller, J.C., Petocz, P. & Farmakalidis, E. (1995). A satiety index of common foods. *European Journal of Clinical Nutrition, 49*(9), 675–90.

Howard, B.V., Manson, J.E., Stefanick, M.L., Beresford, S.A., Frank, G., Jones, B., et al. (2006). Low-fat dietary pattern and weight change over 7 years: the Women's Health Initiative Dietary Modification Trial. *Journal of the American Medical Association, 295*(1), 39–49.

Howarth, N.C., Huang, T.T.K., Roberts, S.B., Lin, B.H. & McCrory, M.A. (2006). Eating patterns and dietary composition in relation to BMI in younger and older adults. *International Journal of Obesity, 31*(4), 675–84.

Howarth, N.C., Saltzman, E. & Roberts, S.B. (2001). Dietary fiber and weight regulation. *Nutrition Reviews, 59*(5), 129–39.

IFIC. (2007). *2007 Food & Health Survey. Consumer Attitudes toward Food, Nutrition & Health.* Washington, D.C.: International Food Information Council Foundation.

Jacobson, M.F. (2005). *Liquid Candy. How Soft Drinks Are Harming Americans' Health.* Washington, D.C.: Center for Science in the Public Interest.

Jansen, A. (1998). A learning model of binge eating: cue reactivity and cue exposure. *Behaviour Research & Therapy, 36*(3), 257–72.

Johnson, J. & Vickers, Z. (1993). Effect of flavor and macronutrient composition of food servings on liking, hunger and subsequent intake. *Appetite, 21* (1), 25–39.

Johnson, S.L., McPhee, L. & Birch, L.L. (1991). Conditioned preferences: young children prefer flavors associated with high dietary fat. *Physiology & Behavior, 50*(6), 1245–51.

Johnstone, A.M., Horgan, G.W., Murison, S.D., Bremner, D.M. & Lobley, G.E. (2008). Effects of a high-protein ketogenic diet on hunger, appetite, and weight loss in obese men feeding ad libitum. *American Journal of Clinical Nutrition, 87*(1), 44–55.

Johnstone, A.M., Stubbs, R.J. & Harbron, C.G. (1996). Effect of overfeeding macronutrients on day-to-day food intake in man. *European Journal of Clinical Nutrition, 50*(7), 418–30.

Kant, A.K. & Graubard, B.I. (2004). Eating out in America, 1987–2000: trends and nutritional correlates. *Preventive Medicine, 38*(2), 243–49.

Kissileff, H.R. & Guss, J.L. (2001). Microstructure of eating behavior in humans. *Appetite, 36*(1), 70–78.

Konturek, S.J. & Konturek, J.W. (2000). Cephalic phase of pancreatic secretion. *Appetite, 34*(2), 197–205.

Kral, T.V.E. (2006). Effects on hunger and satiety, perceived portion size and pleasantness of taste of varying the portion size of foods: a brief review of selected studies. *Appetite, 46*(1), 103–05.

Lawton, C.L., Delargy, H.J., Brockman, J., Smith, F.C. & Blundell, J.E. (2007). The degree of saturation of fatty acids influences post-ingestive satiety. *British Journal of Nutrition, 83*(05), 473–82.

Lee, Y.P., Mori, T.A., Sipsas, S., Barden, A., Puddey, I.B., Burke, V., et al. (2006). Lupin-enriched bread increases satiety and reduces energy intake acutely. *American Journal of Clinical Nutrition, 84*(5), 975–80.

Leidy, H.J., Carnell, N.S., Mattes, R.D. & Campbell, W.W. (2007). Higher protein intake preserves lean mass and satiety with weight loss in pre-obese and obese women. *Obesity, 15*(2), 421–29.

Levine, A.S., Kotz, C.M. & Gosnell, B.A. (2003). Sugars: hedonic aspects, neuroregulation, and energy balance. *American Journal of Clinical Nutrition, 78*(4), S834–42.

Levitsky, D.A., Garay, J., Nausbaum, M., Neighbors, L. & Dellavalle, D.M. (2006). Monitoring weight daily blocks the freshman weight gain: a model for combating the epidemic of obesity. *International Journal of Obesity, 30*(6), 1003–10.

Lucas, F. & Sclafani, A. (1999). Flavor preferences conditioned by high-fat versus high-carbohydrate diets vary as a function of session length. *Physiology & Behavior, 66*(3), 389–95.

Ludwig, D.S., Majzoub, J.A., Al-Zahrani, A., Dallal, G.E., Blanco, I. & Roberts, S.B. (1999). High Glycemic Index foods, overeating, and obesity. *Pediatrics, 103*(3), E26.

Ludwig, D.S. & Roberts, S.B. (2006). Influence of Glycemic Index/load on glycemic response, appetite, and food intake in healthy humans. *Diabetes Care, 29*(2), 474; author reply 475–76.

MacDonald, A.F., Billington, C.J. & Levine, A.S. (2004). Alterations in food intake by opioid and dopamine signaling pathways between the ventral tegmental area and the shell of the nucleus accumbens. *Brain Research, 1018*(1), 78–85.

Marcelino, A.S., Adam, A.S., Couronne, T., Koster, E.P. & Sieffermann, J.M. (2001). Internal and external determinants of eating initiation in humans. *Appetite, 36*(1), 9–14.

Mattes, R. (2005). Soup and satiety. *Physiology & Behavior, 83*(5), 739–47.

——. (2006). Fluid calories and energy balance: the good, the bad, and the uncertain. *Physiology & Behavior, 89*(1), 66–70.

——. (1996). Dietary compensation by humans for supplemental energy provided as ethanol or carbohydrate in fluids. *Physiology & Behavior, 59*(1), 179–87.

——. (1997). Physiologic responses to sensory stimulation by food: nutritional implications. *Journal of the American Dietetic Association, 97*(4), 406–13.

——. (2000). Nutritional implications of the cephalic-phase salivary response. *Appetite, 34*(2), 177–83.

Mattes, R.D. & Friedman, M.I. (1993). Hunger. *Digestive Diseases, 11*(2), 65–77.

McCrory, M.A., Fuss, P.J., Hays, N.P., Vinken, A.G., Greenberg, A.S. & Roberts, S.B. (1999). Overeating in America: association between restaurant food consumption and body fatness in healthy adult men and women ages 19 to 80. *Obesity Research, 7*(6), 564–71.

McCrory, M.A., Fuss, P.J., McCallum, J.E., Yao, M., Vinken, A.G., Hays, N.P., et al. (1999). Dietary variety within food groups: association with energy intake and body fatness in men and women. *American Journal of Clinical Nutrition, 69*(3), 440–47.

McCrory, M.A., Fuss, P.J., Saltzman, E. & Roberts, S.B. (2000). Dietary determinants of energy intake and weight regulation in healthy adults. *Journal of Nutrition, 130*(2 Suppl), 276–79.

McCrory, M.A., Saltzman, E., Rolls, B.J. & Roberts, S.B. (2006). A twin study of the effects of energy density and palatability on energy intake of individual foods. *Physiology & Behavior, 87*(3), 451–59.

McCrory, M.A., Suen, V.M.M. & Roberts, S.B. (2002). Biobehavioral influences on energy intake and adult weight gain. *Journal of Nutrition, 132*(12), S3830–34.

McGuire, M.T., Wing, R.R., Klem, M.L., Lang, W. & Hill, J.O. (1999). What predicts weight regain in a group of successful weight losers? *Journal of Consulting & Clinical Psychology, 67*(2), 177–85.

Melanson, K.J., Greenberg, A.S., Ludwig, D.S., Saltzman, E., Dallal, G.E. & Roberts, S.B. (1998). Blood glucose and hormonal responses to small and large meals in healthy young and older women. *Journals of Gerontology Series—Biological Sciences of Medical Sciences, 53*(4), B299–305.

Melanson, K.J., Saltzman, E., Russell, R.R. & Roberts, S.B. (1997). Fat oxidation in response to four graded energy challenges in younger and older women. *American Journal of Clinical Nutrition, 66*(4), 860–66.

Melanson, K.J., Saltzman, E., Vinken, A.G., Russell, R. & Roberts, S.B. (1998). The effects of age on postprandial thermogenesis at four graded energetic challenges: findings in young and older women. *Journals of Gerontology Series A—Biological Sciences & Medical Sciences, 53*(6), B409–14.

Moorhead, S.A., Welch, R.W., Barbara, M., Livingstone, E., McCourt, M., Burns, A.A., et al. (2007). The effects of the fibre content and physical structure of carrots on satiety and subsequent intakes when eaten as part of a mixed meal. *British Journal of Nutrition, 96*(03), 587–95.

Moriguti, J.C., Das, S.K., Saltzman, E., Corrales, A., McCrory, M.A., Greenberg, A.S., et al. (2000). Effects of a 6-week hypocaloric diet on changes in body composition, hunger, and subsequent weight regain in healthy young and older adults. *Journals of Gerontology Series A—Biological Sciences & Medical Sciences, 55*(12), B580–87.

Murakami, K., Sasaki, S., Okubo, H., Takahashi, Y., Hosoi, Y. & Itabashi, M. (2007). Dietary fiber intake, dietary glycemic index and load, and body mass index: a cross-sectional study of 3,931 Japanese women aged 18–20 years. *European Journal of Clinical Nutrition, 61*(8), 986–95.

Niemeier, H.M., Phelan, S., Fava, J.L. & Wing, R.R. (2007). Internal disinhibition predicts weight regain following weight loss and weight loss maintenance. *Obesity, 15*(10), 2485–94

Orlet Fisher, J., Rolls, B.J. & Birch, L.L. (2003). Children's bite size and intake of an entrée are greater with large portions than with age-appropriate or self-selected portions. *American Journal of Clinical Nutrition, 77*(5), 1164–70.

Ostman, E., Granfeldt, Y., Persson, L. & Bjorck, I. (2005). Vinegar supplementation lowers glucose and insulin responses and increases satiety after a bread meal in healthy subjects. *European Journal of Clinical Nutrition, 59*(9), 983–88.

Petrovich, G.D., Holland, P.C. & Gallagher, M. (2005). Amygdalar and prefrontal pathways to the lateral hypothalamus are activated by a learned cue that stimulates eating. *Journal of Neuroscience, 25*(36), 8295–302.

Petrovich, G.D., Setlow, B., Holland, P.C. & Gallagher, M. (2002). Amygdalo-hypothalamic circuit allows learned cues to override satiety and promote eating. *Journal of Neuroscience, 22*(19), 8748–53.

Phelan, S., Wyatt, H., Nassery, S., Dibello, J., Fava, J.L., Hill, J.O. & Wing, R.R. (2007). Three-year weight change in successful weight losers who lost weight on a low-carbohydrate diet. *Obesity, 15*(10), 2470–77.

Pittas, A.G., Das, S.K., Hajduk, C.L., Golden, J., Saltzman, E., Stark, P.C., et al. (2005). A low-glycemic load diet facilitates greater weight loss in overweight adults with high insulin secretion but not in overweight adults with low insulin secretion in the CALERIE Trial. *Diabetes Care, 28*(12), 2939–41.

Pittas, A.G., Hariharan, R., Stark, P.C., Hajduk, C.L., Greenberg, A.S. & Roberts, S.B. (2005). Interstitial glucose level is a significant predictor of energy intake in free-living women with healthy body weight. *Journal of Nutrition, 135*(5), 1070–74.

Pittas, A.G. & Roberts, S.B. (2006). Dietary composition and weight loss: can we individualize dietary prescriptions according to insulin sensitivity or secretion status? *Nutrition Reviews, 64*(10 Pt 1), 435–48.

Pittas, A.G., Roberts, S.B., Das, S.K., Gilhooly, C.H., Saltzman, E., Golden, J., et al. (2006). The effects of the dietary glycemic load on type 2 diabetes risk factors during weight loss. *Obesity, 14*(12), 2200–09.

Plata-Salaman, C.R. (1991). Regulation of hunger and satiety in man. *Digestive Diseases, 9*(5), 253–68.

Poortvliet, P.C., Berube-Parent, S., Drapeau, V., Lamarche, B., Blundell, J.E. & Tremblay, A. (2007). Effects of a healthy meal course on spontaneous energy intake, satiety and palatability. *British Journal of Nutrition, 97*(03), 584–90.

Porubska, K., Veit, R., Preissl, H., Fritsche, A. & Birbaumer, N. (2006). Subjective feeling of appetite modulates brain activity: an fMRI study. *Neuroimage, 32*(3), 1273–80.

Raben, A., Agerholm-Larsen, L., Flint, A., Holst, J.J. & Astrup, A. (2003). Meals with similar energy densities but rich in protein, fat, carbohydrate, or alcohol have different effects on energy expenditure and substrate metabolism but not on appetite and energy intake. *American Journal of Clinical Nutrition, 77*(1), 91–100.

Raynor, H.A. & Epstein, L.H. (2001). Dietary variety, energy regulation, and obesity. *Psychological Bulletin, 127*(3), 325–41.

——. (2003). The relative-reinforcing value of food under differing levels of food deprivation and restriction. *Appetite, 40*(1), 15–24.

Raynor, H.A., Niemeier, H.M. & Wing, R.R. (2006). Effect of limiting snack food variety on long-term sensory-specific satiety and monotony during obesity treatment. *Eating Behaviors, 7*(1), 1–14.

Richardson, N.J., Rogers, P.J. & Elliman, N.A. (1996). Conditioned flavour preferences reinforced by caffeine consumed after lunch. *Physiology & Behavior, 60*(1), 257–63.

Roberts, S.B. (1997). Human obesity genes. *Nutrition, 13*(3), 236–38.

Roberts, S.B., Fuss, P., Heyman, M.B., Evans, W.J., Tsay, R., Rasmussen, H., et al. (1994). Control of food intake in older men. *Journal of the American Medical Association, 272*(20), 1601–06.

Roberts, S.B. & Heyman, M.B. (2000). Dietary composition and obesity: do we need to look beyond dietary fat? *Journal of Nutrition, 130*(2S Suppl), S267.

Roberts, S.B., Heyman, M.B., Evans, W.J., Fuss, P., Tsay, R. & Young, V.R. (1991). Dietary energy requirements of young adult men, determined by using the doubly labeled water method. *American Journal of Clinical Nutrition, 54*(3), 499–505.

Roberts, S.B. & Mayer, J. (2000). Holiday weight gain: fact or fiction? *Nutrition Reviews, 58*(12), 378–79.

Roberts, S.B., McCrory, M.A. & Saltzman, E. (2002). The influence of dietary composition on energy intake and body weight. *Journal of the American College of Nutrition, 21*(2), S140–45.

Roberts, S.B. & McDonald, R. (1998). The evolution of a new research field: metabolic programming by early nutrition. *Journal of Nutrition, 128*(2 Suppl), 400.

Roberts, S.B., Pi-Sunyer, F.X., Dreher, M., Hahn, R., Hill, J.O., Kleinman, R.E., et al. (1998). Physiology of fat replacement and fat reduction: effects of dietary fat and fat substitutes on energy regulation. *Nutrition Reviews, 56*(5 Pt 2), S29–41; discussion S41–29.

Roberts, S.B., Pi-Sunyer, F.X., Kuller, L., Lane, M.A., Ellison, P., Prior, J.C., et al. (2001). Physiologic effects of lowering caloric intake in nonhuman primates and nonobese humans. *Journals of Gerontology Series A—Biological Sciences & Medical Sciences, 56*(90001), 66–75.

Roberts, S.B. & Rosenberg, I. (2006). Nutrition and aging: changes in the regulation of energy metabolism with aging. *Physiological Reviews, 86*(2), 651–67.

Roberts, S.B. & Williamson, D.F. (2002). Causes of adult weight gain. *Journal of Nutrition, 132*(12), S3824–25.

Rolls, B.J., Engell, D. & Birch, L.L. (2000). Serving portion size influences 5-year-old but not 3-year-old children's food intakes. *Journal of the American Dietetic Association, 100*(2), 232–34.

Rolls, B.J., Hetherington, M. & Laster, L.J. (1988). Comparison of the effects of aspartame and sucrose on appetite and food intake. *Appetite, 11*(Suppl 1), 62–67.

Rolls, B.J., Kim, S., McNelis, A.L., Fischman, M.W., Foltin, R.W. & Moran, T.H. (1991). Time course of effects of preloads high in fat or carbohydrate on food intake and hunger ratings in humans. *American Journal of Physiology, 260*(4 Pt 2), R756–63.

Rolls, B.J., Van Duijvenvoorde, P.M. & Rolls, E.T. (1984). Pleasantness changes and food intake in a varied four-course meal. *Appetite, 5*(4), 337–48.

Rolls, E.T. (2004). The functions of the orbitofrontal cortex. *Brain & Cognition, 55*(1), 11–29.

——. (2005). Taste, olfactory, and food texture processing in the brain, and the control of food intake. *Physiology & Behavior, 85*(1), 45–56.

Saltzman, E., Das, S.K., Lichtenstein, A.H., Dallal, G.E., Corrales, A., Schaefer, E.J., et al. (2001). An oat-containing hypocaloric diet reduces systolic blood pressure and improves lipid profile beyond effects of weight loss in men and women. *Journal of Nutrition, 131*(5), 1465–70.

Saltzman, E., Moriguti, J.C., Das, S.K., Corrales, A., Fuss, P., Greenberg, A.S., et al. (2001). Effects of a cereal rich in soluble fiber on body composition and dietary compliance during consumption of a hypocaloric diet. *Journal of the American College of Nutrition, 20*(1), 50–57.

Saltzman, E. & Roberts, S.B. (1995). The role of energy expenditure in energy regulation: findings from a decade of research. *Nutrition Reviews, 53*(8), 209–20.

Sawaya, A.L., Fuss, P.J., Dallal, G.E., Tsay, R., McCrory, M. A., Young, V., et al. (2001). Meal palatability, substrate oxidation and blood glucose in young and older men. *Physiology & Behavior, 72*(1–2), 5–12.

Sawaya, A.L., Tucker, K., Tsay, R., Willett, W., Saltzman, E., Dallal, G.E., et al. (1996). Evaluation of four methods for determining energy intake in young and older women: comparison with doubly labeled water measurements of total energy expenditure. *American Journal of Clinical Nutrition, 63*(4), 491–99.

Schoenbaum, G., Chiba, A.A. & Gallagher, M. (1999). Neural encoding in orbitofrontal cortex and basolateral amygdala during olfactory discrimination learning. *Journal of Neuroscience, 19*(5), 1876–84.

Schwartz, M.W. (2006). Central nervous system regulation of food intake. *Obesity, 14*(Suppl 1), 1–8.

Sclafani, A. (1997). Learned controls of ingestive behaviour. *Appetite, 29*(2), 153–58.

——. (2001). Post-ingestive positive controls of ingestive behavior. *Appetite, 36*(1), 79–83.

Sewards, T.V. (2004). Dual separate pathways for sensory and hedonic aspects of taste. *Brain Research Bulletin, 62*(4), 271–83.

Simmons, W.K., Martin, A. & Barsalou, L.W. (2005). Pictures of appetizing foods activate gustatory cortices for taste and reward. *Cerebral Cortex, 15*(10), 1602–08.

Small, D.M., Jones-Gotman, M. & Dagher, A. (2003). Feeding-induced dopamine release in dorsal striatum correlates with meal pleasantness ratings in healthy human volunteers. *Neuroimage, 19*(4), 1709–15.

Smeets, P.A.M., De Graaf, C., Stafleu, A., Van Osch, M.J.P. & Van der Grond, J. (2005). Functional magnetic resonance imaging of human hypothalamic responses to sweet taste and calories. *American Journal of Clinical Nutrition, 82*(5), 1011–16.

Sorensen, L.B., Moller, P., Flint, A., Martens, M. & Raben, A. (2003). Effect of sensory perception of foods on appetite and food intake: a review of studies on humans. *International Journal of Obesity, 27*(10), 1152–66.

Stanley, S., Wynne, K., McGowan, B. & Bloom, S. (2005). Hormonal regulation of food intake. *Physiological Reviews, 85*(4), 1131–58.

Stubbs, R.J., Van Wyk, M.C., Johnstone, A.M. & Harbron, C.G. (1996). Breakfasts high in protein, fat or carbohydrate: effect on within-day appetite and energy balance. *European Journal of Clinical Nutrition, 50*(7), 409–17.

Stubbs, R.J. & Whybrow, S. (2004). Energy density, diet composition and palatability: influences on overall food energy intake in humans. *Physiology & Behavior, 81*(5), 755–64.

Taha, S.A. & Fields, H.L. (2005). Encoding of palatability and appetitive behaviors by distinct neuronal populations in the nucleus accumbens. *Journal of Neuroscience, 25*(5), 1193–202.

Teff, K. (2000). Nutritional implications of the cephalic-phase reflexes: endocrine responses. *Appetite, 34*(2), 206–13.

Vinken, A.G., Bathalon, G.P., Sawaya, A.L., Dallal, G.E., Tucker, K.L. & Roberts, S.B. (1999). Equations for predicting the energy requirements of healthy adults aged 18–81 y. *American Journal of Clinical Nutrition, 69*(5), 920–26.

Wadden, T.A., Butryn, M.L. & Byrne, K.J. (2004). Efficacy of lifestyle modification for long-term weight control. *Obesity Research, 12*, 151–62.

Wansink, B. (2004). Environmental factors that increase the food intake and consumption volume of unknowing consumers. *Annual Review of Nutrition, 24*, 455–49.

Wansink, B. & Kim, J. (2005). Bad popcorn in big buckets: portion size can influence intake as much as taste. *Journal of Nutrition Education & Behavior, 37*(5), 242–45.

Wansink, B. & Sobal, J. (2007). Mindless eating: the 200 daily food decisions we overlook. *Environment and Behavior, 39*(1), 106–23.

Ward, A. & Mann, T. (2000). Don't mind if I do: disinhibited eating under cognitive load. *Journal of Personality & Social Psychology, 78*(4), 753–63.

Weiss, F. (2005). Neurobiology of craving, conditioned reward and relapse. *Current Opinion in Pharmacology, 5*(1), 9–19.

Westerterp-Plantenga, M.S., Smeets, A. & Lejeune, M.P. (2005). Sensory and gastrointestinal satiety effects of capsaicin on food intake. *International Journal of Obesity, 29*(6), 682–88.

Williams, G., Noakes, M., Keogh, J., Foster, P. & Clifton, P. (2006). High-protein, high-fibre snack bars reduce food intake and improve short-term glucose and insulin profiles compared with high-fat snack bars. *Asia Pacific Journal of Clinical Nutrition, 15*(4), 443–50.

Williamson, D.A., Geiselman, P.J., Lovejoy, J., Greenway, F., Volaufova, J., Martin, C.K., et al. (2006). Effects of consuming mycoprotein, tofu or chicken upon subsequent eating behaviour, hunger and satiety. *Appetite, 46*(1), 41–48.

Wilson, D.A. & Sullivan, R.M. (1994). Neurobiology of associative learning in the neonate: early olfactory learning. *Behavioral & Neural Biology, 61*(1), 1–18.

Wolever, T.M., Jenkins, D.J., Ocana, A.M., Rao, V.A. & Collier, G.R. (1988). Second-meal effect: low Glycemic Index foods eaten at dinner improve subsequent breakfast glycemic response. *American Journal of Clinical Nutrition, 48*(4), 1041–47.

Wynne, K., Stanley, S., McGowan, B. & Bloom, S. (2005). Appetite control. *Journal of Endocrinology, 184*(2), 291–318.

Yao, M. & Roberts, S.B. (2001). Dietary energy density and weight regulation. *Nutrition Reviews, 59*(8 Pt 1), 247–58.

Yeomans, M.R. (1996). Palatability and the micro-structure of feeding in humans: the appetizer effect. *Appetite, 27*(2), 119–33.

Yeomans, M.R. & Gray, R.W. (2002). Opioid peptides and the control of human ingestive behaviour. *Neuoscience & Biobehavioral Reviews, 26*(6), 713–28.

Yeomans, M.R., Jackson, A., Lee, M.D., Steer, B., Tinley, E., Durlach, P., et al. (2000). Acquisition and extinction of flavour preferences conditioned by caffeine in humans. *Appetite, 35*(2), 131–41.

Yoshioka, M., St-Pierre, S., Drapeau, V., Dionne, I., Doucet, E., Suzuki, M., et al. (2007). Effects of red pepper on appetite and energy intake. *British Journal of Nutrition, 82*(02), 115–23.

Zandstra, E.H., De Graaf, C., Mela, D.J. & Van Staveren, W.A. (2000). Short- and long-term effects of changes in pleasantness on food intake. *Appetite, 34*(3), 253–60.

Zandstra, E.H., Stubenitsky, K., De Graaf, C. & Mela, D.J. (2002). Effects of learned flavour cues on short-term regulation of food intake in a realistic setting. *Physiology & Behavior, 75*(1–2), 83–90.

General Index

Recipe Index

Recipe Index

Acknowledgments

We are deeply grateful to the many fine professionals and volunteers who helped make this book possible. First we'd like to thank all the people at Tufts and elsewhere who have contributed to the research or made other important contributions, and especially Ed Saltzman, Cheryl Gilhooly, Megan McCrory, Taso Pittas, Lisa Robinson, Sai Das, Kimberly Smith, Izzy Greenberg, Russ Kennedy, Helen Rasmussen and others who helped—Mary Rose Dallal, Michael Garshick, Margaret Hagen, David Linz, Janet G. Marks, Lisa Marks and Lorian Urban. Also, lab members Paul Fuss, Maria Berlis, Nick Hays, Manjiang Yao, Gaston Bathalon, Rachel Cheatham, Julie Golden, Dan Hoffman, Kathleen Melanson, Vivian Suen, Julio Moriguiti and Guansheng Ma. And thanks to my wonderful colleagues on the Tufts faculty—Simin Meydani, Gerard Dallal, Tammy Scott, Roger Fielding, Alice Lichtenstein, Katy Tucker, Miriam Nelson, Parke Wilde, Andy Greenberg and Ernst Schaefer—as well as the directors of the Tufts centers, Eileen Kennedy, Rob Russell, Irwin Rosenberg and Paul Summergrad.

Then there are the nutrition scientists worldwide who are working on the science of weight control and weight-related topics, and we would like to thank all of them for their important work, especially Arne Astrup, Leanne Birch, John Blundell, George Bray, Kelly Brownell, Adam Drewnowski, Leonard Epstein, Bill Evans, Gary Foster, James O. Hill, Susan Jebb, David Jenkins, Nancy Keim, Sam Klein, David Ludwig, Rick Mattes, Xavier Pi-Sunyer, Barbara Rolls, Edmund Rolls, Frank Sacks, Dale Schoeller, Anthony Sclafani, John Speakman, Angelo Tremblay, Tom Wadden, Don Williamson, Walter Willett and Rena Wing.

Thanks also to the National Institutes of Health and U.S. Department of Agriculture (USDA) for their generous research funding and, on a personal level, to Heidi Wyle, Ellen Richstone, Debbi Darling, David Gifford, Jonathan Lurie and Henry Roberts for their love, friendship and good-humored feedback as well as recipe testing.

And thank you to Wendy Weil, our extraordinarily smart and talented agent, who believed in this project and was clever enough to put us together in the first place.

We'd like to thank Peter Workman, who we think is by far the most talented publisher in the business, and Susan Bolotin, our gifted editor, whose passion, commitment and brilliant suggestions are reflected in every page of this book. Our heartfelt thanks, too, go to the rest of the amazing team at Workman: manuscript editor Lynn Strong and recipe editor Barbara Mateer, both of whom went far beyond the call of duty, as well as book designer Janet Vicario, production editor Carol White and director of publicity Kristin Matthews. What a privilege and pleasure it has been to work with all of you.